CONTENTS

ACKNOWLEDGEMENTS

Particular thanks goes to my wonderful husband David Slee who has supported, sweated and nagged me over this work and most of all provided me with endless material and technical support. It has been hard for him to read my honest articles about living with him and it also has not been an easy task for him to open up about his own feelings on the subject. I really could not have done this without him.

Many thanks to my friends and colleagues, particularly my supervisors, Dr Dawn Benson and David Littlefair from Northumbria University, who encouraged me to expand on my dissertation; "An Autoethnographic Account of Married Life to a Man With Suspected Asperger Syndrome" and create this book.

Also thank you to my friends and clients who have agreed to let me use their experiences as material. They know who they are.

PREFACE

What is this Book About?

This book aims to help the spouses or partners who are married to or in a long term relationship with someone diagnosed with Asperger's Syndrome or more likely, suspected Asperger's Syndrome (AS).

This is an honest account of what my life has been like with my husband David and how his Asperger's has affected our marriage. We have had many crisis moments over the years but most of these have been through joint ignorance of my husband's condition. With realisation came a long 'getting to know you' process and learning more about the condition and David's idiosyncrasies.

I want to share with you the everyday, nitty gritty, details that most people outside of your family would miss, that really affect you as a couple. I have gone into detail about these and explained why these behaviours happen. Not every man with AS is the same but you will recognise some of these behaviours in your partner.

I graduated with a Masters in Autism from Northumbria University in 2013 and used my then 18 years of experience (research) of living with David to write my dissertation about our marriage. I couldn't help but be worried when he read through my dissertation as I was concerned that I may have misunderstood some things or upset him with some of the detail. I believe it was probably quite hard for him to read how much his behaviour over the years had affected me but all he said after he had read it through was that it was 'very insightful'. I knew then I had done a good job.

Who am I to Author This Book?

I believe I grew up in an Asperger family though we did not know it. Instinctively, I recognised many signs in my husband when I met him, though I was not overtly conscious of it. I was actually comfortable with much of his behaviour.

I have a first degree in English and Communication and worked in publishing, and later Child Protection, before giving up work to have my first child. That child, a boy, was diagnosed in 2009 with Asperger Syndrome and that is when our family life began to change for the better. Reading all I could on autism and Asperger Syndrome, I realised that it described my husband and, what little was written about AS/NT relationships, described us exactly. I began to understand the world that my husband and children live in. I started a three-year Master's degree in Autism in 2010, initially so I could help and understand my son more. I gained great insight and great friends on this course but the best thing I gained from it was deeper understanding of my marriage.

It is inevitable that some subjects will overlap but, as this book is designed for you to dip in and out of, there will be some repetition of subjects in some areas.

Asperger men are very difficult to categorise. They are not a species that we can entirely predict. Each man is made of tens of thousands of genes and each partner will present differently.

PROLOGUE

"Apache Wedding Prayer"

Now you will feel no rain,

For each of you will be shelter to the other

Now you will feel no cold,

For each of you will be warmth to the other.

Now there is no loneliness,

For each of you will be companion to the other.

You are two bodies,

But there is only one life before you.

When evening falls,

You'll look up and there the other will be.

He'll take your hand,

You'll take his and turn together

To look at the road you travelled to reach this

The hour of your happiness

It stretches behind you

Even as the future lies ahead.

Go now to your dwelling place

To enter into the days of your togetherness

And may your days be good and long upon the earth.

(After Arnold (1947), *Blood Brother*)

HOW TO USE THIS BOOK

Your Journey

This book is designed with alphabetic navigation in mind. You can read it from start to finish, or you can dip in and out of it when necessary. Think of a situation such as Anger and turn to that page. I will mostly likely have written about it.

Terminology

Throughout this book I will be referring to people on the Autistic Spectrum in a number of different ways. There are of course, clinical terms, there are affectionate terms and there are ways in which people on the spectrum like to refer to themselves. None of these terms are wrong though some are growing in popularity.

Within our household and amongst most our friends we refer to people with Asperger Syndrome as Aspies. Firstly, it is an easy, roll off the tongue abbreviation. Secondly, it is an affectionate term and in no way derogatory and has been adopted by those with AS themselves. It gives them an identity and means they can relate and empathise more with their group.

Other terms I have heard is Aspergic which the minority of friends use who are also on the spectrum.

When given a diagnosis these days, clinicians do not give a diagnosis of Asperger's Syndrome any more. Most of us do not agree with this and think it is unfair for everyone on the Autistic Spectrum to be lumped together as everyone has different needs that should be identified.

The title that is given is Autism Spectrum Disorder (ASD) which you will see referred to a lot in this guide. There is growing concern amongst many on the spectrum and their supporters that ASD has negative connotations and the use of the word 'Disorder' is more than implying that there is something wrong with them.

We know now that most forms of Autism are genetic and deep within our complex DNA. Autism and Asperger's have been shown via research and fMRI brain scanners to be a different wiring in the brain compared to Neurotypical people. Therefore, this shows that autism is not a sign of a disorder or something broken but of a difference.

Yes, our Aspies do have trouble fitting in socially at times but this does not mean they are any lesser than the majority of the population. This is why a growing cohort are keen to refer to autism as an Autism Spectrum Condition (ASC).

What is an Asperger Marriage?

An 'Asperger Marriage' is when one spouse has or is suspected to have Asperger Syndrome (AS). This is no ordinary marriage. There is no balance between the partners. There is no predictability even though predictability is craved. There is never a day when the wife doesn't wake up wondering what mood her husband will be in or how events of the day might change that mood and what proactive measures she can take to ensure it is a positive one.

The 'normal' or neurotypical (NT) wife, particularly if unaware of AS, even if she has lived with and experienced AS behaviour her whole life will still, at times, be faced with a situation so displaced from reality, she is left doubting her own sanity. An innocent conversation about an everyday event could turn into the wife's whole existence being questioned and denigrated.

These traumatic, seemingly abusive events need not be deliberate. The wife is left feeling stupid, worthless and trampled upon by her husband's overpowering and fixed opinions. She is left dumbfounded and bereft by an unexpected verbal attack. A sincere discussion with the man she loves can inexplicably turn and leave her wondering whether he ever respected or valued her efforts at all.

This is a devastating and lonely situation for a woman to deal with, whilst her husband shows a strong, calm and intelligent face to the outside world.

David and I have been married now for 18 years and together for 20. Though, in some ways, we have a very strong and faithful marriage, in others there are many communication difficulties and misunderstandings. Realising that my husband is on the autistic spectrum has saved our marriage and we have established ways to avoid certain triggers that lead to meltdowns and I have developed strategies for both my family and myself to cope with difficult situations.

I would like to take this opportunity to share my experiences and to show that divorce is not always the answer.

Who are the Asperger Wives?

You are most likely an Asperger wife if you were swept off your feet by an intelligent and interesting man, who thought you were perfect and treated you like a princess. He would have wanted to do everything for you and nothing you said was wrong. He was generous and kind and sweet and innocent. He was quite likely to be hard working, successful and possibly even travelled a lot. He had an interesting life style.

Once you were married to this perfect man it would have all changed. Maybe not overnight, but gradually. He would be less sociable than he used to be. He would get angry with you for no reason. He would start arguments in inappropriate places and accuse you of doing things you were sure you hadn't done. Your once idyllic relationship changed beyond all recognition.

Your self-esteem may well have plummeted and you didn't know who to tell about all the petty little arguments. You found yourself tip toeing around him not wanting to bring up difficult conversation topics in case he overreacted. You started dealing with problems by yourself as much as possible to keep the peace.

You became lonely, disillusioned, possibly depressed at the thought of living this life with the man you thought you loved. It felt like there was nowhere to turn as who would believe you that this articulate, successful man was incapable of having a successful marriage or taking the joint responsibility of children. Maybe it wasn't your husband's fault at all but your own? Perhaps you had changed?

You would have been full of self-doubt and lacking in confidence. Then one day you were watching the television or reading an article about autism or perhaps one of your children got diagnosed with Asperger Syndrome, when suddenly light dawned on you and you realised that he was the problem. Your husband has Asperger's Syndrome.

Who is "The Husband"?

The husband in this guide is a real person - David, my spouse. He has an insight into being on the spectrum and in a relationship with me and has felt able to share how he feels and if my advice to you seems to ring true with him. From time to time you might see a comment from him marked like this:

The Husband Says:

My words: "The Husband Says:", will appear in italics, like this, and under my own heading.

Who is the Advice Targeted at?

Throughout this guide, where advice is given that best benefits a particular person or group, an icon code is used to show the 'target'. Insight into the advice might well benefit others however, so groupings are by no means exclusive.

AS — Aspies, often the male partner in an Asperger Marriage.

NT — Neurotypicals, often the female partner in an Asperger Marriage.

To both partners in an Asperger Marriage.

To males, usually the Aspie in an Asperger Marriage.

To females, usually the neurotypical in an Asperger Marriage.

The whole family if there are kids in the Asperger Marriage.

- Acceptance
- Acceptance of Diagnosis
- Achievements
- ADHD
- Agreeing
- Alcohol
- Alexithymia
- All Men Are Like That
- All or Nothing
- Amygdala
- Anger
- Answering the Phone
- Answers
- Anticipation

- Anxiety
- Appearing to be 'Normal'
- Arrogance
- Asperger Syndrome
- Aspies
- Assigning Blame
- Atelophobia
- Attraction
- Autism
- Autism Heroes
- Autism Quotient Test
- Autistic Spectrum
- Avoidance
- Awareness

Acceptance

What do Aspie men want most in life?

Acceptance.

They want to be like everyone else, have friends and a feeling of self-worth. They know they are different and possibly deficient, even if no one else has ever told them so.

Where do you, as their long term partner, come in to all of this? You are the prize they have sought, the trophy after acceptance that they really wanted to achieve. You are the thing that makes them look acceptable. "Look world, I can't be that bad. She loves me."

The Husband Says:

Yes, I crave acceptance. But it can be hard work.

From my viewpoint, struggling to read social cues to see if I am welcome, I feel like I'm a stranger at a party where everyone knows each other and you have formed a ring and you are all facing inwards having a great time. I'm on the outside, I don't know what the convention is to break the circle and get to the inside where I can join the party too. But my Neurotypical (NT) wife knows the secret and she can help me; she can open up the circle to me. I want to be accepted; I want to be in the circle.

But inside the circle is scary too - they will want to ask me all sorts of questions, to check if I am acceptable to them - to see if Karen's recommendation is good enough - I'm consciously using Karen as my neurotypical guide.

*The hard work is worth it. If you want **acceptance**, your behaviour must be **acceptable**.*

AS *Search for the band 'Ocean Colour Scene' and their song 'The Circle' for a bit about how it feels to be excluded from one circle and joining another circle. One of the live acoustic versions with the crowd singing along is particularly uplifting. See also the article on Music.*

Acceptance of Diagnosis

Without accepting who they are and why they are different, your relationship cannot move forward and improve.

Acceptance of the diagnosis means that our partners also accept themselves for who they are. It also means they can forgive themselves for their inadequacies and silly mistakes.

With David, there was never really a light bulb moment. It seemed to be more of a gradual acknowledgement of the possibility until one day Asperger's was no longer a possibility but just something that was part of him.

For if there was no acceptance of the diagnosis, whether formal or otherwise, we would have to accept that there was a serious problem with our marriage. Which is the scarier option for an Aspie man, a confirmation that you are a little different to the norm or that your whole life is going to fall apart when your wife gives up on you?

It is often the way that having a child diagnosed first, paves the way for introspection and even empathy and gradual acceptance that the apple doesn't fall far from the tree. Being able to recognise in your child traits which you also had at that age is undeniable evidence.

Yet, there are couples who are in limbo because at least one of them is in denial that there is a problem and that the problem is one of autism. Autism has had such a negative press that sometimes it is easier to live as a fake than to come out of the closet. These are often, sadly the couples that end up divorcing because they cannot confront the problem and instead blame each other or the stress of having autistic children.

The Husband Says:

Acknowledging that I'm "different" goes a long way to understanding and acknowledging the differences in my behaviour compared to you NTs. Karen hits the nail on the head above - "...a little different..."; I don't mind being known as a little bit different. I'm acknowledging that I need a bit of help to come closer to the norms - to the expectation of the majority.

*I would worry if I was labelled **VERY** different - I'm not that broken.*

It's probable that I had a diagnosis of something mental health related before I was a teenager. This was back in the days when neither ADHD nor Asperger's was a recognised diagnosis. I think, having seen the benefits of a label for my son, that a formal diagnosis label for me might be quite beneficial. There's nothing our health service would do with an adult Asperger Syndrome diagnosis (shame on the current state of UK mental health practice), but I'm coming around to the idea that I'm not "broken- different", just "English- eccentric- different"; there's no harm in that.

AS
*   So embrace the diagnosis (official or unofficial) - it's a step along the way of moderating unwanted behaviours that can damage adult partnerships.*

A

Achievements

On the whole I have noticed Aspies falling into two camps in this area. Those that want to achieve and are proactive about it to the point of obsession and those who would like to achieve but don't know how to.

Over Achiever

Those that set their sights high tend to want to prove themselves and be the best at everything. They work extremely hard and put in far more effort than most people.

There are several reasons for this:

- Wanting to be the best to bolster their self-esteem.

- Proving to others that they are not "just as good" as them but "better"! This may seem arrogant but it is their way of finding their way in a world they don't understand.

- Not knowing when enough is enough. They find it hard to judge when they have done sufficient amounts of work to do what is required. Therefore, they keep going or even repeat themselves in several different ways.

To this Aspie, the achievement is everything. It is not about the taking part. It is about the winning.

Is this something we need to change? Well, it depends on your own relationship and whether you are both happy about his behaviour or not.

NT If you see that he is putting in too much work, it may be worth asking him to précis it for you or asking to look at the work - if it is an area you are familiar with. He may of course not want you to see it until it is finished or he may possibly be condescending about your own abilities. You must be prepared for this but you will know what type of man you are married to.

NT However, if possible, it is worth pointing out to him that he has at least done enough for the day and he will probably only get paid the same amount of money, no matter how much time and energy he puts into it. Sometimes with an overachiever it is best just to give him space and let him do what he needs to do. He will be poor company until he decides that he is finished.

Underachiever

Then there are those who are very unsure of themselves and don't really want any attention, but to do well would be rather nice.

These Aspies have as much potential to achieve as the former. However, quite often they have not had the support from family or they do not have enough executive function in order to mobilise and achieve their wants. They have as much desire to achieve as the over achieving Aspies but these tend to hide away in their rooms and play on their computers in the hope that something good will eventually happen.

These boys and men lack the maturity and confidence to go out and get what they want. They are terrified of making mistakes and find it is easier to just withdraw from society. These men tend to live with their 'heads in the sand'.

Sometimes however, they manage to meet a woman who encourages and supports them and gets them motivated enough to go out and get a job and achieve a 'normal' life. For a while, this makes your underachiever Aspie happy as he can show the rest of the world that he is just like them.

Bitterness of the Underachiever

Unfortunately, with a relationship comes responsibility which all people on the spectrum find very hard. However, this can be particularly hard for your underachiever. This is the kind of man who, instead of being pleased that his child has a good school report, is actually jealous that she is doing well. It is irrational, and he will probably not admit it to himself, but his wife will be able to tell he is not giving a normal parent reaction to his child's achievements. This man can become very bitter and very hard to live with.

Another example is when the husband refused to go to university following his wife's successful graduation: he did not want to celebrate the fact that his wife was more qualified than he was. Rather than seeing this as an achievement that the whole family could celebrate and be pleased about (given that this is regarding the person he loves most) all he could think about is what he had not achieved. The fact that he had not gone to university and that he was in a dead end job.

What is the solution?

NT

The answer is to bolster his confidence. Remind him of the things he is very good at. His hobbies and obsessions. Where he achieves heights that no one else can. Point out that even though he is a mature adult it is not too late to further himself academically. Universities welcome mature students as statistically they are hardworking and high achievers.

This man needs to feel wanted and well thought of. He may not want to get himself a Master's degree and walk across a stage to shake the Chancellors hand to feel better about himself. He may just need some help and support and encouragement in his hobbies.

A

The Husband Says:

I sound really arrogant if I call myself an over-achiever. These are labels to be provided by others; not yourself. As Karen says, beware the trap of over-delivering compared with over-achieving. You can go too far in an effort to impress.

ADHD

Attention Deficit Hyperactivity Disorder

Asperger's syndrome (AS) is often a stand-alone condition but it is not unusual to find that it comes hand in hand with ADHD. It is much harder for professionals to diagnose AS when ADHD is also present. This is because the patient can present in more unpredictable and hyperactive ways, often a typical person with AS will be much less outgoing, more cautious and wary. Many of these character traits are subsumed by the ADHD and often a patient will go completely undiagnosed with the second condition (co-morbidity).

An experienced mental health team will be able to see past the most obvious character traits of the patient and recognise that actually, behind the outgoing facade, is someone who is very unsure of themselves and their place in the world and who craves stability, predictability and routine in order to control their environment.

The latest research suggests that though some children grow out of ADHD, there are still many adults with the condition. Brain scans done at MIT suggest that like those with Asperger's, people with ADHD have a lack of executive functioning. This means that they find it hard to concentrate and focus for long periods of time, despite often being highly intelligent, they cannot hold down a job, they get bored very quickly and their time management is poor.

Adults with AS and ADHD who go undiagnosed quite often get diagnosed with depression and start on a cycle of medication which may be hard to get off. These people, though often very intelligent, find it hard to finish education or hold down a job for long. They find that they can start with a huge amount of enthusiasm but when things stop going their way they find it difficult to cope and often retreat, mentally and physically, considering themselves failures.

NT
It is perhaps more important for those on the spectrum with a co-morbidity to be diagnosed and have their feelings recognised and supported with understanding and perhaps the right medication.

There is currently much research into how diet can help both children and adults with ADHD concentrate better and for longer.

Agreeing

Agree to Disagree

Arguments are inevitable in any marriage, but misunderstandings and lack of communication in an Asperger marriage provoke so many more. In an (idealistic) NT/NT marriage, couples will have varying views on finances, how to bring up the children and so on, but to promote harmony, they will learn to play to their strengths and know when the other is talking sense.

The NT partners will be able to see the other's point of view and even if they don't agree with it, or feel disadvantaged by it, they will at least agree to disagree and not carry on arguing.

Not so with the AS/NT couple. Unless the woman is completely submissive and actively agrees with her partner at all times, there are going to be explosions where differing opinion occurs. Even when the NT partner realises that she is not going to have her way (and is okay with that), often her AS partner will still not understand her point of view. Unless she completely agrees with him, she must be "wrong". He can't settle until not only he is proved "right" but that his partner totally agrees with him. He is unable to appreciate her perspective and in addition, he cannot see that she is allowed her own point of view.

This puts the woman in an untenable position. She knows what she feels is right but she also knows that, to keep the peace, she is going to have to completely agree with him to put his mind at rest. This can actually feel very abusive to the woman as any consideration for her independent thought is completely roughshod over.

In the modern, developed world, where women are mostly treated like equals and their opinions valued as much (or more!) than the next man, we are not used to being dismissed. It is rude and it is disrespectful. How can you have a relationship with a partner who appears to think quite lowly of your intellect and opinions?

This is a difficult question and is even trickier to answer.

Agree to Agree

Another scenario of an argument that feels surreal and shouldn't happen at all:

David came to me the other day full of enthusiasm about an article he had read in the New Scientist about lactose intolerance. Now I have suffered from lactose intolerance for many years and have only in the last few years realised it. Once I recognised the problem, this changed my life and I managed to change the whole household to lactose free milk without much challenge. I tend to stay away from dairy products (as they don't like me) but I do not deprive the rest of the household of them as they have not been tested for intolerance - though I have my suspicions!

... Anyway, so David knew I had an interest in lactose intolerance and he started talking to me about the article. I was really interested and asked him lots of questions. He started saying, "I don't know. Read the article," to my every question. I was peeling potatoes for dinner at the time so wasn't able to read the article there and then. Because he approached me, I thought he wanted to discuss it with me and I made the mistake of asking him more questions. Some he answered but mostly he got frustrated with me and told me to "read the article."

I realised then, by the tone of his voice, we were somehow getting into an argument where we both agreed with each other! I found this utterly ridiculous to the point where I felt a little hysterical. No matter what I say or do - agree with him or not, he was unhappy.

The Husband Says:

Having a debate or a discussion with an Aspie can be quite hard work. We have a standard of proof or satisfaction with the outcome of the argument that is almost forensic at times. Even the most superficial discussion can turn into a finely balanced debate over the merits of some point which is, in the cold light of day, irrelevant. It's a failure to communicate properly and adequately that is at the root of this.

In Karen's "agree to agree" situation above, I had got myself into an expectation trap. I'd skim read the article and found the content interesting and wanted to go back later and read it in depth. But the content was so relevant to Karen's interests that I thought she should know about it straight away. My enthusiasm for her to read the article came across as an expectation from Karen that I would precis the article to debate then and there; what I had intended was to give Karen the magazine for us both to look at it later, but with some urgency.

Sometimes I think NT's should fly a little flag saying "I'm Busy" or "What I am Doing is Tedious, Feel Free to Interrupt". That way we would get on the same wavelength much more quickly.

Alcohol

Using it as a Crutch

In western society, the use of alcohol in a social situation is perfectly acceptable. It eases conversation and relaxes you. Inhibitions are lowered and people, on the whole, are less easily offended by social gaffes. Those who are socially awkward lose their inhibitions and can even become the life and soul of the party.

So alcohol definitely has its uses but it is so easy to fall into the trap of relying on it to oil the social wheels and subsequently end up drinking too much on a regular basis.

Using Alcohol to Reduce Stress

We fell into the trap of using a glass of wine to help us unwind after a stressful day. Before I met David I drank socially but not very often in the house. Drinking was for pubs and nightclubs and parties and as I wasn't a big social animal and also couldn't afford it, it was never a problem.

Drinking at home became a fairly regular occurrence once the children were born. Like many parents you can't go out but you would like to unwind after a very difficult day. A glass of wine lets you feel like an adult when you have spent the day on the floor picking up jigsaws or cleaning banana puree out of your hair. After the wearing bedtime routine and the house is quiet, you feel like you deserve it.

We didn't drink every night but when we did share a bottle of wine it was rare that it wasn't finished. I wonder now whether that regular bottle of wine stopped us having to talk to each other and facing our marital problems?

Health Issues

The health issues of drinking alcohol are well documented but also confusing. I have a friend who drinks two glasses of red wine every evening as it was recommended to him by a health professional after he had some heart trouble.

NT **AS** The best way to deal with alcohol is in moderation, it seems, or perhaps not at all. Some Aspies have addictive personalities and will become reliant on the social benefits of drinking.

The Husband Says:

With new guidance having me on a par with Karen on 14 units per week maximum, I've carefully weighed up my excessive alcohol intake. I've come to the conclusion that my life might be shortened by alcohol and its consequences, but I'm so much more relaxed and able to enjoy my leisure time at the end of the working day for so many years, that the slight shortening of my lifespan seems worthwhile.

I know Karen worries about my health, but it's a delicate line between alcohol, exercise, eating for calories, eating for enjoyment and lifespan. No easy answers here I'm afraid.

The Wife Replies:

What David doesn't seem to understand is that I care about his health and would like him to be around for as long as possible. Not taking care of his health can be quite a selfish action as eventually the onus is on someone else to care for you.

Alexithymia

An inability to identify and describe emotions. A frequent comorbidity of Asperger Syndrome. Don't mistake this very specific condition with the more common problem of recognising emotions from facial expressions.

All Men are Like That

You will have heard this so many times. Perhaps you were chatting to your friends over a coffee. You may have tentatively dropped into the conversation one of your husband's many foibles. Your friends will have laughed and compared him to their own husband and pronounced "All men are like that."

Believe me, not all men are like that. If you feel there is something 'wrong' with the way your husband interacts with people or reacts to situations on a regular basis, then you should trust your instincts. The problem with Asperger Syndrome is that each little difference can be so subtle that it can easily be dismissed and forgotten about at first. Other people may think you are making a fuss about nothing. What they do not realise is that you have to live with every one of his differences, all of the time. It becomes a chore and you don't even realise how it happened. I have had other long term, 'normal' relationships and I know that not "all men are like that".

The Husband Says:

I had mixed feelings when I first read this article. There's a body of opinion, especially on the Internet, that takes the phrase "all men are like that" and spins it rather negatively and seeks to end that phrase with something derogatory; "all men are like that ... a bunch of %-£!@%s". That starts to look like a militant feminism school of thought.

And on the face of it, men, like any other species, can be divided into broad classifications each with similar behaviour patterns, so it is a truism that "All men (in particular groups) are like that." It doesn't take much coincidence in the groups of spouses getting together talking about their relationships before coincidence in their husband's behaviour is interpreted as pattern.

Odd behaviour stands out. What defines "odd" behaviour? Behaviour is measured against social norms and social norms are very much "of the time" - they change rapidly, even more so in this multi-cultural and technical age. I think Aspies like me are strongly influenced by tradition. I also think that Asperger Syndrome runs genetically, so there are likely to be strong rules-bound matriarchs and patriarchs in the familial line handing down the guide-lines of social norms disguised as absolute rules that must be followed. So these familial hand-me-downs continue to influence the lives of the offspring by restricting the rate at which modern

Aspies can adapt their model of social norms to meet the needs of this modern time. Thus "All (Aspie) men are like that ... a bit behind the times."

All or Nothing

This phrase comes up so often in conversation with wives and parents of loved ones on the autism spectrum.

This comes under the umbrella of extremes, but you will have noticed that your husband is an All or Nothing kind of guy. Examples being:

Noticing that you have changed your hair and not liking it, or not noticing at all, ever.

- Loving spicy food or loving very bland food.

- An exercise enthusiast or can't understand other people's idea of moderate exercise or a husband who is a professional couch potato.

- Always insists on doing the dishwasher as you do it wrong or never doing the dishwasher as he doesn't know when it's loading or not.

- Loves dogs or hates dogs.

- Only believes in the truth of science or is deeply into theology.

- Feels pain acutely and is a terrible patient or never feels pain or illness and is intolerant of other people being ill.

- Had no interest in your project or completely takes it over.

These are just a few examples but hopefully you will recognise at least one in your partner.

We NTs live in a world of moderation, touched only occasionally by the extremes. Our partners only ever feel the extremes of everything. We need to recognise what hard work this is for them and that this is why they cannot understand our 'moderation in everything' attitudes.

Amygdala

Part of the brain that performs a primary role in the processing of memory, decision-making, and emotional reactions.

Cambridge University scientists were the first to discover that the amygdala is under-active when people with autism and Asperger Syndrome are trying to decode emotional facial expressions. This leads to their theory that the amygdala is one of several neural regions of the brain that are abnormal in autism.

Anger

My Anger

I'm a fairly mild tempered person. I am slow to anger. I can take a lot on board and, even when I'm cross or upset, I tend to deal with it quietly. I internalise. I look at the situation from every angle and agonise about whether I handled it right and worry that I did not. I am also very good at seeing both sides of every story.

However, I can be stubborn. When I know I am right I will say so. I am happy to "agree to disagree" but for an Aspie that does not make sense. If he believes that I am wrong, and I am adamant I am right, he cannot leave the situation alone. I have the mature emotional ability to walk away but he will take my disagreement personally.

Just occasionally (and it takes a lot) I will explode! I will freak out and I will let everyone in range have it. This is my secret weapon! I am scary when I am angry but it is like the threat of a nuclear weapon, it keeps them in awe of you and not wanting to upset you.

NT I also know that sometimes you just have to let anger out but I am capable instead of following my baser instincts, of either having a rant online to those in the know, or marching the dog on a very long and fast walk.

The problem with being an Aspie wife is that sometimes you are aware that your own anger is just there, simmering away in reaction to certain persistent behaviour. I believe in picking my battles and not criticising every tiny thing that he does differently to the way I would do it. It's not fair on him and is not conducive to a good atmosphere. So in choosing not to react to the petty things there are times when the anger unhealthily simmers away. I am now more aware of when I'm doing it and try hard not to these days.

My daughter is a fan of the film "Frozen" (though I'll probably have to kill you all now I've told you that!) and she used to obsessively play the song "Let It Go" in our car. At first I thought it was naff but then, when I listened properly to the lyrics, it made me cry. In the car by myself I tried to sing along to it as a stress relief but I couldn't get the words out. They were too poignant.

NT This is what I need to do with my anger. LET IT GO! It isn't really important that he never looks to see if the dishwasher is loading or unloading is it?

His Anger Towards You

His anger towards you can be unpredictable. You will find that how angry he is depends on his levels of anxiety and his lack of control over a situation. Unless you have done something to directly affect his mood then you have to remind yourself that though is anger seems directed at you, it is generally not about you. He is lashing out verbally at the person he loves and trusts most in the world. It may seem paradoxical to do this but this is what young children do to their parents when they are upset. They it is horrible to experience, what they are actually telling you in their distress is that they love you enough to express their real emotions to you. They are assuming unconditional love on both your parts.

Tips to Reduce Anxiety fed Anger

NT
You will know his triggers by now, whether they are other drivers on the road or someone sitting in his spot. It is best to try and avoid certain triggers but we know that sometimes life is just not like that. The key to dealing with triggers is planning. Often, if he knows what to expect then he will feel in control and be much calmer.

Try not to surprise him with anything. Give him plenty of notice of events, especially social ones. Plan holidays and outings in military fashion. It may take some of the spontaneity out of life but it is still far better than sitting by a pool in a foreign country, hating your husband.

There is always a reason for his anger so you need to be an emotional detective and find out what is causing it. It is possible that it is multi-layered and they are just overwhelmed by the amount of 'stuff' they have to do.

If this is the case help them to break each task down to something manageable instead of something looming and overwhelming. A chart with categories of importance and a time frame is useful for this. Don't forget they are visual thinkers, so once they are able to see what is needed and rationalise it they will start to feel in control again.

The Husband Says:

Anger. A difficult subject to talk about.

Where does it start or come from? For me, the principal causes are:

- *Having my personal space invaded - or my perception of what "space" is mine. There are variants:*

- *Having the space around my car invaded by other motorists with their unexpected behaviour.*

A

NT

Karen is good at checking this behaviour in me by reminding me just how childish that would be. The insult snaps me out of it, but it takes a little while to cool down.

- Having my time (like space) "stolen". My time is precious to me and I don't want it wasted on doing the same things over and over if I can avoid it. Some chores are necessary and I want to do them as efficiently as possible. Anything else just compounds the annoyance and anger.

- Failures in communication. I get noisy then I get angry if I believe that I'm not getting my point across by "winning" an argument. Is there ever a "winner" of an argument between partners, or are there just two losers?

- Aspies like to win at what they think they are good at. It gets messy if an Aspie thinks arguing is a talent - only in very narrow circumstances, like the legal profession, is this true.

NT

I struggle to read emotions from facial expressions, so I think I've failed in my communications with you, and that leads to anger. Defuse this by confirming back to me your impression of what you heard; iron out any misunderstanding before doubt and anxiety can take root. Karen is really good at "echoing back" stuff to avoid wrongly interpreted communications.

NT

Karen is really very good at closing down an argument by pouring the cold water of silence into it. But then I get anxious that my anger has caused permanent offence and that anxiety can turn into another cycle of anger about how I found myself in this situation.

AS

Having seen how Transactional Analysis might help me understand how to communicate effectively, I want to try to work with Karen to see how arguments could be cut short and the dialogue started very quickly afterwards with the adult ego talking to the adult ego rather than the crossed egos that led to the argument.

- Being challenged on my specialist subjects (obsessions). I'm right. I know I'm right and see, now, you're wasting my time, and now I'm getting angry...

NT

Karen is getting good at avoiding sparking debate on specialist subjects. Father-in-law has been warned off certain subjects after some bad experiences in the past.

AS

I try not to tell people I'm employed in renewable energy - that immediately kicks off a debate that no-one can "win". The job description Management Consultant does just fine, and that sounds so tedious I can bridge to another subject for conversation...

- *... but that means I'm having to learn how to make small-talk and coming up with a few "canned" anecdotes and lines of conversation that are safe. It's tough. It requires more of that putting on an act for the public and that public includes your social friends.*

Note from the Wife

NT Arguments should not be about "winning". It is about showing the other person your point of view and vital information and about getting to a resolution where everyone can be happy. I am happy to "lose" an argument on subjects of little importance. I will stand my ground where it is vital and I know I am right. It is not about winning.

Note from the Husband

This back and forth looks like an argument. It isn't! But it does prompt...

Aspie Hints & Tips

This is hard for an Aspie to say and even harder to put into practise, but:

- *Choose to debate and even argue (don't fall into it by accident);*

- *Be prepared to be wrong; and*

- *Don't argue so hard that it is necessary to apologise afterwards. If it's getting that heated, LEAVE IT.*

Answering the Phone

When we first started living together I noticed that David would answer the phone like this:

"Hello, it's Dave Slee"

Pause

"May I ask who's calling?"

Pause

"What is it in regard to?"

Pause

Then he would hold out the phone to me.

"It's your mum."

A

When friends called they got the same "I'm at work mode" style of answering the phone. It took many months for regular friends calling for him to actually move on from the necessary. One day I actually caught him in light conversation with my friend before he handed the phone to me. This was progress.

I think it all stems from anxiety of not knowing who is on the other end, though these days with Caller ID it is much simpler but it gives his conversation structure which the other person then has to adhere to until they are trusted to free style.

He often sounds very defensive and interrogative on the phone when people are calling for me. I know he wants to protect me from bad calls. The only ones I need protecting from are cold callers. I have no interest in them but he loves to wind them up.

Taking a Message

This seems such a simple thing: when I am not in, please take a message for me. He is not very good at it and, if it is to do with the children, he immediately tells the caller that I am the expert in that area and will ask them to ring back. He's probably right. I would be cross if he got it wrong but sometimes it is annoying to then have to chase someone through a telephone maze when he could have just answered a simple question on the spot.

The most memorable time when he should have taken a message was when I was actually in the house. I wasn't avoiding the phone or incapacitated, but I was in the shower. He barged into the en-suite with his arm outstretched and told me I had to take the call. I can't remember who it was but it certainly wasn't a life or death situation. I rang them back later.

Of course sometimes he is very good at taking messages and I come home and find little post it notes on my monitor. Other times he takes a message but doesn't remember to tell me until it's too late!

The Husband Says:

Ah, the telephone, sometimes 'The Great Leveller'.

On the one hand, as an Aspie, you can train yourself to pick up on the verbal cues, including the absence of speech, that can give some vital clues as to what is happening at the other end of the 'phone. This levels the playing field. Perhaps the NTs aren't as good at picking up those hints-in-sound and they are cut off from their non-verbal body language cues that they normally depend on.

But it's the anxiety as to the purpose of the call that us Aspies struggle with. First of all, we don't do 'small-talk' very well. Each statement needs a purpose - we like to think we are all killer and no filler in conversation - every word a gem. But that means that after the NT has waffled on, that the punch-line, the purpose of the call will eventually come around. They are going to ask a question. It won't be an open ended question either - they will want an answer

here and now - no one picks up the phone to warn you that they will want answers sometime in the future - they want answers and now!

There's something else at work that feeds anxiety too. If I'm making a call, there is only so much I can plan, control and rehearse about the call. I don't know if it is true for other Aspies rather than just me, but I struggle with thick accents - face to face I do better by doing a bit of lip reading and assessing the most overt gestures. So that's the main reason I don't ring up the take away and order food - I'm anxious I'll mess up the order or insult the person on the other end of the phone because I'm struggling to understand what they are saying.

Finally, from me - I wonder if Karen was happy or suspicious that I was chatting with one of 'her' friends on the 'phone. Is it my mild paranoia that Karen might think I'm flirting with someone that I shouldn't?

The Wife Says

If you read the chapter on Trust, David, you will realise it is your paranoia.

Aspie Hints & Tips

I find the following helpful:

- *Use a decent mobile phone with higher quality digital sound.*

- *Use a smart-phone linked to social networking so you can see a picture of the person who is ringing you, to give you vital seconds to plan what you are going to say first.*

- *Divert the call to voice-mail if you are genuinely not ready to take a call...*

- *... But get a reputation for ringing back the moment you are able.*

- *Conversation with a 'phone in the way will be slower than face to face for both the Aspie and the NT. Slow down, don't gabble and use this to your advantage.*

Anticipation

It is most noticeable in young children with ASD that unlike your NT child they do not enjoy the feeling of anticipation at all.

They feel their emotions so intensely it is hard for them to control them and their thoughts and worries take priority before anything else. The overwhelming thoughts and feelings are one of the many reasons for their egocentricity.

You and I have probably learned to enjoy that feeling of butterflies in the tummy and excitement about a long awaited event but the adult Aspie can react quite differently and negatively, spoiling it not just for themselves but for everyone.

They so desperately want things to go right they spend their time anticipating and ruminating on all the things that could go wrong. They cannot help but dwell on the negative side of this at times and in fact, because they are so negative it becomes a self-fulfilling prophecy but at least they were proved right!

The Husband Says:

That rumbling you hear in your tummy before a big event? That's adrenaline triggering fight or flight. It's also the sound of an Aspie's plans being torn to shreds by happenstance.

Anxiety

An Aspie's level of anxiety is naturally higher than ours. The only time they truly relax is when they immerse themselves in their special interest. I know what I am like when I am anxious, about maybe singing a solo or a job interview. I get easily irritated and my levels of tolerance in other people plummet. Imagine being in that state all the time.

From my observations of my husband and my children, though they deal with their anxieties in different ways, I can tell they are all affected and this has changed and grown as they have changed and grown.

Certainly in the history of courtship, I was not particularly aware of David's anxieties. He hid them well. In fact, to me, he mostly came across as reassuring and confident. It was a very attractive quality. Was this how he felt at the time or was it just a facade, motivated by his love and obsession for me?

Motivation does not reduce anxiety but it can help them push through the pain barrier if they can see the goal at the end and truly desire it more than anything else, even more than fear and uncertainty.

Or perhaps my presence was particularly calming? I'm not a loud person. I'm quiet and a good listener yet I often have things to say. I just pick and choose what I say as I am not one for pretending I know something when I do not. Perhaps my simple, non-threatening attitude was actually calming for my (future) husband.

In recent times when he has had severe meltdowns and I have not (outwardly) reacted to the situation, he has later thanked me for being there and for staying calm. Believe me, in the incident I am thinking of (when he was freaking out driving the car back from Liverpool at a crawl) I was not at all calm. I was so anxious I was almost to the point of self-harming to relieve the tension I was feeling. But he didn't know that.

NT Try to stay calm in the face of your partner's anxiety driven irrationality.

The Husband Says:

Anxiety. The Devil on your back, weighing you down. Anxiety fuels adrenaline, one more step and we have anger.

For me, anxiety stems from never quite knowing if I'm living up to the social norms. I can't measure the extent of emotions and their external effects on the person right in front of me in the way that a neurotypical "just does". On emotional topics I don't know if I've done enough or worse still, gone too far and stepped over a social norm line.

I get performance anxiety, but I can control that with forward planning. Planning is the antidote to anxiety for me. But there is always the nagging concern that I might have to go "off-plan" or worse that I will read a situation so badly that no plan can help. That sums up the Liverpool trip - I had lost confidence in the car and my ability to drive that car safely in the face of the behaviour I sensed in people around me, but I had no choice at all other than to drive it back home. It took weeks to gain confidence in that car (and what it means socially) and I'm still not wholly comfortable with it.

NT
Karen has a good strategy for reducing my anxiety. She want's spontaneity, so we aim for planned spontaneity as the next best thing. If that works out and is fun, we can repeat it either by plan or in true spontaneity.

Appearing to be 'Normal'

Many men with Asperger Syndrome are extremely good at appearing to be normal. Many of my friends and acquaintances have been shocked and surprised to hear that David has social difficulties. Some in fact do not believe it. 'But he is so normal and articulate,' they have said.

Yes, but he has had to work extremely hard to appear like that and finds the whole thing exhausting. He is putting on a show with learned behaviour that he knows is expected of him. He does not want to be thought of as socially awkward or stupid so he will do his best to prove himself and other people wrong, though he is the only one aware of this.

Your Aspie partner is using his other skills and talents to compensate for what is lacking. He is using his extensive memory and intelligence to work out what the rest of the world does instinctively. This is why he will appear social and even charming in public and why he fooled you in to marrying him in the first place. He worked hard on it. You were worth it

Much of his charm is learned behaviour and memorising what has been successful and what has not. When on his best behaviour, his every word and action is considered carefully.

A

However, he can't keep this facade up for ever and this is why when he gets home he retreats to his comfort zone and does not want to speak.

The Husband Says:

*This "appearing to be normal" cuts to the very heart of the difficulties us Aspies have with modern life. For some freak of nature reason, perhaps 4% of the population is wired up a bit differently in the brain department and instead of reacting instinctively in social situations (which is what you neurotypicals do), our Aspie brains are wired more for analysis. So we either react **before** the event (because our analysis says something bad is going to happen if we continue down this path) or we react **after** the event (trying to save a bad situation from getting worse). When we react before the event you wonder why I'm doing it - the reason isn't obvious to you yet. And quite often when reacting after the event the response can be too late and thus judged inappropriate for reasons of timing.*

Where we have time to plan, this analytical approach can be very successful - us Aspies put on an act - we pretend to be the person that society expects us to be (the social norm) by acting like we think a neurotypical would. But this takes a significant amount of effort. The mask of the actor can slip perhaps due to higher priorities (in our minds of course - our list of priorities not your neurotypical list of priorities), through sheer exhaustion with "being on best behaviour", or through boredom and lack of perceived reward for keeping up the act.

*And of course sometimes we guess what a neurotypical would do (remember we don't intuitively **know** what you would do), and we guess wrong, either because logic doesn't apply to a given situation or our analysis turned out to be wrong for some reason. When we get it wrong, it is usually a complete mystery to us as to why, and that just makes things worse.*

Arrogance

This is not an attractive quality in anyone. I do not like people being rude and showing off and I find it embarrassing when it is my husband. I have walked out of shops leaving David arguing with the staff because I cannot bear to be associated with it.

I know the arrogance stems from insecurities and his need to show off is to prove he is better than them. He does not like being patronised by shop staff, especially in his speciality areas of technology and computing. He always does his research before he goes into a shop to buy anything and he knows when a member of staff tries it on. Most NT's just put up with this politely but he does not, despite the fact he knows the guy is just doing his job.

What advice can I give to help you in this instance?

Perhaps the two of you can devise some going shopping rules. IF you promise only to buy what you went out for rather than impulse buying, perhaps he can reciprocate by considering your feelings and not being rude to the shop staff. It's worth a try.

The Husband Says:

*Oh yes. I just **know** I'm right. Even when I'm wrong.*

Over-confidence on a specialist subject is the undoing of the Aspie. Expertise becomes arrogance.

AS *If you are brave enough to make an unusual and specialist point on your specialist subject the principle of a public discussion or professional argument, check, check and triple check that you are, in fact, right and not just winging it. Humble pie tastes very bitter.*

Asperger Syndrome

This is a form of autism that is classed by many people as 'mild'. However, if you have Asperger Syndrome (AS) or live with someone with AS you will realise that it is not a 'mild' condition at all.

It is often said that when you've met one person with Asperger's you have met one person with Asperger's. This is because like every 'normal' person we all have different personalities. We all have a different genetic makeup and upbringing. You cannot get to know one person with AS well and assume that you now know everything there is to do about Asperger's. In fact, I would say that though I know David very well now, he never ceases to surprise me.

I have friends who also have husbands (undiagnosed) on the autism spectrum. I have met them all and not one is alike. They have very different personalities and outlooks on the world. Some come across as very negative about everything and others come across as very sociable and normal. Others are very quiet and intense. Yet when I have sat and had coffee with my friends, at some point over our latte's we will all burst out with 'Oh yes! My husband does that!'

The Husband Says:

I'm an officially undiagnosed person with Asperger Syndrome. I'm an Aspie. I've grown reasonably comfortable with this label if that is how you want to categorise me. It is a reasonable indicator of some parts of my character. With close colleagues I use this term to help explain my behaviour and how I can be of great help in business.

- *I don't ever want to be compared with Dustin Hoffman in Rainman.*

- *I'm not catatonic.*

- *I'm not an idiot savant.*

- *On some topics I just think a bit different from you.*

Oh, and I have a talent for writing lists.

Aspies

"Aspie" is a slang term for a person at the Asperger Syndrome part of the autism spectrum. It is a reasonably well accepted term used to describe themselves by those with an autism spectrum disorder (ASD).

Someone who isn't an Aspie is often described as NT - neurotypical.

A level of caution is required; there is a more militant group of persons on the autism spectrum who dislike the term "Aspie".

The Husband Says:

I don't mind being called an Aspie. It can be a term of endearment e.g. "My Aspie husband". "I'm an Aspie" is certainly much better for conversation than "I have an autism spectrum disorder." I quite often describe myself as an Aspie and then talk about Baron-Cohen's ideas of brain function - the brain wiring not being somehow 'incorrect' in Asperger Syndrome, just different from the so-called neurotypicals, sometimes beneficially so.

Assigning Blame

This is very common in an Aspie/NT marriage and can result in the woman beginning to think that perhaps she is going mad. His need to blame the wife for everything that goes wrong feels like psychological warfare. He does not, however, have any idea what he is doing to his marriage and to his wife's self-esteem and happiness.

So why does he do this? He finds it hard to admit that he may be at fault. He doesn't want to be at fault as that would be admitting weakness and blowing his cover of being 'normal'. He is not emotionally mature enough to deal with negative situations and needs to take his frustration out on someone. Unfortunately, that someone is you. The person he loves most.

I am his Emotional Sponge.

The Husband Says:

Not being "normal" is not fair. I want somebody or something to absorb my feelings of unfairness so that I don't have to carry them around, damaging me. Karen, you are in the tricky position of being close to me and having an understanding of me and so you are a convenient container to allow me to transfer this blame. And that, in itself, is unfair.

Can we find a container to hold this blame? An inanimate object, or even a concept? I wonder if channelling it into this project and writing about it is a beneficial form of therapy?

Atelophobia

The fear of not being good enough. This is the source of many of your partner's anxieties. He wants to be accepted and acceptable but he cannot judge when he has reached this point.

NT To help him judge when he is done enough you should tell him what most people expect from his actions. Point out what is too much and what is too little. Having something to help him gauge his actions will reduce his stress and maybe even make him come home a little earlier from work because he knows he has done enough.

Attraction

One of the questions that is frequently asked is "What first attracted you to your husband?"

Well, I immediately liked him - though I wasn't immediately attracted to him - because he was the most talkative, friendly and helpful person I met at work that first day. I was completely ignored by the one other person I had been put in the office with (but that is understandable as he, like David, was an engineer and a likely Aspie!).

David told me to come to him if I needed help with anything, and I could tell that he meant it. It turned out he had a great sense of humour and I was made to feel very welcome by him and most of the other male staff. When David asked me out, I was a little hesitant. Though I had officially ended my previous relationship, it was very early days and still very raw. There was always that possibility that we might get back together. However, since the ex was still pretty much AWOL, I decided I had nothing to lose and would at least get an enjoyable evening out of the date.

On that first night, David was very attentive and wanted to know everything about me. He insisted on buying the drinks and eventually driving me home. He was easy to talk to. As the weeks went by, he was still very generous, considerate and thoughtful. More significantly, something that I had missed for a while in my last relationship but had never realised, this man was proud to be with me and to be seen with me.

A

There was another level of attraction, a baser one if you will, and I don't actually mean sex. Deep down, every woman (even if she doesn't admit it to herself) wants a man she can rely on. David had reliability and stability written all over him. He wanted to provide for me. He had laid the foundations by buying a house, having a good job and now he wanted to settle down.

He was a little older than me and I had just left university so it wasn't really what I was looking for at the time. I insisted on being as financially independent as I could but he would often win "spending arguments" by pointing out that he had more money than me. It could be annoying at times, but there are many worse things to be annoyed about than your other half's generosity. It took a couple of years of courting but eventually we decided to marry and, though we have our ups and downs, I have no major regrets.

The Husband Says:

They say that Aspies are late developers and that was true of me. I was attracted to only a limited number of women at university and they were all "taken" usually by someone else in the small social circle I was in who was more confident. Once I graduated there was more attraction to the opposite sex, but so many people who I considered out of reach. Karen appeared where I was working and like in Goldilocks and the Three Bears she was just right.

What is Autism?

If you are anything like me, the most you knew about autism was from the film "Rainman" starring Tom Cruise and Dustin Hoffman. Hoffman played Cruise's older brother Raymond (Rainman) who had been living in a nursing home for most of his life as he was considered a danger to society and unable to live by himself. Raymond had many peculiar behaviours and affectations and found it very hard to communicate or even speak. He was also a savant. This is actually a very rare and severe form of autism.

Leo Kanner came up with the term autism.

Classic autism and Asperger Syndrome are at extreme ends of the Autism Spectrum, depending on your view of the autism spectrum.

ASD is a pervasive development disorder that is thought to affect 62 in every 10,000 children and until recently these are mostly boys that were diagnosed. Of every child diagnosed with ASD only one in four are girls. The main developmental effects are difficulties in socialisation, communication and imagination. The presentation and severity of effects can vary from child to child but most obvious to observers are lack of eye contact, seeming to be "in a world of their own", hypersensitivity to stimuli and repetitive behaviour. Those affected by ASD have a different view of the world from the average or 'neurotypical' person and can interpret situations very literally, which can make them seem quite rude at times. ASD covers a wide range of abilities from the severely autistic person, that prefers not to speak at all, to the child with Asperger's who cannot contain his excitement about the workings of the fridge in the supermarket. Hans Asperger considered that 'the characteristics could be identified in some children as young as two or three years, although for other children, the characteristics only become conspicuous some years later.' (Tony Attwood, "The Complete Guide to Autism", 2007).

Autism Quotient Test

The AQ test was devised by Simon Baron-Cohen at Cambridge University.

This can be easily found online or in an App and though not a diagnosis is a very good indicator of whether the person taking the test is on the autistic spectrum or not.

The Husband Says:

AS
Don't set any store in these Facebook type "10 Questions to see if you are Autistic" so-called tests. Fill in the diagnostic level questionnaires issued by professionals honestly, and with the first thing that comes into your head (if in doubt) to get a proper opinion that will be genuinely helpful.

Autistic Spectrum

The autistic spectrum is a range of conditions characterised by difficulties in social interaction and communication and will affect different people in different ways.

The Husband Says:

*There are lots of definitions of **THE** Autistic Spectrum. There are lots of attempts to measure how far along The Autistic Spectrum a given individual might be.*

In reality, since we don't know the root cause of Asperger's and Autism and characterise them by the collection and severity of symptoms, then the Autistic Spectrum is the composite position of an individual along a number of scales, one for each recognised symptom of Asperger's or Autism. These scales cannot be numbered for severity, only that each scale has a mild and a severe end. Everybody is on each of the scales somewhere; only when there are a significant selection of "high" scores on each scale is it considered that a spectrum condition exists.

A

Avoidance

Avoiding doing something means that the Aspie is usually too scared to do it or they really have no interest in it. Lack of empathy means they often cannot predict a scenario that they have not been in before. They find this uncertainty and lack of clarity worrying if not terrifying. If it is not essential to do something, why put yourself in that situation?

This is true to some extent but an AS man and his wife should learn to choose their battles rather than avoid them completely. Sometimes it is worth going through the pain and anxiety of a difficult situation to come out victorious on the other side. The pros and cons have to be weighed up.

NT Be aware not to give in to these scenarios too often as it can become habit to just avoid everything that makes your partner uncomfortable. You will be dragged down by their thinking and also start to avoid these types of situations yourself.

Never be afraid to attend an event by yourself. It can be quite liberating to turn up at a function as you will often get to talk to and know people you would otherwise not have met.

Procrastination

This is the avoidance of doing tasks by delaying them and finding other priorities (distractions). Your Aspie knows these tasks have to be done but he likes to put them off for as long as possible. I am a little guilty of this myself (as are most people) and in the modern age of 24/7 television and social media, it is easy to distract oneself and pretend to be busy.

David however, is a master at this, see also Diesel Jenga and Putting Out the Bins.

The Husband Says:

Yes, avoidance does fall into those two categories, either causing so much anxiety that it must be avoided for mental and physical health, or avoidance stemming from laziness, boredom or perceived irrelevance when compared with all the other things an Aspie could be doing.

I don't get much enjoyment out of large social gatherings. Being judged by so called peers in a social situation makes me anxious. And they take so much forward planning - rehearsing some anecdotes and lines of conversation that are non-confrontational, learning the names of distant family members you are unlikely to see again and so forth. Small gatherings of friends are good, but I want a sense of purpose, so I like to cook or serve drinks.

I'm pretty clumsy - it is an Asperger Syndrome comorbidity - and I don't have a great opinion on my body image so I have never (other than my wedding day) wanted or tried to dance.

Scottish country dancing at school scarred me for life. You won't see me going to a dance with Karen.

Here is pretty much the line between anxiety avoidance and laziness avoidance:

~ ~

I hate ringing up the Chinese takeaway and placing an order. I'm happy to do the 10 mile round-trip and wait for the take-away, so laziness is not the whole story, but any anxiety of being misunderstood on the phone is really a poor excuse rather than a genuine fear. I guess it is just the communicating with strangers thing.

Awareness

Awareness of Self

Your Aspie partner is generally less aware of how they present themselves to the world than you. They will often rely on and appreciate your opinion on the lighter subjects such as style. They will generally have no opinion on the latest fashion unless it involves something that has particularly appealing textures.

David tries harder with his clothes these days but rarely does he get 'casual' right. He will wear dress shoes with jeans or trainers with his smart trousers. Basically, he goes for whatever feels comfortable to him and who am I to criticise?

There is a formula to work clothes, so he mostly gets it right.

He is not a judge of subtle, and fashion is not about subtle and is forever changing, so if you learn the rules for one season they will have changed by the next. It is best not to care about these things.

See also Spatial Awareness for the topic of awareness of self in space.

Awareness of Difference

People often ask me what the difference is between an Autistic person and someone with Asperger's Syndrome. I do have a radar for this. It is hard to put your finger on the difference at first. Having one title is not better than having the other. Asperger's is still an autistic condition; it is just slightly different from classic or high functioning autism. Like apples, Granny Smiths are green and rather tart, whereas Pink Lady® are pink and sweet, but they are still apples!

I cover this in more detail elsewhere. One of the main differences that I notice between those with AS and Autism is that Aspies have great awareness of being different and therefore they are acutely aware of making mistakes.

My family have always known they were different. They didn't know there was a label for it at first but, once our son found out that 'it wasn't his fault', his relief was

A

palpable. Being told he had AS validated his feelings of being different. He knew he wasn't imagining it. Generally, but not always those who are Autistic are less afraid of making mistakes because they are less likely to be aware enough to be embarrassed by those mistakes.

This is a sweeping generalisation as everyone on the autistic spectrum is different but, as a rule of thumb, Aspie's are very hard on themselves when they have made a mistake and will do anything they can to avoid doing that again.

A

B

- ✧ Back-Handed Compliment
- ✧ Behaviour
- ✧ Behaviour in a Crisis
- ✧ Being a Single Parent
- ✧ Being Honest
- ✧ Being Taken for Granted
- ✧ Being Tricked into Marriage
- ✧ Being Useful
- ✧ Bereavement
- ✧ Body Language
- ✧ Bonio® Moment
- ✧ Boundaries
- ✧ Brain Function Theories
- ✧ Breaking Point
- ✧ Breaking Up
- ✧ Brokering

B

Back-Handed Compliment

David is a master at the back-handed compliment. Some of them could be construed as malicious but I (now) believe that it is not on purpose. Most often he says what he thinks without any filter. Other times he believes he is being funny but has completely missed the mark. Very occasionally he can be quite amusing. I don't mind being the butt of a joke sometimes.

For example, when he talks to people about my Master's degree, he will refer to my academic writing as 'a good journalistic style'. He's basically putting me down for not using overly academic language but at the same time making my writing interesting and easy to read and understand. I know what the big words are I just don't see the need to use them all the time. It is intimidating to some people.

I had my hair cut and coloured recently and though David knew I was going to the hairdressers he was too busy with work to say anything when I got home. The following morning when he got up, over a cup of coffee he blearily blinked at me and said, "Your hair looks so much better this morning now it's disorganised. You look more like you." Err, thanks dear. This may be related to his hate of change.

AS However, all Aspies should remember that if they are going to abuse someone's efforts they need to be prepared for a backlash. It goes both ways. You can't play the Aspie card all the time!

This doesn't mean they don't have a good sense of humour.

The Husband Says:

Many of them weren't meant to be back-handed. You fished for a compliment and me, being quite poor at the whole comparison, metaphor and simile thing, and under pressure to reply, went for a straight-forward and truthful statement. The thing is, a compliment needs a level of hyperbole and "buffing up" otherwise it comes out back-handed; a compliment that is not quite as good as it could be.

AS *Aspies, exaggerate a little bit when giving a compliment to avoid it coming out back-handed.*

The Wife Replies:

I don't fish for compliments.

Behaviour

It is very easy to fixate on autistic behaviours, meltdowns, repetition, echolalia etc... but really, these are unimportant. These behaviours are signs that something is wrong and causing them anxiety.

NT YOU NEED TO TURN DETECTIVE AND WORK OUT WHAT THE TRIGGERS WERE FOR THAT BEHAVIOUR IN THE FIRST PLACE.

You must always ask yourself, "Why is he doing this?". Do not take his behaviour towards you or other people personally.

The Husband Says:

Very little of my behaviour is malicious unless directed at PPI claims specialists or solar power salesmen. What looks like unwanted behaviours to you neurotypicals is me being logical in the face of a tangle of perceived social rules and doing something unexpected - unexpected by you that is.

AS *You can do worse than adopt the mantra "What would the NT do?" to give you an opportunity to stop and plan rather than blindly apply logic when choosing tricky courses of action.*

Behaviour in a Crisis

This is often a "personality plus" as your Aspie can be a great leader in a time of stress. He is organised and prepared and has already gone through worst case scenarios in his head, if he hasn't drawn up an entire risk assessment.

As long as the crisis is not personally his own but other people's, he is happy to take charge, be useful and have a purpose.

The trouble can come when you yourself are seriously ill or in an accident or perhaps one of your children. This is often something he is not prepared for as his emotions are strong and overwhelming where you and the children are concerned. He may shut down in inexorable ways. He may act like he doesn't care or he may freak out. You will know your Aspie best.

The Husband Says:

Being good in a crisis because as an Aspie you have a contingency plan and have been quite dispassionate about the outcome of the crisis can back-fire spectacularly when the crisis falls close to home.

B

Our daughter nearly lost her life through a medical condition. In the hospital, Karen was beside herself with anxiety and worry that she would lose a daughter. Meanwhile at the height of the crisis I went out for a walk and to get some food because my assessment was that I could not continue to function without eating. I miss-calculated; I forgot to factor into my assessment that I should have been being supportive to Karen - she needed me to be there for her showing loyalty not somewhere else fending for myself. It just did not cross my mind.

NT

So for partners - when your Aspie is in crisis management mode, don't be scared to load additional requirements and constraints on him to add to his deliberations on emergency action. He is good at keeping lots of plates spinning for a short length of time until the crisis abates. But be prepared to support him at the end of the crisis - he will crash exhausted after all that can be done is done.

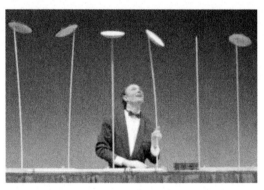

Being a Single Parent

It is hard to describe your relationship to someone outside of the marriage who may be a single parent or in a typical sharing marriage where each parent does their part. I'm sure they wouldn't agree if they had not experienced this type of relationship.

On the face of it, he is there and he is jointly responsible. The reality of the situation behind closed doors is very different, especially when the children are young.

As the mother of your new baby, you are naturally the one that does the majority of the caring for the child, especially if you are breast-feeding.

As you are the one on maternity leave, it makes sense at first for you to do night feeds when the husband has to go back to work. Everyone expects young mothers to be tired. Yet, he never offers to get up when the baby cries, even when you go back to work - and this is often when resentment starts. Even when you ask him to help he will resist or play the part for a few days before slipping back into his normality, as if the child hadn't been born.

B

As the child gets older and you go to birthday parties or to the park, you notice other dads dandling their babies on their knee or pushing them on the swings and you realise that your husband never does that. There is never any spontaneous interaction. In fact, if the toddler hurts themselves he may even walk off in the opposite direction.

So regardless of how hard he works outside the house and how much money he brings in, you still feel like a single parent.

Why?

Remember he married you for your loving, caring side. It is almost like he searched for and employed you to carry out the skills he does not have. He has no innate ability to tell the difference between a happy and a sad cry. He is scared if he picks up the baby that he will hurt it. He can't bear the smell of a dirty nappy and would rather put up with your wrath that the baby has been left in its own mess than have to deal with such a disgusting thing.

Babies do not come with manuals. No matter how many Toddler Taming books you buy there is not specifically one for your child. He feels out of his depth and feels that you have the ability to do what is best for your child. It isn't that he doesn't care. It's almost that he cares too much.

Yet that doesn't help in the middle of the night as you exhaustedly pace up and down with a colicky baby and he is selfishly getting his sleep in the spare room.

As They Get Older

I remember very clearly when my husband sat on the sofa holding our son who was just a a few months old. He said to me 'I can't wait until he has homework'. I remember staring at him in disbelief and wondering why he could not just live in the moment.

The reason, I realise now, is that he loved his child but didn't know how to communicate with this squirming bundle. As our children grew and were able to verbally communicate with him, his bond with them became less tentative.

Tips to Ease the Burden of Child Rearing Alone

NT If you have never told your husband how you feel about being the main carer to your children, then don't assume that he already knows. All he knows is that you do a much better job than him, so why would you want to hand responsibility over to him?

Be careful not to be critical in any way, but tell him you would like him to share more responsibility with the children and that it would be nice for him to bond with them more, especially now that they are getting older.

B

Identify the areas where you need help such as taking a child to swimming lessons on a Friday night leaving you to get on with the tea and bathe the younger one. A task that has a routine to it should definitely appeal to your husband. Make sure that you don't just tell him that this needs to be done and then leave him to it. He may know where the leisure centre is but he will panic about dealing with the right people, changing rooms etc. Try and go with him at least once and show him what your child also expects. Also show him he can sit in the cafe and watch through the window rather than going to sit in the car. He won't necessarily think of these details. He may even think he doesn't belong and that people won't want him there unless you tell him in no uncertain terms that he is perfectly entitled to have a cup of coffee whilst waiting for his child to finish their lesson.

Don't load him with too many tasks. I would gently build them up.

He may be worried about this at first but slowly his confidence will build in this area. He'll probably even start enjoying it and dropping into conversation at work how he has to leave to take his child swimming. It helps him feel normal and he will like that.

The Husband Says:

I agree with all of Karen's points above.

The bodily fluids involved in child-rearing or puppy ownership have a unique odour, colour and texture that just sets off the whole Aspie sensory overload thing in me to the extent that I just have to vomit, further adding to the pile of bodily fluid involved in the clean-up. That's genuine avoidance not the lazy-avoidance alluded to in that article.

Analysing my lack of interaction in my children's early years reinforces the Transactional Analysis theory view of how neurotypicals and Aspies communicate differently; my child-ego voice is pretty broken so the most successful path of communication open to me and my young kids of "child ego to child ego" never really gets started. I couldn't see the point in goo-goo-gah-gah bonding noises. I remain worried that I've damaged my kids by not providing the right types of interactions with them in their early years and that's why they might be growing up like me.

In the last few weeks, I feel like I've started to pay back some parenting-debt with my son. He has been revising for GCSE exams and it's been the first time that I feel I've been able to give him something that he wanted from me: my knowledge; approach to learning and exams; my time and emotional support. He seems genuinely grateful for my involvement - not that he would say in so many words. I feel like I've sat every exam with him in spirit. Let's not get too smug however; this is as much about him developing his own unique Aspie coping strategies than the type of communications we have shared together.

B

Being Honest

Your husband is a literal thinker. He finds it hard to 'read between the lines'.

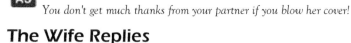 Honesty often is the best policy when trying to communicate with your Aspie. However, I do use this with discretion as sometimes there are things that David just doesn't need to know. At least for the time being, if I can deal with them by myself then everyone is the happier for it.

Having said that, recently, with David and I being more honest and open with each other and our feelings, writing this App has certainly helped, I don't always hold information back, but I do judge when it is a good time to tell or not.

The other reason I am more open with him now is that his reactions tend to be less dramatic and paranoid than they used to be. I put this down not just to our enhanced education and understanding but a lot is down to his diet of reduced gluten and regular intake of Vitamin D3 and other supporting supplements. I wouldn't say he was a changed man, but a more balanced, less moody man.

The Husband Says:

*...or not; the little-white-lie that can be so beneficial, but watch for the little white lie that becomes the all-consuming big black lie. Fundamentally you have to be honest - because you **ALWAYS** get caught.*

I'm getting better at spotting that Karen is omitting the whole truth or using the little white lie with our daughter, and slotting into place in the story that is being told.

AS *You don't get much thanks from your partner if you blow her cover!*

The Wife Replies

That's what he thinks anyway.

Being Taken for Granted

As wives or long term partners, we are often taken for granted. Our partners are not in tune with their feelings at all or, on the other extreme, they feel too much and try to block those feelings out. Probably, if you left him, he would realise that he loves you and needs you and misses you. It's a bit like they don't know they need the toilet until the last minute and they have an accident. They literally do not know what their mind and bodies are telling them until it's too late.

B

I see it in mine and my friends AS children all the time. Why should it be any different when they grow up? To be an AS wife, sometimes we have to just accept that they think and love differently from the rest of us. We just can't expect them to be like us. Accepting that, however, is like going through a form of bereavement for your marriage and for your future life. It is hard.

Perhaps I find it a little easier as I now recognise that I come from an AS family myself. I wasn't short of love but I remember the rare moments my dad said it to me. We never make a big fuss of birthdays or other events. We don't see each other very much but we do stay in contact. For those wives who have come from a more open family I think it must be particularly hard to bear the lack of affection and remembering of birthdays etc. I can see how real resentment can build up.

The Husband Says:

I see what you are saying about "being taken for granted", but that's not what I'm intentionally doing. I'm slow to recognise that what you are doing in the here and now deserves thanks and praise, and by the time I form a plan to thank you and recognise your efforts on my behalf, the "moment" has long since passed.

So it seems to me that in an Asperger marriage, the non-Aspie might need to have the patience of a Saint to wait for their "reward" or even just reciprocation. Perhaps that's the key to not breaking up - being prepared to be patient and to coach your partner for your desired response. Not very spontaneous I know, but could you sacrifice spontaneity for everything else to come good?

Please don't mistake my slowness on emotional topics for an absence of emotion. It's there, just delayed. So I realise after your birthday that I should have gone out with the kids and bought you cards and flowers. Would a pre-planned family meal out do instead?

Being 'Tricked' into Marriage

We dated for over two years before we got married. We must have lived together for over a year and a half all told, as I spent a while living and working in London. There were moments when I thought he was a bit odd and a bit sensitive but all of his other positive assets overrode any doubts I had.

I thought I didn't have any illusions about him. I knew he was obsessed with his work and that he only had a few friends (whom I had never met) and that his parents described him as 'not taking fools gladly'. He only ever showed me his positive side. Before our first date I think he must have even cleaned the toilet in case he got lucky!

He was outgoing, articulate, clever and funny. He had a good job and education, was respected, well-travelled, had his own house and car. He thought the world of me and spoiled me rotten. What was there not to like?

B

I had no idea that I was his special interest, his obsession. I wasn't daft enough to think that marriage would be all rainbows and unicorns but I thought I knew the man I was marrying. How could I have been so wrong?

In some ways it is very flattering to find out that I was worth all that effort. He tried hard to get me and keep me. I'm not sure how honest he was with himself about all the effort he was putting in to our relationship. Did he consciously decide to relax once he had me sign the marriage contract? To many people this is just a legal document and part of the wedding ceremony. To him, my signature meant he had got what he wanted and he didn't have to try so hard any more.

I had my first doubts I had done the right thing on our honeymoon. It wasn't the first time we had been away but this time it was different. Suddenly he was on edge and we didn't always have anything to say. I didn't realise then I had been "deceived" but that was when the first cracks started to show.

The Husband Says:

I've read this article through a few times before commenting. It is interesting to see in print a different view of what happened nearly twenty years ago.

Yes, I set out to find a partner. All the NTs around me were doing that by instinct, so I set out to do it by plan. These were pre-internet days; I've never told you before, but I did try a small ad in the local paper, but that didn't work out - respondents were universally twenty and thirty-somethings with at least one failed marriage behind them and kids in tow.

Aspies seem to look for partners close to home - I suppose it is the familiar environment and the ability to study the target of potential affection from a little bit of a distance before plucking up the courage (and this may take weeks) to approach someone to just hold a conversation, never mind ask for a date.

So, plan in place, I courted you - balancing (or so I thought) my responsibility to work (my enduring obsession) with a new obsession - you. All went to plan until the honeymoon. You wanted Bali, after all the trips to and from London and with my somewhat variable income (would I get a bonus or some lucrative foreign assignments? - no certainty), all I could afford was Ireland. In Autumn. Not ideal. This was not what you wanted and probably the first time I had disappointed you. It sticks in the mind even now.

So if I follow conventional expectation, it just gets worse - Two obsessions now - career and wife; now we add a third - our son. Don't forget in each of these three domains I'm having to plan ahead and act responsibly - I can't rely on NT instinct - I just started to run out of bandwidth to process all these calls on my time and prototype-emotion.

So I hope I didn't "trick" you. My intention was genuine and now I'm disappointed that I'm still failing to deliver what you expect of marriage. Someday we will 'do' Bali.

For an amusing fictional version of this I recommend reading this book The Rosie Project, by Graeme Simsion

B

Being Useful

Your Aspie likes to have a purpose, it is just that quite often he doesn't know what that purpose is. There is nothing more that David likes than being asked to research, procure and set up a gadget for someone. For our son's sixteenth birthday, Morgan decided he wanted to upgrade his computer to "super gamer" quality with his screen refreshing 150 times a second and with an expensive graphics card. I was instructed by David to go and buy numerous magazines for him to do his research. Nothing makes him happier. Also it gives him a chance to talk to his son and bond a bit.

I have learned over the years to filter out and narrow down the areas where David wants to be involved in. Initially when I was on the PTA at the kids First school, I would rope him into helping out with the band nights. I soon realised how miserable he was. He would refuse point blank to dance or even enter the hall where the music was playing and would just hang around aimlessly with a beer in his hand criticising the music he could hear. However, he was in his element when I roped him in to man the bar and he became the absolute personification of helpfulness and charm. He would go out of his way for the demands of every customer and he wouldn't take a break all night. This was because he knew what he had to do and the conversations were predictable and safe. If he was going to be barman he was going to be the best barman he could possibly be.

So when events happen in the village now I quickly calculate what sort of demand will be placed on David's social abilities and I either decline or accept an invite for him. There have been a number of large celebrations in the village recently but these would have meant him doing chit chat for hours with local people. On the surface he is very good at it but really he hates it.

NT If you want your Aspie to participate in an event important to you then give him defined roles and things to do, even if they seem mundane.

The Husband Says:

This is the single thing that can make a social gathering bearable.

AS *But don't take over someone else's event without permission. Ask if you can help and you will probably be met with the desired invitation and even a 'thank-you'. **Don't just assume!***

B

Bereavement

In mourning for your marriage? See the article on Stages of Grief.

Bereavement in the Traditional Sense of the Word

My mum died very suddenly from secondary cancer. I was there at the time as my dad had managed to call me. It was a terrible shock for all of us but David was definitely my rock at that time. I know he was as upset as everyone else as he was very fond of my mum, but he dealt with it in a different way. He made himself useful.

I don't know whether David entirely understood my grief and how I felt but he was definitely there for me, my dad and little sister. I rang him at work when I was in bits and he dropped everything for me. He knew it was not a time to be selfish. I will be forever grateful.

He gave me time to grieve and didn't make me feel silly when I cried. At times he just held me. He didn't give any platitudes but I was grateful for that. We were actually about to move house at the time and he just took charge. I couldn't have asked for anything more.

Supporting your AS partner through Bereavement

We hadn't been married long when David's father died from Type 1 diabetes complications. It wasn't unexpected but his father was not even sixty. Our first baby, Morgan, was less than a month old at the time and I was still in the blur of early motherhood.

David and his younger sister supported their mother as best they could but I think David also took pains to protect me too. I think it was his way of coping with his loss by not concentrating on what had happened but concentrating on what he could do.

I never saw him cry though he tells me he did when he wrote his father's eulogy. He told me he got it out of the way. I was so impressed with him on the day of his dad's funeral as he got up and gave a reading, calmly and with dignity.

I think where death is concerned that some Aspies can come across as very dispassionate about it. I don't think this is true at all, but because they are composed on the outside they can seem as if they don't care.

I think that David had spent much more time thinking about all the implications of his father's illness and discussing with his sister who was a junior doctor as the time, very pragmatically, that he had long come to terms with the situation. He had

B

already considered the most morbid factors and come to terms with them. in some ways, the actual death was just another step in the process. He was sad, but he had prepared himself and it wasn't the shock that some people might have expected from him.

I was concerned about it at the time but he didn't want to talk and so I had to let it go.

I don't imagine for a moment think that he would react the same way over a sudden death of a close family member.

I have witnessed my Aspies different reactions to the sudden death of one of our beloved dogs. She was only a year old and she was run over. Our daughter who was about seven at the time immediately burst into tears and was inconsolable. Our son who was nine reacted very differently. He was quiet for a bit and then started to laugh at his sister. He came across as quite mean but I knew that he just hadn't processed the information at all. He didn't know how to react.

My daughter went to school and told all her friends who immediately crowed round and consoled her. It wasn't until the following morning while I was driving Morgan to school that I noticed he was silently crying. I realised that it had been this journey twenty-four hours before when he had last seen her and it had suddenly struck home.

NT However they react you must be patient and try and understand and support them. Some will just bury their heads in the sand and act as if they don't care so they don't have to feel anything whilst the other half will be completely overwhelmed with their grief and be inconsolable for some time. I think perhaps the second option is healthier.

Body Language

Interpreting Body Language

There was a time a few years ago that I had eaten something that really didn't agree with me. I was standing in the kitchen bent over and David got cross with me because I wasn't talking to him. I'm sure my face had gone very pale and I was sweating but he could not see it at all. Moments later I was violently sick but made to the downstairs toilet.

In the right context David feels he is very good at working out body language. He often tells me that he likes to place himself in a certain way in a meeting in order to make certain people comfortable or uncomfortable. He thinks it through thoroughly.

B

What he can't do is work on the fly in unexpected, unpredictable and unknown situations. He hasn't seen or read about a particular situation and therefore it is not in his mental catalogue to refer to. He either completely gets it wrong or ignores it.

He and the children generally only recognise the extremes of body language and indeed they only display these extremes themselves.

Is this why cartoon characters and particularly Japanese, Anime and Manga are so popular with their large round eyes and expressive mouths?

For your Aspie the large grey area of emotion is often an unknown, unidentified void.

See Meh

'Bonio' Moment

When our son was about three he asked if he could give our dog a biscuit. I said "Yes, of course," and told him where the box of biscuits was. Morgan went into the dining room and found the box. I heard more noise than I expected and followed through moments later. Now we shop at Costco and had bought an enormous box of Bonio® dog biscuits that had only just been opened. Instead of taking one out of the box and giving it to the dog, Morgan had tipped all the contents out onto the floor. The poor dog couldn't believe his eyes and was paralyzed with indecision, stunned by the mountain of Bonios he was presented with.

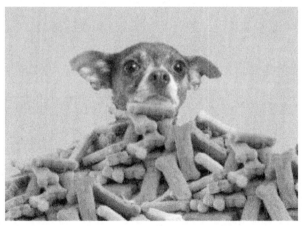

Since then this moment has gone down in family legend as being a 'Bonio Moment'. It is particularly significant due to the way the overwhelmed dog reacted in exactly the way many people with Asperger's react when presented with too many choices.

B

Traditionally, choice is looked upon as a good thing but actually, for the Aspie who has problems weighing up his choices, this can be overwhelming. In fact, with an Aspie, often less is more.

Your average Aspie is good at seeing the detail in things and is not very good at filtering out the unnecessary. He can do it, but it can take time as every option has to be analysed carefully. We NT's who can do this in a split second become very impatient with our poor Aspies and don't understand why they take so long to come to a decision. Surely the answer is simple?

They do not have the mental filtering facility that we have to quickly choose between the good and the less good. To them, particularly when under pressure, the amount of choice can become overwhelming and induce a meltdown or worse, catatonia.

NT At times like this we must be patient and not pressure them into making a decision.

Ways to help your Aspie make a Decision:

- Make a list of the pros and cons

- Give them plenty of time. Depending on the importance of the decision this could take weeks.

- Let them do their research. This is extremely crucial to their decision making. They don't want to make a mistake, particularly over a large purchase.

- Do not interfere with the decision unless asked.

- **Do not be flippant or impatient and say "It's just a television." NB: It is NEVER "Just a television".**

For a comic take on this see TV series "The Big Bang Theory", Season 7, Episode 19.

Boundaries

Some boundaries are obvious. Fences, walls and signs telling you to go no further. These are boundaries that my husband understands. He can see them physically and he can read them on a map. He is very good at map reading: it is something he has to do as part of his job and he likes to argue with people about boundaries. He is invariably right.

At home, however, not so much. It is those intangible issues that we generally learned as children. The "do's and don'ts".

Understandably, he will have learned plenty of these rules as he fell foul of them as a child as he doesn't like making mistakes - he tries not to repeat them. Yet there are areas in his life as an adult he has not learned to apply boundaries by himself such as closing the bathroom door when there are guests in the house.

I have sympathy as the lines of privacy become blurred when family is involved but nobody informs you if what the new rules are. You are just expected to know and again in each household the levels of privacy are different.

What happens to the boundaries when you get married? After all, now you are legally bound together, sharing a room with the woman of your dreams and sharing her body, perhaps he assumes there are no longer any boundaries to be had. You may be intimate with your partner's body but they may still not want to share the bathroom with you.

There is a crucial mistake that these men make time and time again, and they do so in the belief they are 'helping'. For example, when I was nearing the deadline for my dissertation, it was a stressful time and once I had got the children to school, it was my sole focus for weeks. The idea, experience and research had all been my idea. I knew exactly what I wanted to say and how I wanted to say it. In my head I had it planned, more or less (some things I knew would come to me as time went on). On my computer I had each chapter of my dissertation open but minimised on my screen. I would work between them as I found relevant information or a new thought occurred to me. David on the other hand was getting anxious that: a) I had not finished yet; and b) he did not know how much I had left to do.

Now I am a natural optimist and I am a good judge of how long it takes me to do something. He on the other hand is not, especially when it comes to other people. He kept badgering me, saying that "surely I had finished by now". I needed to take a break and took the dog for a walk. I made the mistake of saying he could look over it if he liked. I got back after an hour and he very proudly announced that he had 'fixed' my dissertation. I looked at him in horror. What had he done?

He had taken all my files and put them together into one document so that he could create a contents page and index. He had done some clever trickery where the page numbers would automatically change if I added to the document or made any other changes. I no longer had access to my chapters conveniently left open at the bottom of the page but had to scroll through or search for the section I needed. I was furious. He had violated my work and, even worse, slowed me down horrendously. He was sitting there really proudly expecting me to thank him for this. Even I couldn't hide the shock on my face.

If he had asked me if he could do the contents page I would have been delighted and I would have let him do it- when I was ready. The worst thing was he had done this all entirely for selfish reasons but presented it as a favour to me.

B

Solution

There needs to be a written book of unwritten rules for people on the autistic spectrum - the social norms.

It's so hard to explain to him and I don't want to hurt his feelings, especially when he feels he is helping.

Aspie Hints & Tips

Never assume just because she is your wife that you can treat her possessions like they are your own. This is not respectful. Would you like your wife to constantly go in your wallet and rearrange your money and bank cards?

Even when you think you are helping, make sure you ask your wife if it okay to change or move her possessions before you do it.

Tips for the Wife

There are plenty of relationship self-help guides out there with tips on boundaries within your marriage. I'm sure these are great for Neurotypical relationships but you cannot apply them to your own different marriage without thought.

Make sure that when you make the rules or boundaries that you do it together. Do not just present him with a fait accompli list and expect him to abide by them. For a start he will feel out of control and he won't like that. He won't necessarily understand your reasons behind the rules so it is best to come up with them together.

Keep the list of boundaries short and simple. Stick with the essentials such as 'Always tell me when you have changed something on my computer. Just because you know you have done it, does not mean that I will know or understand what you have done.'

Breaking Point

Within a number of Aspie marriages there has come a breaking point. The AS husband has reached the end of his tether and just left. Without warning.

On talking to these wives, in hindsight the warning signs were there, but they never expected them to take such drastic action. What the wife had seen as a little blip was too much for the AS partner to cope with.

Lack of communication can turn out to be a massive issue on both sides. If the AS partner had just explained to his wife that he was not coping with the family situation then they could have taken steps to resolve it.

It is possible that the AS partner did not feel understood and that his wife would never be able to understand him. I think this happens in many relationships where the AS partner is undiagnosed. They do not even understand themselves and feel isolated from family life. The only solution that they can see is to leave and suddenly.

Breaking Up

This guide has been written to help you prevent this but, of course, that is not always possible. Some situations just get to be so intolerable that they cannot continue.

Sometimes in the heat of the moment you may both decide that it is the best solution to 'uncouple' (as a certain celebrity described it recently) but this does not necessarily solve all the problems that are there, especially if there are children involved.

There have been times when I have literally walked away thinking that I cannot carry on with the marriage but, after time to myself, I have calmed down and gone back. I know he is always glad to see me even if he is not ready to talk to me. I have seen the fear in his eyes when I have got so mad with his behaviour that I too have had a tantrum and walked out. If there was no love there would be no fear.

There have been times, especially when the children were young and we were tired, irritable and impatient with each other, when "to help me" David has suggested us splitting up. He decided that I could do a much better job without him. He felt he was getting in the way and I would be happier without him there.

Again, in the heat of the moment that sometimes sounds quite attractive, but I married him for a reason and that was for his love and companionship. Even though he is difficult to live with (which he acknowledges) he doesn't realise that I want to have him there, that leaving me would leave me hollow and alone. Yes, I would be able to cope, almost carry on as normal (except when we had IT problems) but even though he isn't the most demonstrative of husbands, I still appreciate his presence.

It is a common Asperger trait to offer to remove yourself from the situation and assume the other person will be fine without you. Again it shows a lack of empathy and understanding of your partner.

It is most likely that the decision to leave will be made by you. Very often, regardless of how bad the living arrangements are, it will not occur to them to leave. They cannot see a way out of it and will just bury their head in the sand further.

B

Solution

NT First of all read this App thoroughly and try and make use of all the advice. Try and get your partner to also read it, even if it is only the parts written by my husband. You need to be able to understand each other before you can really make a decision about whether the marriage can be salvaged.

Try and have a sensible discussion about whether you want to salvage the marriage. If you do it may be worth seeking out a counsellor as well as educating yourselves more about AS.

This is very important. Lower your expectations. You are never going to have the magical marriage you see in films and glossy adverts. Life is more real than that. Asperger's is a bumpy ride even for those who know the rules.

Give yourselves some time and don't rush into either decision, whether to stay or go. They are both equally as important and will affect you for the rest of your lives.

Brokering

This is one of my main jobs at home and yet David only put a name to it just the other day. You would think that on the day your child was born, and the midwife passes your child over to the teary-eyed father, that one introduction would suffice for the rest of their lives. Not so.

This seems to be an Executive Function deficiency where David, although he wants to interact with his children, does not know how to approach them. As a family we live quiet and often separate lives coming together for meals, entertainment and taxi duty. The rest of the time when, for example we wanted to help our son revise, David could not organise this himself. He either wrongly assumed that our AS son would instigate the revision time or rightly assumed that I would create a time and a place for them to communicate.

I am expected to micromanage everything. If I am not there, interaction barely happens.

The Husband Says:

Karen has a valuable point here. I've never really had the confidence to approach my kids in a consistent way. I'm not at all sure how they would react. If I had NT kids, then after a while I think I would start to pick out some patterns and gain confidence. But my kids are fellow Aspies. Their problems with emotional responses to my clumsy emotional approaches has the makings of a disaster. So I suppose I haven't tried. That's verging on avoidance.

B

C

- Catastrophizing
- Central Coherence Theory
- Challenges
- Chameleon
- Change
- Changes in Attitude
- Changes in Routine
- Childlike
- Children
- Chit Chat
- Choice
- Choosing to be Alone
- Closure
- Clumsiness
- Co-Dependency
- Coercive Control

- Cognitive Distortions
- Coming down off a High
- Common Sense
- Communication
- Communication Disorder
- Comorbidities
- Compartmentalising
- Compliments
- Compromise
- Consequences
- Consideration
- Constant Feeling of Guilt
- Control
- Cortisol
- Counselling
- Criticism, Concern and Advice

Catastrophizing

It could start with an innocent text while you are out for lunch. It could be the bank sending a solicited update. Unfortunately, he can't read the text and starts to panic that it is the bank sending him bad news. He then leaps to an unlikely, but not impossible, scenario that he may not have enough money in the bank account to pay for the lunch. He immediately starts becoming agitated and trying to get Wi-Fi access in an area where there isn't any. As the bill is brought he is increasingly panic stricken, convinced that his card will be rejected and the police will be called. He is rude to the service staff and rude to his partner. The card payment goes through but instead of calming down and realising the situation is alright he need to get to the nearest cash machine to check his balance. His driving becomes dangerous and erratic. He finds a cash machine and checks his balance. He comes back even more panicked as his fears have come to fruition. There is no money in the account. He starts screaming at his wife for spending all the money or for being careless enough to let fraud be committed. The wife is left confused and abused on the car journey home. Again he checks his online bank balance before he uses telephone banking to find out where all his money has disappeared to. Once he is at his own desk he calms down enough to enter his complicated password on the second try. He looks at his balance and discovers that the money has been there all along and that in his panic he had misread the information at the cash machine. He calms down and smiles, leaving an emotionally and physically exhausted wife still reeling from the assault on her senses.

Many AS individuals can demonstrate an irrational form of anxiety, though not exclusive to Asperger's Syndrome, that is significant to their meltdowns. David's inability in moments of stress to regulate his emotions leads to intense, overwhelming feelings and the tendency to catastrophize. Catastrophizing may lead you to self-pity, to an irrational, negative belief about the situation, and to a feeling of hopelessness about your future prospects. Further, both of these types of catastrophizing will define either the presence or absence of alternative possibilities, and possibly paralyse you from going further with efforts toward your goals in life.

Many people with an autistic condition not only have difficulty recognising the emotions of others, they also have difficulty comprehending their own and their own state of mind. They are however, able to recognise extreme emotions when they are upset or frightened. This agitation, unless addressed, may lead to behaviour problems such as catastrophization.

The Husband Says:

I know I catastrophize. There's not a lot I can do about it. The situation comes on so unexpectedly and suddenly that I have no plan for it. My anxiety at the situation and lack of plan just fuels the catastrophizing. I have to make a plan and quickly. This will be a logical

plan to be executed quickly and it won't be pretty; social norms will have to be ignored and the consequences dealt with later.

Catastrophizing for me generally comes about through what I see as grave peril to me and my family: theft from me like stolen credit cards, medical emergency involving me directly or a threat like an imminent street brawl.

Central Coherence Theory

People with autism or Asperger Syndrome find it very hard to see the big picture. Unlike NT's they tend to concentrate on the fine detail in front of them.

Central coherence can account for some of the patterns of strengths and weaknesses in autism and refers to an information processing style, specifically the tendency to process incoming information in its context - that is pulling information together for higher-level meaning. In the case of neurotypical strong central coherence this tendency would work at the expense of attention to and memory for details. In the case of weak central coherence (proposed for autism and Asperger's) this tendency would favour piecemeal processing at the expense of contextual meaning.

Put another way, the weak central coherence theory is that some people have a limited ability to understand context and 'see the big picture' and that this is central to the condition of autism and Asperger's. Having a weak central coherence can explain why many people (not all) on the autism spectrum are good at logical subjects like maths and the sciences but have great difficulty with language and communication.

The Husband Says:

The authors of the various papers on this subject find that the results of their experiments are somewhat contradictory. There might be some crumb of truth in this theory, but it does not seem to address root causes of autism and Asperger Syndrome, and feels like an attempt to fit facts to the symptoms. I think this theory will fade in time.

Challenges

NT Never set your Aspie a challenge unless you really want him to carry it out. What I mean by this is be careful with throw away comments. We NT'S are guilty of doing this without thought or awareness of the consequences.

Remember you are married to someone who only does literal thinking.

C

Every day Challenges

A major part of being an Aspie wife is knowing your own strengths and weaknesses. The reason for this is if you are not able to carry out a task or fix something, the natural course is to ask your partner to carry it out if at all possible.

The problem with this is down to their mood, ability and executive functioning. Timing is everything. If at all possible if you would like your husband to carry out a task you need to be prepared for him to insist on carrying it out there and then, regardless of time constraints. It is possible to try and prepare him in advance but on the whole his executive function difference will not let him put that thought to one side for later. He will generally insist on doing it there and then.

Reasons for this are:

- You asked him to do it, therefore he thinks you want it done NOW!

- He cannot in his mind see past what you have asked him to do. It is in the forefront of his mind and to get rid of it he must do it now.

- You have set him a challenge and he likes a challenge.

We have been in this situation so many times. Something has gone wrong in the kitchen just as we were about to leave the house for an appointment and I have made the mistake of telling him about it. It is more vital to get to the appointment on time but in his head it is more important to fix the dishwasher there and then. This is where arguments start. He cannot prioritise situations.

Over the years I have learned to say nothing about the problem until a more convenient time. I have, even though he is an engineer and keen to fix things himself, on occasion got someone else in to fix the problem.

Daring an Aspie

NT This is not something I recommend you do too often, however, the results can be pleasing.

New Year's Day 2011 it had snowed overnight, very heavily for Britain. Our son had had a friend to sleep over and we had to take him home. David was secretly pleased as we had a newly acquired four-wheel drive which had never seen the snow before. He was quite happy to drive ten miles in the snow to take this boy home.

The roads were obviously very quiet as it was the morning after major celebrations plus the 'bad' weather. We passed a few abandoned vehicles on our way. Once we had dropped Morgan's friend off I assumed we would be going home but David wanted to go home via the 'scenic route'. We were all up for this and as we were in a little rural town it didn't take him long to find the scenic route. After a few miles of gentle driving we came to a crossroads. Right would take up home quickest, straight ahead would be an interesting route home and left would take us up a very steep hill to a tiny hamlet where our friends were snowed in.

I pointed left and said "You'll never get up there." Well this is when I discovered don't challenge an Aspie. "We'll see about that," he said and turned the car left. There was a fair amount of slipping and sliding and a few worrying moments but our new car made it up to the top of the very steep hill. We crawled cautiously into our friend's yard and parked up. The look of astonishment on their faces when we knocked on the door was amusing but the look of satisfaction on David's for getting there was very memorable. We stayed for coffee and then headed slowly home. It had him on a high for the rest of the day and if, on occasion, it is mentioned he always has a big grin on his face.

Though this is a cautionary tale, all ended well and it often gives us something to laugh about. Never Dare An Aspie!

Chameleon

David has a chameleon like personality. He has consciously evolved this to the point that he has different names at work from home. At home he is very much David or Dad, but at work he is Dave. Even though I met him at work I refer to him as David. I think, at the time this was an unconscious effort to lay claim to him and separate our relationship from work.

I have noticed over the years how his personality changes depending on whom he is spending time with. When he is in the workshop he uses a lot of colloquialisms and Geordie slang. His accent becomes rougher and his grammar appalling. This is very different from the refined northern accent I first associated with him, though I wonder now which is his true accent. Perhaps he doesn't even know.

As a freelance consultant, this often means he mixes with everyone from small community groups to government ministers. He has appeared on television talking about projects and has never seemed daunted or out of place. He makes it seem natural and effortless but I'm sure it involves a lot of mental work behind the scenes.

Other times he can be in a screaming rage and the phone will ring and he will change immediately to business-like Dave without a hitch.

He also loves to wind cold callers up on the phone, sometimes pretending he is very old or very stupid. It is one of his small pleasures in life.

Change

I remember during our son's visit to the Consultant Psychologist for his assessment, she asked me whether he got upset if he came home and I had changed the furniture around. I laughed and said "No, he wouldn't notice, " but then pointed at my husband sitting quietly next to me, "But he would freak out".

David and I had been living together for a few months and I would often get home from work first. Well before the days of internet, life was a bit dull, so I decided to move the chairs and sofa around in the living room. I was very pleased with it. I did not expect the reaction I got from David when he came home. He stood there his mouth moving soundlessly like a goldfish in stunned silence. He insisted I move it all back immediately. Now I know that he tried really hard not to freak out and was trying to be as calm as possible but I don't think I took it well.

Even Good Change is Change

A recent occurrence was when David had agreed to pick up our son from college to get him home for a tutorial on time. Morgan actually finished college early and texted his dad to tell him he would get the train home, so no need to drive a 40 mile round trip to pick him up.

Now, most people would see this as a positive thing. It saved, time, fuel and effort. He didn't have to put his shoes on and leave the house, interrupting his work but have an extra hour to either relax or concentrate on work.

Not so in this Aspie household. David had known all day that he had to make this trip into the busy town, full of roadworks and annoying people. He had psyched himself up to do this and kept an eye on the clock to make sure he did not miss his appointment. Instead at feeling relief at the news he became much more anxious and started to find all kinds of problems with it instead, being concerned that Morgan would have missed the train and would therefore be late for his lesson. The problem here is partly theory of mind because he could not put himself into his son's shoes and see that he had already worked out the pros and cons of his actions. He also could only see the problems and hadn't worked out that in fact the worst case scenario was that our son would miss the train and David would have to leave the house at the same time he had originally planned to do anyway. It took some time after I had pointed this fact out for the information to sink in. He was still anxious and on edge until Morgan materialised thorough the door.

NT I learned that I would have to inform him of any future spontaneous behaviour.

The Husband Says:

The thing about change is that it disrupts the carefully laid plans. I've got enough on my plate implementing my coping strategies that all require careful planning to have to worry about changing the plan to accommodate all the furniture having been moved.

Is this because I'm a predominantly visual thinker and like to have certain things in certain places to act as 'anchors' that don't move over which I can spread a more complex canvas of thought? These things aren't necessarily physical objects in a geographical landscape (but that's an obvious example); they may be abstract thoughts that I've grouped together and 'parked' in a specific place in a specific list to come back to together. Change in the widest sense means that when I come back for these thoughts they have moved and I will have to work hard to recall them from their new location.

Aspie Hints & Tips:

AS **NT** Try Planned Spontaneity if the full fat variety of spontaneity is too much.

Changes in Attitude

If you love your husband and you want your marriage to succeed then change is necessary. Assuming that you are the NT in an AS/NT relationship, then you have the ability to make the change for both of you. This could be looked upon as making a sacrifice of yourself for your marriage; for example, not being able to express your personality as fully as you would like, but if your marriage is worth it then this is probably what you have to do, if just for the short term.

NT You are the one with the fully functioning 'normal' brain and therefore you have the ability to ask yourself whether you want your life to change for the better and whether you have the strength and determination to carry this out. What you have to realise is that you may want your husband to change his ways but that you have to be strong enough to change yours first. He will most likely follow by example.

NT **AS** If you do not bring up stressful situations constantly, then he most likely won't. If you are calm and organised then he will be less anxious and influenced by his calmer surroundings, possibly even following your organised example.

NT If you stop shouting, you are most likely not giving him a reason to shout back.

Hopefully you are not reading into this that I am blaming you for his anxiety and attitude. What I am saying is that over the years you have made each other increasingly upset, anxious and defensive about issues in your marriage. Why should you back down if you are wrong? Why should you not retaliate if he has been particularly rude and patronising to you?

The answer is because he doesn't mean to do these things, or at least not at first. He doesn't know what he has done wrong, all he knows is from your reaction is that you despise his actions and that he is not worthy of your love (in his eyes). He gets more defensive as time goes on and views every criticism as a personal attack on him. He knows he can never reach your standards.

The Husband Says:

Perhaps I come across as weak-willed. But I am perfectly happy to follow an example set by Karen. It is logical; it makes sense. Karen's calming of situations by taking the moral high ground does work.

Changes in Routine

His routine is there for a reason. He finds it very hard to predict what NT people will do and therefore he finds it hard to predict the future. To have some control over his life he craves routine and tries to implement it as much as possible.

He is happy as long as everything is going the way he expected it.

The moment something unpredictable happens, and this does not have to be a negative change, he will most likely react badly to it. It is an Expectation Violation. It was not in the plan and is therefore disconcerting.

No matter how practical and obvious the change may be it will upset him for the rest of the day. Change has to be planned and in advance.

The Husband Says:

Detailed planning can help avoid the worst parts of many situations. But it is, of course, impossible to plan for every eventuality. I only have the bandwidth to deal with the ones I feel are most likely to happen. Routine saves have to re-plan over and over again. Change means mental effort and tiredness to modify all the plans that depended on that stuff I thought wasn't going to change.

Childlike

The majority of people I have counselled who are in an Asperger Marriage have at some point said to me (usually accompanied with tears) that it is like having an extra child to care for. A child that is not going to grow up.

Now, every wife in a typical marriage will have exclaimed this at some point about her husband as we all have an inner child. We can be messy, or sensitive or excited about life and we are just showing an uninhibited side of our personality to the ones we love. The difference between the NT husband who still thinks his farts are funny and an AS husband (who probably doesn't) is that the NT husband after his moments of down time will step up and support his wife with the running of the household or the bringing up of the children. They will not expect their wife to be their constant emotional sponge and they will reciprocate in kind.

The AS husband will always need their hand (metaphorically) holding over many and the same issues. They will never learn to provide the emotional support that you need. They will always love you unconditionally.

The Husband Says:

It is interesting that Karen sees my rather broken child ego (see Transactional Analysis). That's the one I try to push to the back and be less noticeable. Perhaps that's the hardest of the ego states to predict and put on a convincing act for?

Children

Making the Decision

Before we married we did not really discuss if we wanted children, it was too scary a subject. It was almost unspoken when we did decide to try for a baby. We just stopped using contraception. I think it was easier for both of us it was just too big a decision to put in to words. When I discovered I was pregnant I was a little terrified but at the same time overjoyed as was (I think) David but he will have to tell his side of the story.

NT With hindsight my advice would be to make clear to each other where you both stand. The last thing you want to do is get pregnant when he is totally against it. Yes some men may come around, but others may be resentful towards you or even the child. Remember your Aspie man is less mature emotionally and does not have the ability to adapt his feelings easily.

C

NT
He may be very keen to have children, and that is wonderful. However, if he has not considered it before, you should be clear about your wants and needs (but not forceful). Gently introduce the subject but don't expect an immediate answer. This is an enormous, life changing decision that is worthy of much thought. When he comes to the conclusion by himself, and he is likely to be positive in this area, he will have made the decision to be the best dad in the world and will dedicate himself to that.

Parental Roles

I was young and still naive. I still made a lot of assumptions in those early days of marriage. I assumed that, though I would be giving up work to look after our child full time, David as the father would want to play an equal role. I assumed he would occasionally get up in the night to comfort the baby and occasionally let me have a lie in. I thought he might come home from work at a reasonable hour in time to bathe his son.

None of these things happened.

Solution

NT
Now I know I should have talked to him about his role as a father. He didn't know what to do. I didn't tell him what I wanted him to do. He assumed the role of overall protector and provider and went out caveman style to kill the digital dinosaur and bring it home. I as a tired, lonely and tearful young mum felt unsupported and unloved and I worried that he didn't love his son too.

The Husband Says:

If Karen had asked my opinion on having a baby, then I would have immediately refused. That's simply an enormous change to the lifestyle that I was beginning to enjoy. Here's the start of a list of excuses:

- *How much will this cost? I'll have to work even harder to pay for this*

- *Karen, you are mine; I don't want to share you with someone else*

- *The dog will eat the child, or the child will eat the dog and the dog poo*

- *We will need a bigger house, we will have to move house; I'm just getting comfortable here*

You see how they all revolve around change? In reality, now that I am a (sort of) parent, I realise that the vicar was right to re-edit my edits to the wedding vows to reflect a biological duty to produce a family. I see a few friends that haven't married and haven't started a family and the peer and family pressure on them to conform to what is a social norm.

C

So Karen did the right thing. I knew that contraception had stopped, but I suppose I consciously chose not to think about the inevitable consequences. In the end I'm very, very happy to try in my own unusual way to be a parent and to have my son and daughter in my and Karen's lives.

I'll leave it to Karen, now in the role of Counsellor, to choose whether would suggest springing a proto-family on an Aspie or if full and in-depth planning is the 'correct' way to proceed. With hindsight, her bringing a dog into the 'family' before children was just a way of softening me up. Perhaps this is the right middle ground?

Chit Chat

There have been a number of large celebrations in the village recently, but these would have meant David doing chit chat for hours with local people. On the surface he is very good at it - but really he hates it. I was trying to explain to my twelve year old daughter what "chit chat" was the other day, why we do it and how we do it.

I said it is there to fill uncomfortable silences and to get to know people. Making chit chat with someone you don't really know is quite a technique that I hadn't really thought of before but realise we NT's do it all the time. My daughter and I had just been roped into making up the numbers of a choir for a wedding and I was talking to one of the girls there. I thought my daughter would have been able to have a short conversation with her as they were in the same choir at the Abbey but it appeared not. I realised that my technique to make everyone comfortable was to dredge up what little information I knew about the girl and relay it back to her. I had just heard that this sixteen-year-old girl who was very talented was not going to be joining us at the wedding, so I relayed this back to her with a sad face. She then told me what she was doing the following day and I remembers my friend's daughter was also doing that so I asked her if this was true. On the way home I explained it to my daughter what I had done and I have to say, even though it is completely true and we NT's do it all the time, I can see why it can seem quite odd and completely pointless from an AS point of view!

The Husband Says:

What is it with you NTs and your need for chit-chat?

Information theory says that if you are not transmitting new information on a channel then you are wasting its bandwidth. I can see what the weather is outside; I can guess your political affiliation and I don't need to know your whole family tree - but that seems to me to be about 90% of NT conversation at events. What about the things going on around us: the opening of the new meeting room or the charity we are supporting or how good (or bad) the music has been at the concert.

This is a closely related subject to answering the telephone; the Aspie approach is to transmit the maximum information in the shortest space of time then clear

the communications channel for others to use. We don't wiffle on unless the NT sends a VERY strong cue that they NEED this pointless conversation to continue.

I suppose it's a social norm so I'll just have to play along.

Choice

This is not considered a good thing. Too much choice in particular. You can't just choose by intuition you have to know the ins and outs of everything you need to choose between. This is why it can take weeks to choose the correct television as everyone is slightly different from the other and they would kick themselves if they made the wrong choice.

Your Aspie's difficulty in choosing comes from his inability to filter out the unnecessary information. See Top-Down Modulation for more in depth understanding.

For understanding overwhelming choice, see Bonio Moment.

Hints and Tips to help them Choose

1. Do not spring surprises on them.

2. Give them fair warning and let them do their research.

3. Do not pressure them.

4. If you also have to make a decision e.g. from a menu, let them know what yours is early on

5. Try and limit the number of choices.

6. Once he has made a decision try not to change it.

Choosing to be Alone

For Him

For the Asperger man, alone time is essential. Coming back in from an exhausting day at work to his safe haven, he just wants to have time to himself to not think about other people and their needs for a short amount of time. To recharge. This may mean playing mindless games on the computer or pottering in his shed.

This is a time when, even though he loves you, he is not yet ready to deal with you and all that happened in your day. You should not take this as an insult. He is taking a small amount of time away from the world so that he can recharge in order to then give you and the family his undivided attention.

NT
It is very hard to stand back when he comes in from work and not to bombard him with questions and information. I do try and stand back or even just stay in the kitchen when I hear the car draw up on the drive. He will come to me when he is ready.

On the other hand, if my husband has had a good day, he will immediately come in and talk to me about it and that is fine. Hugs are not necessarily exchanged until I can see he is ready for them.

For Her

NT
Why should he be the only one to choose to have some time and space? Choosing to be alone is not loneliness. It is quality time with yourself where you can relax without any outside stress from anyone else. You have probably felt this when your husband and children have left the house whether to go to work and school and you are left to your own devices. You can relax, be yourself, have your music on as loud as you like and sing along where no one can hear you.

The Husband Says:

The title of this article is quite emotive for me. I've never really truly been alone for any great length of time. About a week is the longest I've been away from friends and family; any longer than that and I start to despair and will jump on the nearest train, plane or automobile to get back home. Work colleagues are a poor substitute - I need space away from them every day to collate my thoughts and be ready for the next day.

I think that's one of the reasons I set out to find a partner - I wanted someone to talk to and impress with what I achieved and for them to be proud of me since it is rather self-centred and conceited to be too proud of yourself.

Karen's thoughts are about being alone as in having "me" time; time and space to contemplate. The idea that I need time on arrival at home to recharge is more or less correct, but bear in mind that I am an actor in two personas - the husband at home and the executive at work, so I need time to change the costume, mask and disguise. I'm getting better at doing this in the car after work, but the petty distractions of driving behaviour can get in the way of the transition.

Sometimes I want to bury a disaster of a day. Other times I want to whinge about it to someone who will listen (sorry Karen!). I expect my tales of business woe are quite tedious, but it is important to leave them behind to try to give my family "the other David".

C

My current 40 minutes each way commute in the car is good therapeutic "me-alone" time. Music turned up very loud and the only time I sing along because no one can hear me, and I'll never see that person staring from the other car in the queue ever again...

Closure

Seeing a task through to the end. David finds it most irritating to not be able to finish a task. He won't start a task if he is not sure of finishing it. It would probably keep him awake at night.

I often make the mistake of asking him a question or suggesting a task for an alternative day just as he is about to leave for work or he is in the middle of another task. He will get very irritated with me as he now cannot concentrate on anything but the question I have just posed. When I realise my NT mistake, I try and backtrack but it is too late. Regardless of what it is, he will insist on doing it and completing the task that I had casually mooted moments before. Recently I asked him if it was okay if I moved a wardrobe while he was a work. Normally I wouldn't even ask him (I would just do it) but I was trying to be considerate about his hate of change. Instead of him saying as I expected, "Please don't" or "wait until I get home", he suddenly insisted on doing it there and then. Of course the wardrobe needed dismantling and he ended up being quite late for work and also making me late for my meeting that I had planned that morning.

I must learn to keep my mouth shut. He can't let things go. It didn't make sense for anyone to be moving wardrobes at the time but he insisted on doing it there and then because he believed I wanted it done.

The Husband Says:

It's part of the psyche of us Aspies to crave closure. Especially closure where the task will not "bounce back". By that I mean that quite often you NTs say you have fixed something but what you have done is dealt with the superficial symptoms. The root cause of the problem has not been addressed and it is likely to recur. Us Aspies hate having to repeat a task so we crave the closure of a proper solution so that "fixed" stays fixed.

For a good example see The Big Bang Theory episode "The Closure Alternative".

Clumsiness

One of the triad of impairment when diagnosing a child with Asperger Syndrome is their motor skills, or usually lack of. Many children or autistic adults will be diagnosed with Dyspraxia but some are less affected and may only have minor problems which just look like clumsiness.

What are the Signs?

Fine Motor Skills

One of the signs that was picked out in our son's report when he was first diagnosed with AS was his terrible handwriting. It was definitely as if a spider had run over the page. I realised shortly afterwards that I had hardly ever see David write with a pen. When he does it is to sign his name, which is a well-practised Flourish or he writes lists in capital letters. Looking back to our early days of courting the signs were already there. I didn't get many love letters but it was before the days of email and for a year we had a long distance relationship. They were all written in capitals. A little odd to say the least.

Gross Motor Skills

Surprisingly these are often not affected with AS. You will often find that those with AS are actually very good catchers of balls (though terrible runners) or excellent car drivers.

Stress

One noticeable point which is not often mentioned is the effect of stress on their abilities. For example, one day when I was sorting through a box of old school work I came across a poem written in lovely handwriting and lovingly coloured in. I immediately assumed it was my daughter's work as she has neat handwriting. Looking closer I noticed it was my son's from when he was in First School. He had mostly been a happy and relaxed child in his small village school and it wasn't until he went to middle school with all the change and added responsibilities that his autistic traits really started to show. All his school work is badly written to the point that he often has to use a laptop for exams so it is legible. Surprisingly, when he wants to and it is important to him, he can write a very neat letter of birthday card.

Likewise, in situations where they are normally capable, Aspies' skills can deteriorate under stress. I can tell if my husband is upset about something as his driving becomes affected. He is hesitant or even aggressive depending on the situation. He will even become paranoid about other drivers having a go at him.

NT
I have learned in these situations to keep calm and not say anything as it just aggravates the situation and could even make it dangerous.

The Husband Says:

I subscribe to the theory that a level of dyspraxia is a comorbidity of Asperger's. I do think I am clumsier than my peers. But beware that being over-weight also changes the body's centre of gravity making elegant activity more difficult. So my apparent dyspraxia might just be me acting like a bull in a china shop.

On handwriting: I agree with the theories on fine motor skills. To produce elegant calligraphy requires the muscles in the lower arm near the hands to work hard against each other in continual tension; the more control, the higher the tension. I make a trade-off between handwriting (almost never, too tiring, too slow for it to be legible) and a stylised capitals writing that is not in any particular font, but chosen to be legible and fast to write. Of course these days, my two fingered typing in Arial or Cambria is how most people see my written communication.

Tools are very important when fine motor skills are impaired. Reducing the drag across paper or the general energy required to perform the action improves the appearance of the final product.

AS

Aspies - choose your weapons:

- Pilot Hi-Tecpoint V5 wet ink fine tipped ballpoint pens. Some people like the V7, but for me these drag across the paper. The V5 is just perfect. The Uni-Ball Vision Elite is in a distant second place. My son likes the Stabilo B 10 point 88 Fineliners, but they are too slow for me since they are felt-tips.

- Sharpies - genuine ones, not the knock-offs

- Pentel 0.5mm propelling pencil (the classic black plastic and metal body) with HB leads. The clutch wears out in time.

- Steel rule, scalpel and surgeon's straight blades

- Genuine Stanley knife and Stanley blades - replace frequently

- Dressmakers scissors

- In general: the correct tool for the job at hand without dangerous improvisations of the type you NTs are fond of making

Somewhat bizarrely, I am ambidextrous. Perhaps this means I am equally bad with both hands. I spent a lot of my years growing up in my dad's car repair garage, so I think I have a tremendous muscle memory for operating certain tools in particular directions.

Note that Aspies usually have a strong eye for detail so we will spot our own mistakes caused by poor control and berate ourselves about them. DIY thus involves lots of cursing and swearing about our own limitations.

C

Co-Dependency

Situation

I can pinpoint certain times when I was under a lot of stress and I had turned to my husband for sympathy. Instead of reassurance and platitudes, David would become so concerned by the situation, his paranoia would become contagious. Now I see that what I really wanted from him was reciprocation. Someone to listen to me and tell me it would be alright. That my worries would come to nothing. Instead, my stress levels rose as did his anxiety for a social situation.

I would often describe this to my friends as 'a trouble shared is a trouble doubled'.

I slowly learned from my experiences and I made a conscious effort not to tell him about any problems unless it was completely necessary. Having moved into a village with a strong community I was lucky enough to find some good friends whom I was able to talk to. Yet the one problem I could not talk to my friends about was the biggest one in my life, which was the dire communication with my husband.

What is Co-Dependency?

Co-dependency is a condition very common in men with Asperger Syndrome as they willingly become dependent on their partner's ability to deal with the social, emotional and communication difficulties they find hard to deal with. In an AS/NT relationship this can slowly creep up on the emotionally strong partner (generally the wife) and before she knows it she is taking responsibility for all social, emotional and communication situations that crop up. This can be mentally exhausting for the NT partner, particularly as she has no one else to lean on and make decisions together.

Solution

NT First of all you need to realise that you are in a co-dependent situation. If you find yourself keeping information to yourself in order not to upset the equilibrium you are likely in a co-dependent relationship.

Secondly, if you are dissatisfied with this situation you need to gently discuss it with your partner. It may be that all you need to do is redefine your roles. It is quite possible he has left certain responsibilities to you because he feels you are better at it, but it may be with a little coaching that he too could take on this responsibility.

Due to his reduced executive functioning, despite his eye for detail he cannot see that you are struggling with the onslaught of family life and need help. This will be particularly true if you both work.

C

To begin sharing more responsibilities, draw up a short list of what you would like him to help you with. Explain with bullet points what the job consists of e.g.:

- Wednesday is bin day
- Empty all the bin in the house and put in wheelie bin outside.
- Put wheelie bin in street before midday when the rubbish is collected.
- Retrieve bin and return to yard.

This can work quite well as a social story since in a conventional relationship these things are social norms. See for example 'Putting out the Bins'.

I admit it is additional work in the short term, but once he understands you are struggling and is fully aware of what you need, he should make more of an effort for you. My warning is this will only be successful if you don't overwhelm him with too much. Take it slowly.

Coercive Control

Coercive Control is a term used to describe what used to be called domestic violence but is now more commonly known as domestic abuse. Domestic abuse is now considered more than a physical fight; it is a pattern of behaviour which seeks to take away the victims freedom and their sense of self.

This has now become an offence in the UK.

Coercive Control is a concept developed by academic and activist Evan Stark. He explains "Coercive Control is like being taken hostage; the victim becomes captive in an unreal world created by the partner/abuser, entrapped in a world of contradiction and fear'.

I find this statement worrying on several levels because in some ways being an Asperger Wife can be like this. Does this mean we are suffering abuse? Do we need help to get out of our situations? Are we abused and in denial of it?

Certainly at times, if your AS partner is controlling over a distinct area of your marriage such as finance or the state of the house this can cause huge conflict and upset.

My feeling is that most men on the spectrum are naturally gentle, caring souls but they are struggling to deal with the unpredictability especially of life.

Before he met you he didn't have a joint bank account and he knew exactly what went in and out of it. Now it feels like he has no control over his finances and to him in his panic and negative thinking the next logical step is losing the house and bankruptcy.

You can see why he is trying to be controlling. As supportive partners we have to be able to see the intent behind the behaviour before we cry abuse.

I worry because of this new law that more Aspie men may end up in prison classed as abusers.

The Husband Says:

If Karen finds this worrying, then as an Aspie I find the subject extremely alarming. I believe, like Karen that the vast majority of Aspies are kind and caring and that any coercion is not intended and planned. I would dread the idea that one of my socially clumsy actions might be misinterpreted, perhaps by a judge resulting in punitive action.

So strong is the sense of avoidance of this situation in me that I go to extreme lengths to make sure that my actions can't be misconstrued. I held the door open at a train station yesterday for a particularly beautiful young woman who thanked me. So great is the fear of the wrong type of social interaction that I quite consciously made sure that I joined the train in a different carriage to her to make sure that the social interaction ended properly and my actions were beyond reproach.

This just sets up more social barriers for us Aspies. What are the social norms at this precise moment in time? I believe my actions to be too strong a response to perceived threat, but we must not probe the boundaries to establish what the rules actually are. The consequences of one step too far are just too grave.

Cognitive Distortions

From Cary Terra's article: Ten Cognitive Distortions and Asperger Syndrome:

American psychotherapist David Burns published 'Feeling Good: The New Mood Therapy'. The book details the relationship between thoughts and mood. Burns identified ten common 'cognitive distortions' being exaggerated and irrational thoughts, which can negatively affect mood:

1. ALL-OR-NOTHING THINKING: You see things in black and white categories. If your performance falls short of perfect, you see yourself as a total failure.

2. OVERGENERALIZATION: You see a single negative event as a never-ending pattern of defeat.

3. MENTAL FILTER: You pick out a single negative detail and dwell on it exclusively so that your vision of all reality becomes darkened, like the drop of ink that discolours the entire beaker of water.

4. DISQUALIFYING THE POSITIVE: You reject positive experiences by insisting they "don't count" for some reason or other. In this way you can maintain a negative belief that is contradicted by your everyday experiences.

5. JUMPING TO CONCLUSIONS: You make a negative interpretation even though there are no definite facts that convincingly support your conclusions.

a. Mind Reading. You arbitrarily conclude that someone is reacting negatively to you, and you don't bother to check this out.

b. The Fortune Teller Error. You anticipate that things will turn out badly, and you feel convinced that your prediction is an already established fact.

6. MAGNIFICATION (CATASTROPHIZING) OR MINIMIZATION: You exaggerate the importance of things (such as your goof-up or someone else's achievement). Or you inappropriately shrink things until they appear tiny (your own desirable qualities or the other fellow's imperfections). This is also called the "binocular trick."

7. EMOTIONAL REASONING: You assume that your negative emotions necessarily reflect the way things really are: "I feel it, therefore it must be true."

8. SHOULD STATEMENTS: You try to motivate yourself with shoulds and shouldn'ts, as if you had to be whipped and punished before you could be expected to do anything. "Musts" and "ought's" are also offenders. The emotional consequence is guilt. When you direct "should" statements toward others, you feel anger, frustration, and resentment.

9. LABELING AND MISLABELING: This is an extreme form of over-generalization. Instead of describing your error, you attach a negative label to yourself: "I'm a loser." When someone else's behaviour rubs you the wrong way, you attach a negative label to him: "He's a damn louse." Mislabelling involves describing an event with language that is highly coloured and emotionally loaded.

10. PERSONALIZATION: You see yourself as the cause of some negative event which in fact you were not primarily responsible for.

Cognitive distortions are characteristic of depression and anxiety. Adults with Asperger's are especially vulnerable to adopting distorted patterns of thinking.

The Husband Says:

I think that over the years I have been guilty of each of these classes of distorted thoughts with the exception of 7.

Coming down from a High

Avoiding the High

Have you ever noticed that your husband not only avoids difficult events but he can also avoid going to things that you know he will like?

It is understandable if he doesn't want to go to a surprise birthday party, there are so many things that could go wrong and so many people to be avoided but what about if you book him a show about something he is really obsessed about? Has he ever tried to duck out of it? Or has he been in such a bad mood beforehand he has managed to make you too late to go?

You have to feel sorry for them in this event. They may have built the longed for event up so high in their mind that they are worried that the reality will not meet their extremely high expectations. They end up being too scared to go in case they are disappointed or have a major Expectation Violation. They would rather not go and therefore not be let down. Of course, how do they verbalise this to you? They don't want to seem ungrateful for the present or they can't verbalise their feelings. All they know is that they don't want to go and so they catastrophize sufficiently to stop the event happening.

Coming Down

Sometimes the draw to go and see such events, the comedy show for example, is too much and they manage to look forward and motivate themselves to get there. Sometimes this is managed because they have been before and know what to expect.

If all goes well at the venue and the show, your loved one will be on an enormous high. Or if he was worried that the car is about to be clamped, not so much. He might enjoy the show but all the while in the back of his mind he is worried that he won't be able to drive home or that you will miss the train. The moment he comes out of the theatre he may come down with a tremendous bump and get very agitated. He may not calm down until he sees that the car has in fact not been clamped and the car park is still open.

NT To avoid this, even though he likes to be in control, it may be good for you to be in charge of all the details (if at all possible). Make sure he knows the details, where you are going to park, what time the car park closes, what time the show finishes. You could stay the sober driver so he doesn't have the stress of driving through night time traffic to get home and he could even have a drink in the interval.

Immersion

I have noticed with my family, that they often get completely immersed in films and shows. It is like they are not just observers but experiencing them for real. They are there. If all goes well they will find it hard to leave it behind. They won't want to lose that feeling and want to stay and live through it all again. Of course, reality hits home and they realise that they can't. They have to leave the theatre and fight their way home through people and traffic and go back to their real lives of money troubles and constant work.

To you and I, the NT's, we are able to put these things to the back of our minds and extend as long as possible the feeling we had in the theatre, whilst at the same time incrementally letting our heart beat settle and our mind slowly detach from our enthralment.

To our Aspies it can come as quite a shock. They can literally go from absolute joy to very irritable within the space of finding the exit door. To us NT's this is quite disturbing and perturbing. We can't understand why they are suddenly, moody and sullen. The journey home can be a very uncomfortable one and you wonder why you bothered in the first place.

The Husband Says:

It's been a really "bad" couple of years for coming down off a high. I blame you Hollywood! You stretched "The Hobbit" over three episodes. You extended the "Star Wars" franchise by at least another three episodes (Spoiler: HAAAANNNN!) and you let J J Abrahms loose on Star Trek. All too much for one Aspie to take, and not just me judging by the responses in the cinema.

Common Sense

In the early days, when I had David on a pedestal, I mistakenly believed that common sense came hand in hand with intelligence. Of course if I'd looked a little bit closer to home at my own family I would have realised that this was not so.

Example: When my sister was little she left the bathroom tap on and it flooded the floor and the ceiling of the kitchen below. This created a bulge in the ceiling. My father in his wisdom, with his doctorate in statistics, decided the solution was to use an electric drill plugged into the wall to drill into the bulge in the ceiling and release the water. How he was not electrocuted I do not know.

David acts so confident even when he doesn't know what he is doing - so that I used to believe he knew what he was doing! After all, he is a highly qualified electrical engineer. When the washing machine broke down mid wash he set about fixing it. This seemed like an achievable thing despite the fact he doesn't know anything about washing machines. The machine was full of water and refused to empty it. David managed to persuade the machine to unlock. He asked me to get him a load of towels. I obediently did as he asked, not totally realising what he was going to do. He dumped the towels in front of the machine and opened the door. The dirty water poured out all over the floor and some of it was caught up by the towels. We were at a stage in our marriage when I had realised that questioning his actions was not appreciated, but I had not learned how to tactfully tackle these anomalies in his practicality. What I wanted to say (yell!) was "Why didn't you ask me for a bucket that would collect the water?" I had assumed that he was going to use a nearby bucket and put the towels around it to collect any excess water that missed the bucket. I did not have enough confidence in my own common sense to stop him before he did it.

NT

If you ask him to do one thing he will only do one thing

Why?

I believe this is called applied common sense. If I ask my son to lay the table he will only lay the cutlery for himself. This looks like an extremely selfish action but he is hungry and not aware that anyone else might be hungry. It stems from theory of mind.

If I ask David to empty the rubbish bin, he will do so. He will not see that the recycling bin is also overflowing and empty that. Most wives would expect both bins to be emptied, despite not asking specifically. It is no help at all if one bin is still full. The reasons he didn't do what I didn't ask? He isn't me and he can't see inside my mind for the simplest of notions and also if he does use his imitative he worries that it might be wrong without direct instruction, so he just doesn't bother.

The Husband Says:

I often say to my legal colleagues, when drawing up a contract, "Well that's just common sense. Can we not just add a term that says Common Sense will apply." The legal eagles just roll their eyes and say "Well, OK, but what exactly is 'common sense' and how do we define it, where is all of 'common sense' written down, so that when something isn't 'common sense' we can call for a breach of contract?" Well they have a point. What exactly is "common sense"?

The Aspie in me has me reach for Black's Dictionary of Law: "Sound practical judgment; that degree of intelligence and reason, as exercised upon the relations of persons and things and the ordinary affairs of life, which is possessed by the generality of mankind, and which would suffice to direct the conduct and actions of the individual in a manner to agree with the behaviour of ordinary persons."

So there we have it. Common sense is something that would be expected of a normal person. So that's something that you NTs would normally do. Us Aspies, well, we are trying to figure it out and we make a lot of it up as we go along - after all, all of the "common sense" isn't written down so that we can crib from it. No wonder we get it wrong.

Now I suppose that's what this Instant Help guide is all about - writing down a small fraction of that 'common sense' so that we all know what that term means - where the boundaries lie.

On the washing machine example - well I am a fully qualified Engineer (yes, capital "E" and everything). Repairing a washing machine is fully within my grasp with the right tools and spare parts. Yes I splashed a bit of water around, but in the end that machine was beyond economic repair. And it took a blood sacrifice from me that caused the worst of the cursing. I suppose, with hind-sight that the

"common sense" thing to have done would have been to explain to Karen my intentions and get help from her.

I hate plumbing.

Communication

It is essential to remember that communication is a two-way thing.

It is also extremely important to realise in an Asperger Marriage that you are both speaking different languages. The wife speaks Neurotypical and the husband speaks Asperger's. It's a little like an Italian and a Spaniard marrying, the languages are both Latin based and there are many similarities but with complacence comes misunderstanding. For example, a family friend who speaks fluent Italian went on holiday to Spain and went into a grocery store to ask for "burro", butter. The shop assistant kindly explained to him that they didn't sell donkeys in their shop. My kids think that story is hilarious.

Presumably, if an Italian and Spaniard got married they would take pains to learn each other's languages fluently in order to enhance communication and matrimonial harmony.

NT **AS** This is what we need to do with our partners. Learn their language. They have done quite well at learning ours but still need some help.

The Husband Says:

That sounds like a good idea, but don't go adding additional words or (worse still) new syntax to your language. I'm still studying the basics and asking to buy a kilo of donkeys to put on my toast.

I think Karen would say: above all don't take things too literally; that's a big Aspie mistake. NTs use a lot of metaphor. A favourite example is that when you toast the bride at a wedding you don't set her on fire.

There are some good "field guides"; a large part of NT communication is non-verbal, so try looking at some books on body language and Neuro-Linguistic Programming. There are some humorous guides to Englishness and etiquette - these give some clues to social norms.

Further Reading

- Peoplewatching: The Desmond Morris Guide to Body Language
- Watching the English: The International Bestseller Revised and Updated
- It's Raining Cats and Dogs: An Autism Spectrum Guide to the

Confusing World of Idioms, Metaphors and Everyday Expressions

Communication Disorder

Asperger's Syndrome is a Social and Communication Disorder. Many people who are unfamiliar with autism and it's spectrum may believe that this is entirely to do with speech. There are some people on the spectrum who do have difficulty with speech but mostly, for those with AS it is more subtle and more complex than that.

It is about not understanding the subtle social signs such as facial expressions, body language and intonation. This creates a myriad of social misunderstandings.

Your average NT has no difficulty in understanding body language and intuitively will know if someone is bored for example. They can tell the difference between sighs. There are many types of sighs but to those with AS they all sound the same and they immediately assume that a sigh is a negative emotion.

The Husband Says:

AS
The only way this gets better is to practise. You can learn the basics of body language (where an NT just 'knows' all of the subtleties). It's going to be hard-work and there are going to be hilarious and embarrassing mistakes along the way.

Co-Morbidities

From a medical dictionary: "Two or more coexisting medical conditions or disease processes that are additional to an initial diagnosis."

From a practical stand-point, co-morbidities of Asperger Syndrome are those symptoms commonly seen that seem to result from Asperger's Syndrome, but are not exclusive to or diagnostic of Asperger's Syndrome by themselves - the symptoms are in common with other conditions.

Also be aware that Asperger's and autism is about not being 'normal' in respect of these symptoms of feelings or states, so that can mean being hyper-sensitive (super sensitive to the symptom in question) or hypo-sensitive (barely affected by or not registering the symptom or feeling).

ADHD

It is fairly common for ADHD to be a comorbidity with Asperger Syndrome and for both ADHD and Asperger Syndrome to share a lot of symptoms.

The latest research suggests that though some children grow out of ADHD, there are still many adults with the condition. Brain scans done at MIT suggest that like those with Asperger's, people with ADHD have a lack of executive functioning. This means that they find it hard to concentrate and focus for long periods of time, despite often being highly intelligent they cannot hold down a job, they get bored very quickly and their time management is poor.

Alexithymia

Alexithymia - or low emotional intelligence

Bipolar Disorder

There are many people with Asperger's Syndrome who have wrongly been diagnosed with Bi-Polar or manic depression as it used to be called. Much of the symptoms are steep mood swings which can be seen in AS.

Be aware that Bi-Polar is considered a mental illness whereas as autism and AS are considered as a condition or a different way of thinking. Bi-Polar moods last longer and are harder to change than everyday emotions.

Signs to look out for in Bi-polar Disorder

Mania

1. Feeling overly happy or elated for long periods of time.

2. Feeling easily agitated e.g. jumpy or twitchy.

3. Talking super-fast with racing thoughts.

4. Extreme restlessness or impulsively.

5. Impaired judgement.

6. Unrealistic over-confident in your abilities or powers.

7. Engaging in risky behaviour, such as gambling with savings or having impulsive sex.

Depression

1. Feeling sad and hopeless.

2. Lacking energy.

3. Feelings of guilt and despair.

4. Feeling pessimistic about everything.

5. Being delusional.

6. Lack of appetite.

7. Suicidal thoughts.

Many people think this is part of having Asperger's Syndrome but it is not a pre-requisite.

Dyspraxia

People with autism often have difficulties with motor coordination e.g. tying their shoe laces, if they are significantly affected they may be given a formal diagnosis of Dyspraxia.

Gastrointestinal Disorders

These are extremely common in people with ASD but there are ways to improve health, mind and behaviour with good diet and the right use of vitamin supplementation.

General Anxiety Disorder

General Anxiety Disorder is a long term condition that causes you to feel anxious about a wide range of situations and issues.

Personally, I believe that most people with Asperger's Syndrome have this and many autistic people too. See Anxiety

Obsessive Compulsive Disorder

Though many people with AS appear to have this disorder you will actually find that they enjoy putting order and routine in their life unlike people genuinely afflicted with OCD.

Sensory Problems

This may be co-morbid but I believe that this is also part of the diagnosis for Asperger Syndrome. I don't know anyone with AS who is not either Hyper or Hypo with sensory dysfunction.

Tourette's Syndrome

This is considered a neuropsychiatric disorder with onset usually during childhood. It is characterised by multiple physical and some verbal tics. These tics are generally unpredictable their frequency but tend to get worse with stress.

The Husband Says:

So here begins the alphabet soup of what kind of Aspie I might be. I don't really care that much - Asperger Syndrome as a label is both small enough to capture "my" population segment and large enough to cover the vast variation in presentation of each of us individual Aspies.

There is no need for the question "What Type of Aspie are you?" Further sub-divisions of the label aren't helping. Now coping strategies for each of the symptoms - well that's a different matter - click on the links; go and look them up...

Compartmentalising

Although we Neurotypicals do this to a certain degree in our lives, we don't have difficulty "crossing the streams". If our work life overlaps into our home life, this may be annoying but we deal with it or possibly even embrace it.

Not so for our Aspies.

With our Aspie Children one of the hardest things to get them to do is homework. There are many reasons for this, like any child they are reluctant to do schoolwork, but our Aspies have another reason which they cannot help.

Compartmentalising means that Work should be done at work (or school) and home life should be kept at home and never the twain shall meet.

Being forced to take school work home is very confusing to an Asperger child and they will resist this terribly. It does not compute in their brains. This leads to tantrums, avoidance and meltdowns which parents have great difficulty dealing with until they get a diagnosis and put strategies in place such as extending the school day.

What happens to the adult Aspie who still compartmentalises his life in this way?

It is obvious to me that I am in the neatly labelled "Home" box in David's head. Once he sweeps off the drive in the morning I am put out of his mind and he starts preparing himself for the day ahead whether it be planning how to deal with the NT's he has to work with or some technical problem that needs to be solved.

He doesn't look at his phone for text messages from me and he does not answer phone calls from me either. This is very annoying for a wife when there is a family emergency.

To him it is logical and keeps everything pure and using his ghostbusters reference not "crossing the streams".

So I am wondering how he manages when he is in his home office. What are the thought processes then?

The Husband Says:

To start to answer your question about the home office; the threshold of the separate room we use for a home office is in "Twilight Zone" styling the threshold to another dimension - that of work. Answering the 'phone is in my work style. Interruptions like the postman should really be handled by the receptionist. The bins are put out by the cleaners. Swapping back to

"home" mode takes time and doesn't happen instantly back at the threshold either. In the transition period I swap from my work e-mail program to my home e-mail.

I do, however, keep a common list of web-site favourites that apply both at home and at work. And whilst my 'phone is on silent-vibrate at work, my mobile phone rings in my home office. Voicemail after 4 rings still applies though.

Compliments

We can't deny it. We women love a compliment but it is often missing from our marriages. To be fair I do get the occasional compliment from David though sometimes they are back handed. I'll take what I can get!

Types of Compliments

A compliment isn't just for the way you look. It can be for the way someone has washed up or driven a car or handled a difficult situation.

When you see your husband has done something well, it is worth telling him as he won't be able to judge for himself. If he is confident in his abilities and he knows you like what he does then there is a good chance he will be happy to do it again. Possibly without you asking.

The Husband Says:

Reminder: It's The Little Things.

Compromise

He was probably prepared to compromise in the early days to do anything to keep you happy. You are probably feeling cheated right now that he never compromises on anything.

NT It might be worth considering that you need to show him the way and tell him when you are compromising.

I suspect you already make compromises every day to keep the peace, but maybe he is not aware that you are silently and automatically doing this. It can often feel oppressive and definitely taken for granted.

If a decision has to be made, no matter how large or small, it could well be worth writing down the pros and cons of the decision and also why you would like to do it a certain way. Don't forget to include and consider his argument. Try and find a common and acceptable ground between the two of you. Let him see that you are openly working towards a harmonious marriage. All that effort you thought you were putting in by keeping silent, by silently seething inside, is not healthy for you but he would be also unaware of the sacrifices you are making for him.

Remember this man lives on his self-esteem. Let him know you care enough about him to make compromises and give up something or part of something that you like or want. Let him know that he is worth it. He will follow by example and, if he doesn't, you are in a good position to remind him that it is his turn now.

The Husband Says:

Compromise. Now there's a difficult subject.

Compromises seem to hint at a list of demands. My list of things to do or achieve doesn't match with yours so we need to compromise - your list is more important than my list. Why isn't the point on my list good enough? For beneficial compromise to happen we need to get away from the lists.

Compromise means going against the plan I've probably already formed, or making me have to come up with a new plan.

NT *So start your approach to a compromise with a thought out plan of what this compromise will mean to me, not only "selling it" with the advantages of this compromise, but the nitty-gritty of what will need to change in order for this compromise to be a success. This change of plan will make me look stubborn because I will test you on the compromise to make sure you are sure that this is now the right thing to do.*

But if it makes sense to me on my terms, I'll go with it. I might even adopt it and pass it off as my own. That's another topic...

As I read and review my comments just before publication, I realise just how one sided the advice in this "compromise" article is. I stand by my thinking that compromise is best led by the NT in the relationship; but the Aspie needs to spot (or be told) what is going on and join in.

Consequences

This has a large effect on Aspie behaviour, from when they are very small and into adulthood. Being able only to see the detail and not the bigger picture makes them wary of things going wrong. They concentrate on the negative side of any event. This means they are generally safer than the average child growing up as they are much less likely to cross the road without looking, but it also means it is so much harder to get them to do anything even vaguely dangerous/risk taking as they grow up.

Throw into the mix the co-morbid condition of ADHD though and you get a child completely unaware of consequences. These are the ones you can't take your eyes off and, as a parent, you have to lock all the doors and windows and keep your passwords safe.

If these children survive into later life they often become very interesting and successful adults who take many risks in life. Some of the risks may even pay off.

The Husband Says:

I seem to have side-stepped any significant ADHD component of Asperger's. I still retain my caution in what I consider dangerous situations. I may have a fear of heights, but I don't think that is true vertigo, as in a disturbance of my balance system related to height; more a worry about the pain involved in the sudden stop at the bottom.

Consideration

This is one of the crucial things missing from an Aspie marriage. This is a sweeping generalisation but usually the NT female partner is considerate to her husband's needs. She will surprise him with thoughtful gifts at birthday and Christmas and often in between. She will think ahead and consider how her actions may affect her partner at home or when they are out. These will come naturally and easily to her and will often be appreciated if somewhat taken for granted.

This subject is close to but different from reciprocation.

Consideration is when the male partner is putting the washing on, reading the label of his wife's new expensive jumper and not putting it in the general wash or the tumble dryer.

The Husband Says:

Whoops...

Constant Feeling of Guilt

David will regularly apologise for things he does not have to apologise for. On a quiet Sunday afternoon when he is relaxing on a well-earned break, watching one of his favourite, undemanding TV programmes, he will take any glance in his direction from me as a look of criticism. He will defensively explain why he is having some leisure time and will justify that actually it isn't really leisure time as he has set he computer running on a task and he is waiting for that task to finish. He seems to think that if I catch him not doing anything then I consider him a bad husband.

C

He has no concept that I have his best interests at heart. I want him to be able to relax. After all if he is relaxed and happy then the whole household can relax too. His not being able to relax makes me not able to relax as I have to constantly second guess his moods or mop his fevered brow to calm him down and tell him that it is okay. He is filled not just with anxiety but with feelings of guilt. He is aware of his communication failing so he is constantly trying to second guess what I am thinking. Unfortunately, as he has a very low opinion of himself, and his lack of empathy gives him the impression that I am thinking what he is thinking, he therefore believes that I have a low opinion of him also. However, add into the mix that he absolutely hates criticism and to be wrong, he automatically gets defensive about something he has completely created in his head - all because I have walked into the room with an expression he cannot fathom and immediately assumed the worst. It is exhausting emotionally for both of us.

AS Note to the AS Partner: We married you because we love and admire you and we are still here after all these years so you must be doing something right.

The Husband Says:

Thanks. Those feelings are Cognitive Distortions numbers 1 and 5.

Control

Aspies like to control the environment around them and that often means the people in it. This does not necessarily mean that they dictate what other people do but they certainly like the people around them to stick to routines and not do anything too unpredictable.

Feeling out of control leads to extreme anxiety but being in control can lead to satisfaction and even pleasure.

For our daughter's fourth birthday party we decided to "go traditional", we hired the village hall and introduced her and her classmates to retro party games. This was relatively successful until it came to musical chairs. None of the pre-schoolers had ever come across this game before and had been brought up so far in a non-competitive environment. After some confusion and direction from parents much hilarity ensued and also a little bit of crying. Our daughter very quickly dropped out of the game even though she had not lost a seat. She insisted on taking charge of the CD player herself so that she could dictate to her peers when the music would start and stop. At four she was taking control of an uncertain situation.

C

The Husband Says:

Allowing an Aspie to take control is a double edged sword. In an environment when no-one is quite sure of the social rules, then the Aspie will apply logic and figure out some rules. It is easy, though, to take this to excess and apply rules when it is intentional that there are none.

In my professional life, I control things so that they follow my rule set which is an adaptation of what I perceive "the rules of business" to be. When laying out the room for a meeting, or coming into someone else's meeting, I'm looking for the correct seat for me - in an adversarial negotiation I want to be on the opposite side of the table to the "other side". I'll generally line us up by rank with the principal negotiators at the middle of the table facing each other. I'll be on the right hand of my principal and nearest the computer screen to display documents and evidence.

I don't like being out of my own control. I have very seldom got so drunk that I can't remember how I got home, and I don't like that dizzy feeling of drunkenness. I've tried, but won't 'do' illegal drugs for much the same reason - to the point where if prescribed some classes of drugs by a doctor that I wouldn't take them either. I won't go on a roller-coaster until I can have seen all of the track and what it does and imagine what it would be like to ride it. I'm OK with heights, but only as long as I've rigged my own rope and harness. I'd like to meet the pilot of my plane where at all possible.

Cortisol

Cortisol is a naturally occurring steroid hormone released in response to stress and low blood glucose levels. Long term high cortisol levels are implicated in insulin resistance and the onset of Type 2 Diabetes. Cortisol seems to help forming short term memories but hinders retrieval of long term memories and general learning.

People with autism or Asperger Syndrome may have levels of cortisol very different to the norm. This is likely to be as a result of the long term stress of anxiety.

Counselling

For You

If you can find a counsellor who will listen to you and understand your situation, please tell me where you found them!

In all seriousness, even if a counsellor has never come across an Asperger Marriage it is still worth talking to them about your situation. They may learn something and you can offload in a safe, compassionate and confidential atmosphere.

Counsellors in the UK with relationship and Asperger's expertise:

- Maxine Aston

- Barrie Thompson

(Not an endorsement; correct at time of writing)

I am currently taking training for giving counselling and am also contemplating being able to diagnose so keep an eye out for my Facebook pages and website. Asperger Relationship Consulting.

For Him

It is very much a case of whether he has accepted his diagnosis. He may accept his diagnosis and feel he now knows enough about it that he doesn't need to see a counsellor. It's possible he doesn't want to open up about his childhood and talk about traumas he has managed to hide away all these years.

Recently, our son was having a hard time settling into high school and we contacted a private psychotherapist that specialised in Asperger Syndrome and school problems. It turned out to be very helpful for our son. We were not allowed into the sessions and he was told he didn't have to discuss it with us if he didn't want to. Apart from the frustration of being a mum who wants to know everything that goes on in her child's life, this worked out very well for him and he was able to tell the therapist lots of things in private and build a relationship with him. During our first session however, when we went as a family to discuss therapy, David became quite tearful as he realised that some of the questions the therapist was asking our son brought up a lot of past memories of bad times at school. He had never relayed these to me and had obviously bottled them away. Afterwards David wondered whether he would benefit from some therapy himself. So far he has not done this but I still believe it would be beneficial to him like it was to our son.

Together

In the UK we have what used to be called the Marriage Guidance Service but is now called Relate. They do not specialise in counselling for people with AS. In fact there are only a handful of people in the country who do specialise in this area. Going to a Relate counsellor who is not trained in AS will most likely be damaging for your marriage. If the counsellor does not understand the way your husband processes his thoughts and how AS makes him react to certain situations they will more than likely give the wrong advice. Without expert AS knowledge when a NT wife and an AS man talk about their marriage it can come across as being abusive.

The Difference between Criticism, Concern and Advice

This is a distinction that has to be made clear in an AS/NT relationship between criticism and advice.

NT First of all, the wife should carefully consider her words whether she is giving either of these things. You must give your husband notice that you would like to speak seriously to him and you need to consider how to clearly and tactfully phrase and deliver your criticism or advice.

When giving advice to your husband or partner, one should actually consider whether it is criticism of advice.

1. What is the purpose of your advice? You may want to start off by telling him why you are giving him this advice in the first place so that he knows why you are saying these things.

2. Are you giving him guidance on an aspect of life he is unaware of or unsure of? This is advice. Be aware though that advice is freely given but does not have to be accepted. It is the choice of the person you are talking to whether they choose to accept your advice.

3. An important point to remember is that the AS person needs more time to process their thoughts and take on board another person's ideas and perspective.

Just because they do not immediately agree with you, does not mean that after a certain amount of time, unpressured rumination, and cogitation, that they will not come around to your way of thinking. However, what often happens in my household is that once I have suggested an idea and left it to germinate, he will often come back some time, perhaps days later, with my idea but in the guise that it is his own original idea (he calls this "Not Invented Here"). The question is: are you prepared to let him own the idea? Is it worth the subsequent and quite often irrelevant argument of whose idea it was in the first place as long as the piece of advice or concept has been taken on board? I have learned that it does not matter who owns the original idea. Is pride so important to you? I have often turned his way of thinking to my advantage by dropping little seeds of ideas in to the conversation, such as ideas for holiday destinations and letting them germinate. Certainly, when I suggested the idea of his potential Asperger diagnosis I did not force the issue but let him think upon it without pressure and use his own observations and research to come to the same conclusion. That way, not only does he agree with me but his conviction is solid as he came to the decision by himself and not from any pressure from me.

C

4. It is much easier to dish out advice to one's partner than it is to dish out criticism. They often do not want to hear it, and I am sure I don't have to tell you or you wouldn't be reading this book now, that they take very badly to it indeed.

Now in the basic manual for recognising someone with autism or Asperger's or your one day course 'Introduction to autism' one of the most common fallacies told is that those with autism do not recognise the different tones of voice. This may be true for some but this is a sweeping generalisation and I believe most intelligent people with Asperger's learn on the whole to recognise at least when their loved ones are cross. Sometimes they get crossed wires and confuse certain intonations with others. It often depends how stressed they are. If they are less stressed in a situation they can bring their history of learning NT communication to bear in full and will, on the whole, listen and take on board what you are trying to say to them.

When having to criticise your partner try not to do it suddenly unless it is an emergency and just has to done. Make an appointment and let them prepare mentally for what is to come. Think carefully about your words and perhaps even prepare a script or notes to prompt yourself and keep you on the right course. Try not to use negative language and try not to let them think they are stupid. Explain why you think it would be better if they stopped do the thing they were doing wrong and explain how it would make their life better (and your life better) if they could do it in a different, more positive way. You may want to consider employing what in modern management terms is called a 'Shit sandwich' which is during an employee appraisal, start off by praising them for their good work, then move on to the thing you really wanted to talk about which concerned you, and follow it up by again praising some more of their good work, or at least finishing up on a positive note.

5. Remember that like children and dogs, most people like to be praised, but Aspie's have very low self-esteem and they thrive on praise and success. Being shown they are doing something wrong however trivial is devastating for them (Cognitive Distortion #1). They feel not only failures about that small task but wonder whether secretly they have failed on everything else they are doing and you are just not telling them. They are highly self-critical and to have any of those doubts confirmed is extremely hard for them (Cognitive Distortion #2). It is no wonder they are often depressed. Unfortunately, and generally unwittingly, we are often the cause of this self-doubt as we assume that they can cope with a little criticism, when in fact they can't.

Aspie's find it very hard to find the distinction between criticism, advice and concern. Concern can sometimes come across as a criticism of someone so if you are concerned about your AS husband's behaviour or actions, be very clear that you are not being critical but you are saying this because you love and care for them and want the best for them.

The Husband Says:

Try to always start with advice; that's the least emotional form of criticism or concern. I can take or leave your advice (although I will probably adopt it and take it given some time).

D

✧   Decision Making

✧   Decompression

✧   Defence Mode

✧   Delayed Effect

✧   Delegation

✧   Denial

✧   Depression

✧   Diagnosis

✧   Diagnostic Gap

✧   Diesel Jenga

✧   Directional Anger

✧   Disease or Difference?

✧   Dispelling the Myths

✧   Divorce

✧   Does He Love You?

✧   Don't take it Personally

✧   Double Standards

✧   Doxophobia

✧   Driving

✧   DSM-V and Asperger's

✧   Dyspraxia

D

Decision Making

Every Saturday for years we have dropped the kids off with their grandmother and gone off to do a little shopping and treat ourselves to lunch. The same pattern occurs every Saturday where I would ask David where he would like to eat as we are driving towards town. He always replies that he doesn't know and wants to know what I would like to do. This is very frustrating for me as on the surface it looks like he is being considerate but actually he is passing the buck. I don't mind making the decisions but I feel it is selfish for me to decide where we should eat every week. Though we enjoy the same food we do have slightly different tastes. He doesn't seem to realise that I genuinely want to know where he would like to eat and am not being polite. Plus, if we get to a restaurant and he isn't keen on the food it will be considered my fault as I made the decision.

I have a little more sympathy these days as I realise he does find it hard to choose. We are lucky to have a plethora of good restaurants within a short drive in our region. However, just as I worry that he won't like my choice of restaurant he worries overly about this to the point of refusing to make the decision. He thinks women are complicated and just ask trick questions. Maybe some of them do, but when I ask him where he would like to eat I really can't see any ambiguity in that question. Hence our frustration with each other over the tiniest of things.

Yet, on a good day when he doesn't have any pressures of work, when his mother hasn't said anything to annoy him, and maybe someone he respects has recommended a good restaurant, he will independently come up with a genuine suggestion that he is excited about.

When anxiety takes over even every day decisions become a chore.

The Husband Says:

Decision making should be really easy. It seldom is when the NTs get involved. They say I'm obsessive, but I say my decision making is organised. I make lists; I weigh pros and cons, perhaps with a SWOT diagram; I apply logic. Then I get a different conclusion and a different decision that I would like to make from you. Conflict results unless we compromise; then everyone gets their second best choice and no one gets the best choice.

So if a decision is not going to affect or influence you, do you need to have "your say"?

There's a further trap on the eating out front. I really fancy a pizza but you don't want me to consume too much gluten; I'm leaving you space to allow me to "do" Italian and get my wheat fix. Perhaps I should just ask permission?

D

Decompression

We all get this feeling from time to time, the need to have our own space after spending a lot of time with a lot of people, or to just sit quietly with a glass or wine and relax after a hard day's work. We might sit with a book and try and unwind and take our minds off the events of a busy day. We NT's are good at this and have many tactics that we don't even realise we are utilising. A hot bath, a chat with our best friend, a moan to Mum on the phone. All help us to unwind and eventually help us get a good night's sleep.

This does not come naturally to our Aspies. The tension of the day builds up to such a point where if they don't relieve it they may well have a meltdown. As adults this comes out in different ways. When the children were little I would tell them that dad was feeling grumpy (so that they knew to leave well alone).

An Aspie child, after a very long, mentally exhausting day at school, will often take out their bad mood on their parent who comes to pick them up. There is still a major difficulty in diagnosing young children with Asperger Syndrome as, when teachers are asked about their pupils (especially girls), they generally say there is "no problem at all" and can't understand what the parent is implying about their child.

To your Aspie there is always a refuge, a safe place where they can be themselves. Their parent, their home, their bedroom, a man-cave - where they can go in and shut the door and not have to work hard at being someone they are not. This takes such effort; it is hard to control your emotions when you no longer have to. To avoid a back lash from your Aspie partner, it is best to let them decompress in their own time and space.

I will let David elaborate more on decompression. He is very good at it.

The Husband Says:

Every Aspie should have a way to decompress. But you have to find what works best for you. For me, the following:

- *In the car on the way home from work. Music very loud.*

- *Having a routine when I come into the house - shoes on the rack, keys in the drawer, phone on charge, check the e-mails. Check the post for bad news in brown envelopes.*

- *The lowest dregs of American serial drama - as box set binges. Probably with a law and order twist (more movie physics to roll your eyes at).*

- *Unloading about how bad my day has been.*

Defence Mode

This is put into action when your AS partner feels misunderstood or their actions criticised. He will often feel criticised even when you are just generally chatting to him and get quite defensive. His natural paranoia starts to come out and he may even lie in order to make himself look and feel better.

Delayed Effect

NT This is when you have been in conversation with your husband about something. You may have had a great idea and talked to him about it. He will listen if you are lucky but often he cannot cope with new ideas. It is best to leave him to think about this as it often means a change.

After a certain amount of time, often a couple of days, he will come back to you with the idea and agree with you. The bizarre thing about this is that suddenly it has become his idea and he is now in control of it. Let me tell you from experience, it really isn't worth arguing about who came up with the idea in the first place. If he is in agreement with you, just roll with it.

Delegation

Delegation is the fair sharing out of work to the people who are best suited to it, in order to relieve yourself of an overwhelming burden.

People with Asperger's have a great eye for detail and can often see what needs to be done. They also like to perfect any job they start. Unfortunately, due to their lack of theory of mind, they do not trust anyone else to carry out the tasks that need doing.

This leads to them making themselves unpopular at work and at home, as people don't feel appreciated.

For instance, If I talk to David about something that needs doing, he immediately thinks that I want him to do it. He believes that I am giving him instructions. That is not necessarily so. I believe that asking someone to do something usually begins with the words, 'Please can you do me a favour?' or 'Can you have a look at this for me?' Instead, he gets cross just because I mention that the grass looks like it needs to be cut or the hedge has grown over night. These are just normal forms of conversation that he doesn't allow me to have.

D

He immediately sees it as having a burden put upon him. Now actually, if I had kept a diary of who cuts the grass and drawn up a graph from the results it would look like this.

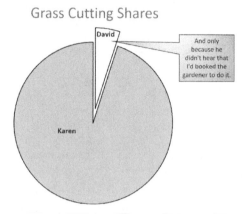

Grass Cutting Shares

Also I am the one that rings the gardener to come and cut the hedge a few times a year. We have attempted to do it ourselves and it took several days and many trips to the tip and it looked terrible afterwards. We had butchered it.

Bizarrely, he rarely asks me to do anything. I'm not sure why.

One of the worst problems with David's inability to delegate is that he ends up taking too much work and responsibility on to his own shoulders. It means he works far harder than anyone else, when he doesn't have to.

After a while, people just take him for granted.

His level of dedication to his work affects the time he has to spend with his family. For example, our daughter asked if he could spend some time helping her with her maths homework. He was very grumpy with her in reply and told her he was far too busy. What he should have done is made work aware that he has a family life that needs attention on the weekends.

Solution

It is hard to find a solution to this one as I am not privy to David's work environment. I only get his perspective and, though I suspect his idea of work and his colleague's expectations are warped, I do not know without interviewing and undermining him in doing so.

The Husband Says:

Delegation should be really easy. It is in business, because there are rules and it can be systematised.

AS The key is in "letting go" of the task. I'm often worried that the task will come back uncompleted or not completed to my standards, so a winning strategy here is to spend time defining what a successful outcome looks like and passing that along with the delegation. As a result, in business, I'm known not only as someone who can make progress in a complicated mesh of requirements, but also as a "finisher" - my tasks stay done and don't pop up again for re-work.

Let's look at the idea that I have mind blindness (the Theory of Mind explanation for some of my behaviours). Whilst I might have poor empathy for the person to whom I've delegated, I will be able to see the tangible deliveries at the end of the delegated activity. So it looks like I'm not very good at continuing to support a delegated activity from the side-lines. This is true. I tend to want to lead by example rather than micro-manage and coach through a delegated task. Bizarrely, in business, my mind blindness might make my few delegations **more** successful rather than less. As long as there is good feed-back at the end.

I work a lot in the public sector where authorities must be respected. Authorities are delegated down the organisational hierarchy. Delegation of activity is thus really simple - if you have the necessary authority, I can delegate the activity to you if I choose to do so.

I spend a lot of time with my clients drawing management organograms and RACI charts to show how delegation works. A RACI chart shows who is **R**esponsible, **A**ccountable, **C**onsulted and **I**nformed.

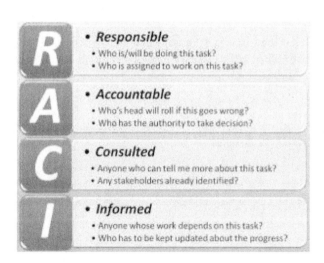

- **R**
  - **Responsible**
    - Who is/will be doing this task?
    - Who is assigned to work on this task?
- **A**
  - **Accountable**
    - Who's head will roll if this goes wrong?
    - Who has the authority to take decision?
- **C**
  - **Consulted**
    - Anyone who can tell me more about this task?
    - Any stakeholders already identified?
- **I**
  - **Informed**
    - Anyone whose work depends on this task?
    - Who has to be kept updated about the progress?

But are any of these things helpful in "real life"?

D

Denial

When life gets too much, the AS husband can completely switch off. He can cope with many a crisis at work because he is doing something he is good at. He can cope with friend's crises because he is not so emotionally involved. He cannot cope with his own and your crises. This is too much to handle.

When my mother died of secondary cancer my father was in such denial, despite calling me to tell me to drive over, and there being two Macmillan nurses caring for my mother, he did not let himself acknowledge the seriousness of the situation. In the last hour of her life he went shopping. Their last conversation was him telling her he was going out. He came back about ten minutes before she died whilst I was holding her hand. When I had arrived at the house, I had not realised myself the seriousness of the situation until I saw the nurses and the state my mother was in. It slowly dawned on me that this was it.

When I knew she was going I persuaded my father to hold her hand. He didn't know why. It wasn't until she took her last rattily breaths that he realised what was happening.

How could this highly intelligent man who had been with her throughout her cancer diagnosis and treatment not realise his wife was literally at death's door? I think, at least partly, my mother had sheltered him from it. Indeed she had sheltered us all. Yet, even when she had said to him that morning to 'Tell the kids I love them', he had told her not to be so silly. He could not face up to the truth of losing the woman he had loved for 40 years. It's very much going back to that childhood behaviour of if you can't see it or hear it then it's not there.

There are other less "terminal" occasions that happen in a family's life where the husband is needed for emotional and physical support. Some women are lucky that their AS men can step up to the plate

The Husband Says:

I'm not sure what you describe is truly denial. Denial would be a deep seated belief that what is happening should not be happening therefore it is not happening at all. The description above is of "giving up", avoidance, or taken to extreme abdication of responsibility.

Us Aspies can hold strong beliefs that we have done enough, or can't do anything else that will improve the situation. We don't do social filling very well (just look at our conversations - factual; no filler). In the absence of something constructive to do, here we will go off and do something else - or tear off the coping mask and snooze to recharge batteries. This is not what you expect - you want social gestures; that's the social norms.

*If my thinking is anything to go by, Aspies deal with grief very badly, so full blown avoidance kicks in. I'm very uncomfortable at funerals and around death. I don't **want** empathy with*

the situation (for obvious reasons), so it is hard to fake the socially acceptable responses that you NTs expect in such events.

The Wife Replies

I feel it is somewhat ironic that my husband is in denial about denial.

Depression

For the Woman

I know I have never been clinically depressed, but a few years ago life got to the stage when I started to wonder if I was. I spoke to my doctor at some length. Possibly he expected me to ask him for anti-depressants but I did not. He did offer me counselling as I explained the pressure I was under in all areas of my life. I felt I wasn't coping very well. I am lucky that I was able to climb out of the mental hole that I was in. Much of what affected me was circumstantial and I felt very alone and tired. I know now this is different from clinical depression.

However, there are many cases of women with ASD men who suffer desperately from depression. They have no support from their partner and have to rely on themselves or medication to get by. These women will be hard to diagnose with depression because one of the signs of depression is often that the depressed person is very good at covering up how they feel and presents a brave and happy face to the world.

For the Man

It is fairly common for those with ASD to be diagnosed with depression. This is because at times they can have very negative thoughts and if things get particularly bad and they feel they cannot cope or explain to anyone else how they feel, they can feel suicidal. Not all diagnoses of depression are correct for people with ASD and it is suspected many of them are medicated when it is unnecessary. Depression is a co-morbidity of ASD not a trait.

If you suspect you or your partner are depressed it is worth seeing your doctor but it may also be worth seeing a counsellor first before you decide to take any medication.

The Husband Says:

I don't think I'm clinically depressed. Depression has so many comorbidities with Asperger's, especially in the area of cognitive distortions that it would be easy to believe that I am.

How can this be? Perhaps the psychologist's theories are not yet sophisticated enough to deal with even your garden variety Aspie.

D

I've just spent a few minutes doing a very silly thing - looking to the Internet for opinion rather than to my direct experiences. The Internet seems to fall into three camps:

The medical profession; seeing comorbidities of Asperger's as symptoms of depression. It walks like a duck, it quacks like a duck, it must be a duck. All people with Asperger's are depressed.

The "advice sector"; These neurotypicals don't live with Asperger's so they can't tell the difference between symptoms of Asperger's (with which us Aspies just have to get on and try to cope) and the clinical depression they have seen in others or may have experienced themselves.

The blogs of Aspies. I think the truth may be found here. We know we might be more susceptible to the symptoms of depression but we believe that our symptoms are the outcome of the tiredness from prolonged anxiety. This tiredness IS NOT DEPRESSION.

Diagnosis

Is it Necessary?

Just the light bulb moment I had when reading about Asperger's, the dawning realisation why my marriage was in trouble, that there was a reason for it was enough to keep me going.

I was reading Tony Attwood's "Complete Guide to Asperger Syndrome" back in 2009 and came across his chapter on relationships. You could have inserted the names Karen and David instead of the characters mentioned. It described our courtship and subsequent marriage exactly. I cried - and I never cry.

I'm not sure if I was crying with relief, or joy or sadness. Possibly, all three.

Is it necessary to have an official diagnosis? I would say it depends on the man. If you are absolutely convinced he has AS but he is in complete denial about it, then perhaps the only way solve the argument is to see an expert.

For our part, David is still not officially diagnosed. He is blatantly Aspie and he himself is now happy to admit it. Both our children are now diagnosed and they definitely have more of their father's traits than my own.

How to Broach the Subject

The next step was to convince David of his condition. I had learned by then after twelve years of marriage not to just jump in with both feet and announce he had a disability or condition. I talked mostly about Morgan, about how AS was considered hereditary and when he showed interest I would gently suggest there may be similarities between his son and his own childhood.

NT

Basically, he had to come around to the idea of his diagnosis by himself. He would resist terribly if I just told him what I thought. He would believe that I was accusing him of something terrible rather than finding a solution to our marriage crisis (and it was in crisis).

Getting a Diagnosis

In the UK you can approach your GP and ask for a referral. It is a postcode lottery and some people do not get funding for this. Before you go to your GP be aware that most GP's are not trained in autism, let alone Asperger Syndrome. Our GP had to go and look it up.

NT

Do your homework. Take a clear, typed list of symptoms and reason. Stand your ground.

Alternatively, there are private practices around the country where you can get a diagnosis. Be aware though, once you have a diagnosis there is no magic wand to help cure your husband's difference. The adult diagnostic process is for clarification only. For funding and understanding is just not there.

The Husband Says:

Time for a bit of controversy.

Asperger's can be seen as a sign of weakness, failure or non-manliness. So many blatant Aspies are never going to acknowledge the condition or seek diagnosis and will just bumble along, sort of coping. This might work outside of a relationship, but inside a relationship will stress it, often to breaking point.

Knowing and believing that I'm an Aspie and that the unfolding story is not all bad, means that Karen can make suggestions for improvement in our married relationship and my wider social relationships, and I can hang them on the scaffold that I know and acknowledge that I'm an Aspie. There is a reason for my behaviour and there is a way to measure our relationship improvements. None of that is really possible without the label acknowledging the condition.

It doesn't have to be worn as a badge for all to see. But the format of this book wouldn't work if I didn't "come out" as Karen's husband.

Diagnostic Gap

Though the idea of autism has been around since the early 1940's, it has been a very hidden and secret condition until recently. Many people had hardly heard the term until Dustin Hoffman and Tom Cruise starred in Rain Man back in 1988.

D

I myself had only heard the term Asperger's mentioned once before and in a very negative context. Many professionals in psychology also knew very little about this condition.

There will have been many children at school who were having problems and referred to the educational psychologist. One of these was my husband. They seemed to recognise that David was different from most of his peers but they did not have the diagnostic tools or terminology for his behaviour. Or at least they thought they didn't. Autism was considered to be so rare that many professionals would not see it in their working lives. Though David did have difficulties at school such as making friends and talking in a monotonous tone, he did not present any obvious learning difficulties. In fact he presented more as a child genius. It was felt he was not being stretched enough at the school he attended in Gateshead and it was suggested he get a scholarship to Kings in Tynemouth where he could fulfil his potential. David decided he did not want to go. Comparing our son at the same age I can see why he didn't go. It would have seemed a very long way to go and entering an unknown environment would not have seemed worth the benefits to him. Better the devil you know.

So David, assessed at 11 as being different and gifted was left to cope in a rough inner city school. No one recognised he was on the autistic spectrum. It wasn't until 30 years later that I realised what the cause of his problems were. He had fallen in the diagnostic gap. I do wonder whether we would have had less problems if his AS had been recognised earlier and he could have understood himself and explained it to me. Perhaps we wouldn't have had those years of utter despair and sought help sooner. I have hope that our son will cope better with future relationships because of this knowledge.

Diesel Jenga

The Husband Says:

"Diesel Jenga®" marks the border-line between laziness and avoidance. It is a game that NTs and Aspies can play.

It is the game caused by the laziness of having to go to the garage in a semi-rural area and fill up the car with Diesel. Laziness leads to the car sitting on the drive with only just enough fuel to get to the nearest garage (if it is open), rather than making a special trip or adding time to another task to leave the car with a useful amount of fuel in it. Diesel Jenga gets to be more fun when you have two cars. I know that Karen has Jenga'd me on the Audi if she takes the Toyota on an errand.

There is a related game: Dustbin Jenga. You can easily guess the rules.

AS

I don't suggest you play either game competitively.

DIESEL-JENGA: HOW LOW CAN YOU GO?	A WINNING MOVE IN KITCHEN-BIN JENGA:

 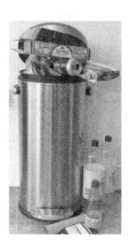

The Wife Says:

Here is a fine example of over thinking. I do not view life as a competition but to be lived as fairly as possible. When I take the smaller car it is to put less miles on the gas guzzler or because I am going somewhere where parking is tight.

It's probably best to find a way to take turns in emptying bins, cleaning toilets and filling the car with fuel.

AS

Don't expect any praise for doing a chore shared by the whole family.

NT

Whilst you shouldn't need to give your Aspie praise for carrying out household chores, a bit of recognition that they have been done might not go amiss.

Directional Anger

When your Aspie partner get frustrated and cross, he finds it very hard to control his emotions and, in fact, gets overwhelmed by the tsunami of feelings that he can't control and doesn't really understand. Some people on the spectrum will shut down

D

at this point, going inward until they can sort their thoughts and feelings. Others will feel a burst of anger and will become verbally aggressive towards whoever is in their way.

This anger is fed by their low self-esteem and their need to be right. They are cross with themselves.

Yet, your AS partner does not have the capacity to process the way his body is reacting quickly enough. The overwhelming feeling makes him verbally (and occasionally physically) lash out to others in his way, regardless of whether they deserved it or not.

The strength of their reaction and how they cope with problems depends very much on their current state of wellbeing. If they are calm, relaxed and happy, they are less likely to over-react. If they are already under a certain amount of stress, it is very likely that their anger will not be contained.

NT In situations like this you yourself must not overreact as you will only escalate the situation. Try to stay calm and if possible walk away to let him sort out his feelings by himself.

Our own breakthrough in this area has been David using a tablet form of serotonin in ever increasing doses. His level of happiness is generally higher and his base line of stress is naturally lower while he continues to take this natural remedy.

I have noticed that he may still get angry or frustrated about annoying things, but he does it less. More importantly, and this I am thrilled with, the direction of his anger has been at the offending inanimate object (that is providing the frustration) and not at me just because I happen to be in the same room. This reduces the tension between us considerably and he is starting to be more like the young man I used to know.

Disease or Difference?

I sometimes come across articles which describe Autism or Asperger's syndrome as a disease. This is not a disease. It does not kill you or make you ill. It is a difference in the way the brain is wired.

The Husband Says:

It is a condition, a state of being, a disorder. There is no cure (as for an illness), only coping. There's nothing clinically wrong with me, I'm just different.

Dispelling the Myths

Autism Spectrum Disorder by its very name is complex by nature. There are many assumptions and misunderstandings connected to it. I intend to analyse and dispel some of the most common myths related to autism:

Eye Contact

Not everyone with an ASD has a problem with eye contact. Some are generally more comfortable than others or are very good at pretending they are making eye contact by looking at someone's eyebrows. It also depends how comfortable they are in your presence. Often with family members, and particularly with AS rather than classic autism there is never any problem with eye contact, except when caught out in a lie. Another misconception around eye contact is that the person with ASD is not listening. In actual fact, they find it much easier to listen to you when they are not forcing themselves to make eye contact and they can concentrate on one sense at a time. Never force anyone with an ASD to look at you.

Lifelong Condition

Autism does not stop when the autistic child reaches eighteen.

Finding a Cure

Autism Spectrum Disorders are neither a disease or needs "curing". Contrary to popular belief, most people on the autism spectrum do not want to be cured. They would much prefer the population to have a good level of awareness and understanding of the condition.

Lying

Again, contrary to popular belief, people on the spectrum are capable of lying.

The Husband Says:

With regard to eye-contact: just over the left or right shoulder of the person I'm avoiding staring at does the job.

On that point of Lying; if Aspie politicians couldn't lie, how could they cope?

Divorce

Many NT marriages have trials and tribulations which are eventually resolved by communication between the partners, including communicating that the relationship should end. In Britain, Relate offers a service to counsel couples in this way if they cannot mediate and resolve for themselves and they can continue to counsel the partners during any decision to divorce. Presumably, NT couples in a troubled relationship either improve their ways of communication and begin to cope with their situation, or they decide to divorce.

During my time at university I would often come across research papers citing statistics about the divorce rates of parents of disabled or autistic children.

I believe many couples will have gone to Relate counselling but not reached a satisfactory conclusion because they did not know that one of them was on the autistic spectrum. Though there is Relate counselling offered for couples where one of them is on the autistic spectrum, this is little known and of limited availability and location. Most counsellors are not aware of the effects of autism on a marriage and are unlikely to be able to formally diagnose or recognise the condition as a prelude to support counselling and therapy. Also, even if they did recognise the diagnostic symptoms of an ASD, is it not their moral place to tell the couple or the husband. Thirdly, unless a therapist was expert in both relationship counselling and on the diagnosis and support of those on the autistic spectrum, it would be unwise to try to render marriage guidance in those circumstances.

One of the main problems affecting AS/NT couples is ignorance. They may know little about autism and in all likelihood, not suspect that this could be at the root of their marital disharmony. I have seen and heard testimony time and time again online or in support groups and it happened in my own case, that I did not suspect my husband had AS until my son's educational psychologist suggested he was on the spectrum.

On forums for parents with autistic children, I frequently see complaints that these Mum's feel like single parents or that they are, in fact, divorced. They blame it on the stress of having an autistic child. However, there are many successful marriages that survive having a severely disabled child. High stress circumstances can often bring the couple closer together, albeit the relationship may work better after some counselling. I have felt that the elephant in the room is often that one of the parents (and statistically it is most likely the father) is also on the spectrum and therefore cannot cope. The wife cannot cope with both his moods and their child's behaviour and may often feel it would be easier to move out or let the husband go.

Divorce may seem simpler and easier in the long run, but David and I have proved that a turbulent marriage can be salvaged with enlightenment and understanding.

The Husband Says:

Karen and I are of one voice on this subject. Don't give up unless the situation is truly, demonstrably hopeless.

Does He Love You?

Well my husband would probably be quite flippant and say, "Well I'm here aren't I?" That to him is a declaration of his undying love. To most NT women, not so much.

It isn't that we want to be told every moment, but we do need to be told more than once. We are aware that love can be tidal, it comes and goes. We need the reassurance that it is still there.

For the Aspie man though I'm not sure love is tidal. He made his decision about you, probably moments after he met you. He knew you were "the one" and he has never changed his mind. That is love. (For those under 40 I would say it is very much like the concept of "Imprinting" in the film Twilight.)

On the other hand, I do believe he needs me to reassure him, every now and then, that I still love him. So he has (and admits that he has) complete double standards in this area.

NT How does He Show it?

By physically showing he loves you in his mind means doing things for you. He won't do tasks for people he doesn't like.

It doesn't necessarily come naturally to want to hug someone. Being touched is a very contentious area.

So lying in bed this morning I gauged his mood which was pensive but good. I asked him how often he needed to be told that I loved him. He considered this and said about as much as I tell him now was about right. This is probably nearly every day unless he is really pissing me off! I then asked him whether he was happy with the amount of times he told me that he loved me. He thought it was fair that he hardly ever said it as basically it was obvious wasn't it? He wants to be able to show me he loves me. Though he then asked me what he should do to show me. So, verdict: I should tell him as often as possible that I love him but he doesn't have to tell me because apparently it's obvious.

The Husband Says:

My conclusion from this is:

AS *You should probably tell your partner you love her more often than you do currently. It seems unlikely that they will complain you are doing this too much if you are sincere.*

D

Don't take it Personally

NT It won't be hard for you to imagine this scenario: You are in the middle of cooking dinner and supervising the kids when the doorbell rings. Your husband is sitting at the computer in the other room. He doesn't get up to answer the doorbell so you raise your voice over the noise in the kitchen to ask him to answer the door. He completely overreacts and roars with rage as he has to leave what he is reading on the screen to go and interact socially with an unknown person. His body language says it all, "This is your fault".

I always advocate not interrupting your partner but life just isn't like that, especially with a young family to deal with.

He will have been prioritising his 'me time' and expecting you to carry on with what he probably perceives as your job: cooking, looking after the children and dealing with communications. He doesn't consider any of those responsibilities to be his and resents being interrupted to do something as tedious as speak to an unsolicited visitor. He hates being interrupted so he demonstrates his frustration verbally - and you are the main person in his life and in his path. It is unlikely he will take his frustration out on the innocent person at the door.

What seems like the slightest interruption or irritation to a NT seems enormous to an Aspie, especially if they are tired and trying to relax. Or worse, if you have interrupted their train of thought. They have great difficulty switching tasks.

This may well depend on your personality and how resilient you are, but try not to take it personally. Remind yourself he doesn't mean it and he would miss you if you weren't there. It does get a little easier with time.

Double Standards

This is something I hear a lot from wives of men with Asperger's Syndrome. Even something as simple as telling a child off for leaving a door open and then walking through it and leaving it open himself. I believe this is a combination of their Theory of Mind deficiency and also lack of self-awareness. The moment they walk out of the room the people within it cease to exist so he is not going to consider whether he is making them cold or not.

Indeed, David does this all the time. He will go into the garden on a cold winter's day and leave the back door wide open letting all the heat out and freezing everyone else. If however, I go outside and do the same thing (possibly because I am invoking my own form of petty, silent revenge) he well protest.

Or, for example, when the children were small (and long before we were aware of autism) we regularly watched TV programmes about improving child behaviour. We would sit there quite smugly in the knowledge that our children were not like that. However, David was most critical of other parents and vocal about it despite having never been involved in the raising of our own children! I used to sit there seething that he was staking claim to all of my hard work. I should console myself that, in some ways, he had a right to be smug as he had laid the way in choosing the right woman to control his children.

Doxophobia

Doxophobia is a fear of being praised or a doxophobic may be someone who is fearful of expressing their own opinion.

David is not one of these! He operates at the extreme craving end of the acknowledgement spectrum and can't get enough praise.

At the other extreme, doxophobia is a fairly common occurrence in our Aspies who either do not like or cannot cope with praise.

Some are simply not interested and others get overwhelmed by the emotions it evokes in them.

Our AS son is very doxophobic, to the point he'd rather be mediocre at something to avoid praise. When he was at Middle School he did very well in a design and technology project but, when he found out there would be a prize-giving ceremony in front of the whole school, he got very anxious and didn't want to win. As it was he got third place and a special commendation but did not have to go on stage to get his prize, so he was happy with the eventual result.

The Husband Says:

I'm not sure that the lines are so clear. I enjoy sincere praise. I can see through someone who is giving pseudo-praise in an effort to manoeuvre me into some unpleasant situation.

Driving

Why does their personality change when they get in a car?

It is like wearing a mask. They can put on a facade and be whoever they want to be, depending on their style of driving and what car they are driving.

D

The Husband Says:

When driving a car my personal space has to expand. It has to be at least as big as the car is (otherwise an invasion of my personal space would also be a collision). It extends at least as wide as from the kerb to the white line. It extends as far in front as I need for stopping distance. It extends as far behind as the distance I think the car behind needs as stopping distance.

Invading my car-space has the same effect on me as invading my personal space. I want to push out my elbows and regain that buffer zone. Too little space makes me anxious.

Cars are status symbols. They are the second most expensive thing you possess behind your home. A car needs to be a projection of the personality that an Aspie wants to be or aspires to be. If Aspie car owners had no aspiration, we would drive grey Ford Focus cars to be as near to the average as we could find. Perhaps a car is the one area where we project an image.

The choice of car is very difficult since as I have said above it needs to project an image. Choices can go one of two ways: either a very bland looking exterior hiding a fun to drive car or an obvious status symbol car that tries on behalf of its owner to send a signal on class-hierarchy and social ambition.

DSM-V and the Disappearance of Asperger Syndrome

Asperger's Syndrome does not exist anymore in the American Psychiatric Association (APA) Fifth Edition of the Diagnostic and Statistical Manual of Mental Disorders (DSM-5) used by American health professionals. Asperger's has been reclassified into 'autism spectrum disorders' so that all people are just part of a very wide spectrum. You cannot just dismiss a large percentage of the population.

Interestingly the British College of Psychiatrists haven't yet followed the APA, so here in Britain AS is still real and separate from autism. Personally (as an academic writing on AS for an MA degree thesis, and with a partner and other family members on the spectrum) I feel the re-labelling will have severe, negative consequences. To label someone as Autistic, without explaining the sliding scale of the spectrum will lead to too many people not recognising it, and therefore not getting whatever support/help/ encouragement they are entitled to. Not only that, but how many people will disclose it on job applications, medical forms etcetera? The risk being that they are making themselves vulnerable to others automatically assuming that the label "autistic" means they are on the highest end of the spectrum, with Low functioning autism?

There is currently research taking place that demonstrates that those who are Autistic, and those who are Aspergic have completely different neurologies, and just share some characteristics. Thus, this re-labelling of Asperger's as Autistic is the same as being told that Sleep Apnoea and ME are the same due to sharing characteristics.

The Husband Says:

I'm with Karen on this one.

I quite often like to point out that the underlying conditions giving rise to these bundles of symptoms are all different. It is convenient for simple studies and diagnoses to acknowledge that the spectra for Asperger's, autism, ADHD and the like all seem to point in roughly the same sort of direction. Everyone is Aspie to some degree; everyone is autistic to some degree; everyone has weight or height to some degree. It is your personal position on each and every one of these spectra taken together that defines the condition in which you are found, and the dominant or more unusual positions tend to be used as a single label to describe what you are and who you are.

Comorbidities are by definition not diagnostic of a state. Neither do they really help understand root cause. If we understood the root causes of Asperger's, autism, ADHD, OCD (and the rest of the alphabet soup) we could separate them by showing they had different root causes. For the time being we are stuck with this tangle.

Dyspraxia

Dyspraxia is a form of developmental coordination disorder (DCD) affecting fine and/or gross motor coordination in children and adults. It may also affect speech. DCD is a lifelong condition and is distinct from other motor disorders such as cerebral palsy and stroke - being of unknown cause - and occurs across the range of intellectual abilities. Like Asperger's and autism, individuals may vary in how their difficulties present: these may change over time depending on environmental demands and life experiences.

Dyspraxia also refers to those people who have additional problems planning, organising and carrying out movements in the right order in everyday situations. Dyspraxia can also affect articulation and speech, perception and thought.

Dyspraxia, Asperger's, autism etcetera all share a group of common symptoms - comorbidities.

Clumsiness as compared to Dyspraxia is more likely to come about through an obvious organic causal mechanism such as a faulty limbic (balance) system, or being over-weight or having restricted joint movements.

D

E

✧   Eating Out

✧   Echolalia

✧   Effort

✧   Egocentricity

✧   Emotion

✧   Emotional Sponge

✧   Empathy

✧   Expert

✧   Environment

✧   Epidemic

✧   Executive Function

✧   Exercise

✧   Exhaustion

✧   Expectations

✧   Expectation Violation

✧   Eye Contact

E

Eating Out

Once you have made the decision to eat out and you make your way to the favoured restaurant, there are plenty more obstacles to consider before you can have an enjoyable meal:

The Staff

David is quite happy to chat to members of staff and is always very forgiving of genuine mistakes on their part, especially if they are new and nervous students. He does however take great exception to rude servers who do not have the time for him. He will not return to a restaurant where he has received bad service. He does not like to be asked how his meal is, especially when he has a mouthful of food. I have often thought about handing out a leaflet to the staff upon entering a restaurant asking them politely to back off.

The Seating

He does not like being squashed in a corner or put on a communal table. I know immediately that he will not enjoy his meal and will not talk to me. In this case we might as well leave, but he will refuse to unless the service is so bad we haven't even been offered a drink after ten minutes. It is always worth ringing ahead and asking for a particular table if you are familiar with the restaurant.

The Menu

This is often a tricky area. I think David likes to decide in advance what he is having and will often look up the online menu. This has both advantages and disadvantages as he knows what to expect and it takes away uncertainty but if the restaurant cannot provide the meal he can get upset or at least a bit disgruntled (expectation violation). Worse, if he doesn't tell me what he is having and then I tell him my meal decision and it clashes with his, he refuses to eat the same meal as me and he refuse to let me choose another meal to let him have his preferred choice. I cannot help but have the same discussion with him every time, telling him I do not mind changing as often I was torn between two delicious menu options.

NT I have occasionally persuaded him that it is a help to me if he takes my first option leaving me able to choose the other option I was considering, but this is only a recent advancement.

Timing

If the staff do not ask us for our order within a certain space of time he is offended and likes to leave. This is extremely rude and extremely un-British and makes me very uncomfortable. I would rather sit and wait longer in a busy restaurant where I

E

have a seat than wander the streets hungry, looking for somewhere else. Usually by this time however, he is so hungry he can't think straight and would rather just go home.

Volume

We much prefer restaurants where the music is just a background noise and does not impinge on conversation, however, in family restaurants the music tends to be much louder to drown out the cries of children. David does not enjoy these restaurants as they attack all his senses at once.

Conversation

I much prefer to go to a restaurant when we have a big issue to discuss as it means we actually have a topic of conversation. David does not do chit-chat and does not seem to understand that I feel uncomfortable sitting in public in complete silence. I have learned to steer away from sensitive topics as the stress of eating out and then the additional stress of difficult topics has meant he has not been able to cope and walked out on me. Not a good situation to be in I can tell you. He also does not keep his feelings to himself and will not keep the volume down when other people are obviously listening. Again, I am typically British and do not like to air our laundry in public. It is much easier when we have the kids with us as I can easily get them on to a safe topic. We had a lovely time on my last birthday when we spent about an hour and a half discussing favourite films and we ended up going home and watching one with the kids. It was a rare, very successful evening. Sometimes I take a pack of playing cards in my handbag or even a pack of conversation starters. Safe ground when it is just David and myself is asking him about work. He always has something to say and even if the topic is a little dry he is always enthusiastic and can tell some really fascinating anecdotes at times.

This kind of behaviour detracts very much from what should be an enjoyable meal out.

The Husband Says:

By now you will have probably read enough of this guide to have been able to predict all of my behaviours above. Now you can test yourself:

- **Asking if the food was OK when my mouth is full** - *I'm sure this is part of waiter training school; that way the 'punter' can't respond that there is anything wrong with the food without breaking a social norm that you don't spit your food out and you don't talk with your mouth full.*

- *Good service deserves a good tip regardless of where you are in the world.*

- *Certain forms of communication would work better with flags on display.*

- **Dyspraxia is no fun in a restaurant** - *I already expect to have dinner*

down my shirt; pack me into a tiny corner and expect to have the whole contents of the table on the floor by the end of the meal

- **Testing The Whole Menu** - *I was brought up that going out for dinner was a very special (perhaps annual) treat. Therefore, the whole experience was pretty novel. Between all the family diners we attempted to test all of the meals by not duplicating what anyone else is having.*

- **Menu choices in company** - *If I think I will not be paying, I won't choose the most expensive item in any category. I'll also avoid the "special offers" because that is being an overt skinflint. I want to demonstrate I have my own personality, so I will always try to avoid duplicating someone else's choices. Welcome to "Aspie Menu Chess".*

- **Waiting for dinner** - *even with the advent of mobile phones, I dine out a lot on my own for work and waiting ages for dinner is really quite tedious. Waiters don't know what to do with a sleeping diner! So I carefully choose places that have swift and efficient service. There is no excuse for slow service other than "We didn't employ enough staff because we are skinflints". Do you want to dine there?*

- **Perfect "background music" volume** - *just enough to drown out other diner's conversation, but not so loud I can't hear **my** guest's conversation. Chain restaurants take note. Brewers Fayre · a duck trapped in an accordion is not "background music"; get it fixed!*

- **Background Music (part 2)** - *Liverpool, I'm looking at you. Restaurants don't need a DJ. Disk Jockey that is not dinner jacket.*

...annnd breathe! I'll put my soap-box away now.

Echolalia

What is it?

Echolalia is strictly a meaningless repetition of another person's spoken words. There are various levels of Echolalia and to some extent we all use it as a social tool.

We repeat back to the person we are talking to the words they have just said to us. It shows them that we are listening.

For those with autism or Asperger's Syndrome it is often a way of filling conversational gaps when they don't have the words or confidence to say something original.

E

Delayed Echolalia

This is part of the long term memory and echolalia can happen even years after the event. Most common might be TV adverts or song lyrics or amusing phrases.

An autistic person often has a very good memory and can repeat many facts and phrases verbatim with little effort. They can derive an immense amount of satisfaction and comfort from this.

The Husband Says:

There is a form of echolalia that is a dead give-away of the Aspie trying to hide in plain sight. With that Tourette's co-morbidity, an Aspie can accidentally find themselves repeating just a syllable of a phrase or a chord of music over and over again. That can be both embarrassing for the Aspie and annoying for the NT, especially if the repeated section is an "ear-worm" that gets inside your head.

I find certain phrases trip lightly off the tongue and in a variation of echolalia I will over-use them for weeks on end. Even inappropriately.

Effort

Unless it is an activity they are particularly keen on they will usually tackle it with the least amount of effort.

This will change if they are keen to please the person who has asked them to participate but otherwise there will be a severe lack of interest or even point blank refusal.

Motivation is very important to get someone with Asperger's to do something. When they are motivated they are often unstoppable.

The Husband Says:

Lots of Engineers are aspies. Engineers are some of the laziest people I know (and I know because I am one). Our role in life is to fulfil society's needs. Usually this involves achieving a goal in the most efficient way possible so as to work with limited resources like time. So time efficiency looks like laziness!

The interesting point here is that the effort goes in up-front - to find generalised solutions that can be repeated over and over again. Once we reach that delivery phase of repeating a minimal activity over and over again the effort looks small.

Don't underestimate, however, how Aspies like me can swap avoidance for reduction in effort. If we can get away with not doing "it" at all, that's got to be the lowest amount of work and the most efficient way of delivering it, right?

Aspie Hints & Tips

NT

To ensure an activity gets done, present it as an impossible challenge; your Aspie will usually rise to the challenge. But watch out that he doesn't go off at a tangent and embellish the solution.

Egocentricity

The word autism actually means 'self' so it should not come as any surprise that our men are egocentric or to put it bluntly, appear to be selfish.

On a bad day and without any understanding of his condition it certainly comes across like that.

Yet, also my husband is the most caring, generous and hard working person I know.

The short temper and selfishness tends to come out more when he is tired and under stress and to be honest we are all a bit like that aren't we?

Emotion

Aspie's are often accused of not having any emotion. My experience with David is that he has far too much emotion that he does not know how to control. He gets overwhelmed with it, be it happiness or sadness. Some men with Asperger's manage to come across as very cold people because they have learned to suppress their emotions as they cannot deal with them. They find it so hard to find the middle ground.

The wives of these men believe that they really do not have any feelings (to the extent of being psychopathic) but I believe that these men have been badly hurt and just find it difficult to relate to other people's high emotions. When an Aspie has worked hard to come across as socially and emotionally "normal" during his early relationship with a partner, it is all the more devastating to her once they have married and the AS husband stops trying.

Emotional Sponge

NT

What is an Emotional sponge?

E

As the NT wife, it is most likely that you are! Not only do you have to deal with all of your emotions alone, but you have to soak up and deal with your husband's emotions as he becomes overwhelmed and can't deal with them.

Like a sponge, you can quickly take on board emotions but it is much harder to dispel them. As your Asperger husband calms down and moves on to his next area of interest, you will notice that you are still reeling from the onslaught of his emotions.

How to get Wrung Out

NT

The best way is to leave the situation calmly and quietly and make sure you have in mind some techniques that you can use.

Suggested Techniques to Dehydrate your Emotional Sponge

1. Go for a fast walk or a run. The exercise will help you release those pent up emotions and tire you out.

2. Get in the car, drive somewhere quiet and scream as loud as you can at the top of your voice. Believe me, that is very satisfying. Beware speed limits.

3. If you can't escape the house because you have young children you cannot leave alone, try starting a diary or a blog. If you are a typist it can be therapeutic to release your angst into the keyboard. Don't worry about spelling mistakes, just type! (you can use spell checker later), or if you prefer something more tactile, use a pen and a notebook. A word of caution about writing things down on paper: you probably want to keep your emotions private and a notebook is easy for anyone to pick up and read, so find a safe place to hide it.

4. Ring a friend and bend her ear if she is sympathetic to your situation. If your friend does not know that your husband has AS, even though she may be sympathetic, she may not really understand your situation. You may end up feeling worse when you get off the phone. Hence, it is useful to confide in trustworthy and open-minded friends about what AS actually is and about being in an Asperger marriage. Then you can judge who "gets it".

5. Join an online forum for people with an Asperger Marriage and have a rant on there. You will get sympathy and understanding.

6. Join a singing group. Learning new music is therapeutic and takes you mind off your home situation for a while. Other hobbies and passions in life will help equally!

E

Empathy

This is often referred to by professionals as Theory of Mind.

This is when another person can relate to you and imagine themselves being in your situation. Those on the autism spectrum find if very hard to imagine what it is like to be anyone other than themselves. They cannot predict what other people will do.

My husband cannot naturally read my intentions. Therefore, he has to work hard to figure out what they are. He is quite often inaccurate. His inaccuracy derives from misunderstanding because he thinks I have intentions when I do not. This can cause stress not just for the AS person but also the NT.

The Husband Says:

Us Aspies are not completely devoid of empathy. It can kick in unexpectedly and the emotions can be quite severe.

Environment

NT It is worth thinking about your home environment and whether it is conducive to a calm atmosphere.

What stresses your husband out about the home? Are the neighbours too close or you have to share a drive? He may never have mentioned these things but they could be on his mind. Every time he gets out of the car in your busy street he may be wondering if he has upset a neighbour by parking where he does. It could be worth thinking about where you park your own car. If you are happy to leave your vehicle further down the street, in order to let him park nearer his own door, it might be worth doing.

Having his own space to retire to can be very important to him, such as a man cave. When you first met you both would have had quality time together but also quality time apart. Now you are living together and probably have children, the home environment may seem loud, cramped and overwhelming to your husband. It may be why he prefers to stay at work late. If he does come home, he will probably retreat to the quietest part of the house to try and have some time to gather his thoughts and prepare himself for the onslaught of family life - some decompression time. Is there a place where he can do this?

This may seem unfair to you if you have been stuck in the house all day with small, demanding children and you feel that you could also do with "some space", but

E

allowing him to recharge his batteries after a demanding day at work will work better for your whole family in the long run.

It is worth discussing or even drawing out with him a diagram of the house and where he feels most comfortable and uncomfortable. What he would like to improve or change? There may be nothing but he may appreciate being asked.

Epidemic

Is there an Autism Epidemic?

It is understandable that the general population believe that there is an epidemic in autism as, indeed, there has been a large increase in diagnoses over the last few years.

When Leo Kanner wrote about autism in the 1940's he was convinced it was a very rare condition and that most practitioners would not come across it in their work lifetime.

The National Autistic Society describes autism as "A lifelong developmental disability that affects how a person communicates with, and relates to, other people and the world around them".

The main reason for the increase in diagnosis is because there is now better awareness of autism and better diagnosis. People are starting to realise that Kanner's classic autism is still actually quite rare but that his parameters in which he judged whether someone was autistic or not were very narrow.

Because of this many people went through their young life without diagnosis even though parents and teachers realised that they were different from their peers. Better understanding from Lorna Wing and Judith Gould with the translation of Hans Asperger's original paper have changed this.

Children and adults who may well have been wrongly diagnosed with bi-polar or schizophrenia are now being correctly diagnosed with an autistic spectrum disorder. The levels of diagnoses in mental health in general have not increased but the type of diagnosis has changed with more understanding.

Wing and Gould set out for there to be a large increase in autism diagnoses. They succeeded and now statistics are showing that the number of diagnoses are levelling off and not rising.

E

Executive Function

Executive Function is an influential theory of autism that is particularly successful at explaining some of the everyday behaviours frequently seen in individuals with autism and which are not successfully tackled by the other theories. The major proponents of this explanation of autistic symptoms have been Ozonoff and Russell and their collaborators.

'Executive function' is traditionally used as an umbrella term for functions such as planning, working memory, impulse control, inhibition, and shifting set, as well as the initiation and monitoring of action. Historically these functions have been linked to frontal structures of the brain, and to the prefrontal cortex in particular, because people with damage in this brain area have difficulties with these executive functions.

The theory of executive dysfunction in autism makes an explicit link to frontal lobe failure. Executive dysfunction seems to underlie many of the key characteristics of autism, both in the social and non-social domains. The behaviour problems addressed by this theory are rigidity and perseveration, being explained by a poverty in the initiation of new non-routine actions and the tendency to be stuck in a given task set. At the

same time the ability to carry out routine actions can be excellent and is manifested in a strong liking for repetitive behaviour and sometimes elaborate rituals. Repetitive actions dominate in the daily life management of many people with autism. It is well known that they benefit from prompts and externally provided structures which initiate new behaviours to replace the repetitive ones.

An NT child is meant to be able to access this executive control ability by 'switching on' their frontal lobe by the age of eight years old. To have a deficit in this functioning means that those with AS lack organisational skills, strategising and spontaneity. NT's are able to respond to a changing situation whereas the AS individual, when solving a problem, has only a one track mind and cannot see through the noise to the solution, causing frustration. This is down to their neurology and not choice.

The Husband Says:

I don't seem to fit to this theory. Am I an outlier? Perhaps the level of impairment of frontal lobe connection and control is at the heart of the difference between low functioning autism and Asperger's?

Perhaps a better explanation might be a developmental delay to the development of advanced executive function? If the Baron-Cohen "extreme male brain" theory is as true as the executive function theory, then the two could work together if male brains tend to be wired to favour single-fixed tracking of task.

E

My personal theory, that would seem to amalgamate all of the work on executive function and central coherence is that mental processing of situation and required response requires engagement across the whole of the brain, marshalled by the frontal lobes. Different pieces of the puzzle arrive for processing at different times and assume different priorities as a result. My Aspie brain wiring is thus fully functional but a bit unusual, since all of the parts of the brain seem to deliver the right parts of the "answer" to my frontal lobes, but they are prioritised 'wrongly' as compared with the wiring and prioritisation demonstrated by NTs. I value single task completion over juggling multiple tasks. I prioritise logic of recalled prior experience likely to be repeated over predictive feeling or emotion of what might be going to happen.

Exercise

There are obvious benefits to exercise, be it gentle walking or high impact cardio vascular. As well as getting the heart pumping, your body gets fit and your mood level is raised. If you are outside you also get the benefit of interesting sights, sunshine and Vitamin D3. Serotonin levels are raised and generally one feels happier and healthier afterwards.

I doubt I would be as fit as I am if I didn't have a dog that insisted on being walked for at least an hour a day. Even if I am not in the mood or the weather is awful, we still have to go for that walk. As long as I wrap up warm I always feel better once I return home.

The Husband Says:

It's difficult for me to comment on exercise without being a bit hypocritical. I wonder how many of us Aspies have body image issues and certainly won't go to a gym or go outside to exercise because people might see us? It might not be a "body image" thing either. Perhaps the last thing we want to do after a hard day at work is to have to deal with a whole other set of social norms to do with dog walking, the public gym and so on.

Karen and I have invested in a decent treadmill and elliptical at home. Now both, as an NT and an Aspie, have to deal with the stops and starts of an exercise regime. It's very difficult to get into the habit of regular exercise and very easy to fall out of the habit. There's a whole chapter on when avoidance turns into laziness.

Exhaustion

For the wife it is often a feeling of emotional exhaustion as she has to keep the whole family on track while no one else is helping her deal with her own emotions.

E

The Husband Says:

Keeping up the act of obeying social norms can be exhausting for an Aspie. Some of the worst "flare-ups" in our relationship come from when I'm dog tired and, instead of thinking, I just Aspie-react to what I think Karen has said, rather than "reading" what an NT would make of what an NT has just said.

It's also easy to feel guilty about stopping because you are tired and exhausted, usually trying to avoid a claim of laziness. That's not a claim our NT partners make of us Aspies very often, but it's something we imagine them doing. We can be guilty of unnecessarily driving ourselves to exhaustion by being stubborn or trying to prove a point.

An exhausted Aspie will behave even worse than normal.

"Expectation Violation"

This is a phrase used regularly by my family when something goes wrong or something unexpected happens. For example, you walk into a room you are familiar with but someone has moved the furniture around. This is a shock to the Aspie system and does not compute for a moment. This is not what was expected and therefore it is a violation to the senses.

I ran out of bread this morning so I gave our son bacon wrapped in a pancake instead. The look on his face showed his expectation violation. He didn't eat it.

The Husband Says:

I love this little phrase. It neatly sums up how I will plan for something, but then a perfectly normal happenstance will occur, and my expectation (my plan) is violated. It has become a popular refrain in our household, to describe when any of us see in any of the Aspie's behaviour a puzzlement about the situation or even circumstances that are heading in that direction.

It works even for NTs! You expect salt and vinegar crisps in a blue packet and cheese and onion in green; you know, blue for the salt in the salt and vinegar and green for the onion in cheese and onion - what on earth are Walkers playing at swapping the two over - total expectation violation when you get the crisps home and find you have the wrong type. This is so much of an issue that Walkers have a FAQ on their website about it; they claim they never swapped!

So it's a great coping mechanism. I am disappointed because something hasn't worked out as planned and Karen cheerily says "Expectation-Violation!" It's just the right amount of levity to break the moment and raise a smile. We should get little flags printed that we can wave!

E

Expectations

This might be a hard chapter for you to read. In this help guide I can provide a lot of the answers and reasons why your chosen lifelong partner acts the way he does. What I cannot do is give you an immediate fix.

NT One of the main things you need to do as the NT partner is to understand things from his perspective and know that this process of learning, understanding and improving your relationship cannot be rushed.

You may start reading this guide with the hope that you can give him a few tips and all will be changed for the better. That is not so and never will be.

The change has to start with you. You have to look at your own behaviour first and see how it is affecting him. Once you start to see ways in which you can change your reactions to stressful situations and you can both see the difference then he is more likely to also want to learn and come on board. Not all men will admit to a problem however, but I hope that by reading my husband's side of the story they may begin to empathise and start to recognise the problems within your relationship and be inspired to implement suggestions.

By all means have hopes and expectations for we cannot live without them but make them realistic ones.

Expert

There are definite advantages to having a man with obsessions. Their hobby can be all consuming for them but it means that they aim to be the best they can be at that subject. He will be the 'go to' guy whenever you need help.

Thankfully David's obsessions are fairly useful ones (if you discount his love for terrible, addictive television). Ever since he was a little boy and his uncle Raymond came back from overseas with a digital calculator, David deprived his uncle of if as soon as he saw it and worked out how to do all the difficult calculations on it that his uncle had not fathomed. His obsession with it was so obvious that his uncle generously allowed him to keep it and bought himself another one. They were very expensive at the time.

So, there started David's love of electronics and anything computerised. He and his dad built his first computer, a Sinclair ZX-80 from a kit as they could not afford to buy one off the shelf. David went on to do an electrical engineering degree at Birmingham University. When I met him, his hobbies were programming and learning different programming languages - just for fun! This didn't seem so strange to me as I come from a family of computer programmers and mathematicians (that gene completely bypassed me by the way). David was the first person I met who had the internet.

Of course our household is full of tech and all our computers are networked to within an inch of their lives. Our kids have no idea how lucky they are having all this technology and someone who knows what to do with it - and be able to fix it straight away.

Recently, our son had a meltdown because his internet went down on his computer. Morgan is a serious gamer and every nanosecond online is important to him. He came to me in great distress that his connection had gone down. He had tried to fix it himself but had not managed to. I made a few suggestions and he did a few diagnostics but we ended up making it worse. In desperation I tried ringing his father who was at work. He rarely answers the phone when he is working with other people, so I was not expecting success. However, he had decided to leave after his meeting and was making his way home. I spoke to him on his hands free kit (another gadget that David insists on) and got him to speak to his son so he could diagnose how serious the problem was. Between the three of us we managed to fix the router problem before he got home and our teenager was happy again. It is good to have an IT expert close at hand.

Eye Contact

It is one of the questions that they ask when diagnosing children with an ASD. Our son when he was being diagnosed had zipped his hoody all the way up and sat slumped with his head down. Not much need to ask the question there you might think. Yet, actually, he doesn't really have a problem with eye contact. Just with other people and how he deals with them. If he likes them and is comfortable with them he makes very good eye contact. This is one of the reasons that Asperger's gets diagnosed so late in life as it doesn't really fit into the neat box of Autism.

Though Morgan had an easy diagnosis at the age of ten, I had to push for our daughter to be diagnosed. People are shocked when I tell them she has Asperger's. They can't understand it as she is so articulate. When during her first assessment with the Consultant I knew he had his doubts as she chatted away comfortably to him. I knew I would have to ask for a second opinion and speak to an expert on girls. Many people with ASD learn to mimic certain NT behaviour and looking at someone's eyebrows gives the same impression as looking at someone's eyes.

The Husband Says:

This is something that is so difficult to get right in the "act" of an Aspie pretending to be NT. The body language books tell you just how important eye contact is to appear sincere. But the timing:

- *One squiff-o-second of eye contact: not enough - the other person didn't*

E

subconsciously notice that you made eye contact, you could have been just scanning the room - your gaze didn't land for long enough

- Half a second of eye contact: feels like forever but possibly the right amount - watch carefully for some reaction... and ...

- One second plus: whoops, over-thought it, now I look like a stalker staring at my prey. They are staring back. Now what do I do?

As an NT, try consciously making eye contact, you will get uncomfortable trying to figure out "the rules" of what is normally second nature for you. For best results try it with a total stranger.

E

F

- ✧ Facial Expressions
- ✧ Facial Recognition
- ✧ Faking It
- ✧ Family and Friends
- ✧ Fear of Rejection
- ✧ Feelings
- ✧ Feeling Overwhelmed
- ✧ Fiction
- ✧ Fidelity
- ✧ Fight or flight
- ✧ Finding Things
- ✧ Fixations
- ✧ Fixer Upper
- ✧ Flapping
- ✧ Forewarned is Fore armed
- ✧ Forgiveness
- ✧ Friends
- ✧ Further Reading

F

Facial Expressions

At times, it is handy that he does not recognise my facial expressions. There has been a few occasions when he has surprised or shocked me or he has asked me a direct question and for one reason or another I have not wanted to tell him the truth. Any NT person would see that I have been caught out and wonder what was going on, but he has not. It might be something as simple as when I have been silently blubbing at something traumatic on the TV and I haven't wanted him to know. Another time I had had such a dreadful day and didn't know how to tell him so when he asked me directly how my day had been, despite the fact I knew my face was an open book, when I dismissively said "Oh fine," he was satisfied.

The Husband Says:

This can be the root of so much misunderstanding and Aspie Angst. I wonder if a much better test of position on the spectrum in adults might be to ignore the usual multiple choice stuff and cut straight to a "can you tell the difference between these two emotions being expressed on a photo of someone's face?" I think I'm probably lucky and lightly affected by Asperger's but my absolute Achilles heel is facial expression.

I can "do" a clown's face doing happy and sad. After that the subtleties are just too much.

Try these for size: they are four of the ten Baron-Cohen/Wheelwright/Jolliffe "basic" emotion test pictures from their standardised test. If you are NT, write down the first emotion that comes to your mind. Now go back and consider that this might be a trick question and decide if you want to change your answer? Beginning to feel a bit Aspie now? Answers below the pictures.

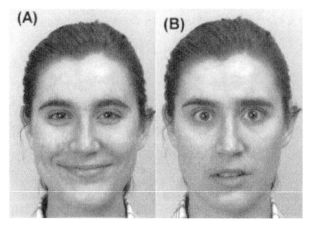

F

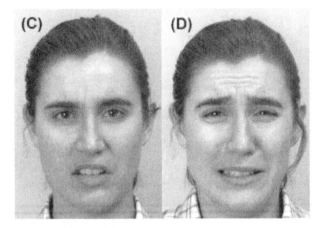

(A): *Happy (as compared with surprised?)*

(B): *Afraid (as compared with angry?)*

(C): *Disgusted (as compared with just sad?)*

(D): *Distressed (as compared with just sad?)*

Go and read the paper and try out the more complex emotions...

Visual Cognition (1997) Vol. 4 Iss. 3, p311 to 331: "Is There a Language of the Eyes?"

Facial Recognition

It is very hard for those on the autistic spectrum to remember the names and faces of acquaintances, though if they are really into you, they will remember every nook and cranny of your face and perhaps idolise it.

The Husband Says:

Perhaps this is another quirk of Aspie-ness or perhaps it is just me.

I'm really good at recognising a face that I have seen before, perhaps only fleetingly. But I'm really terrible at putting names to faces. Is this an Executive Function thing - that the pattern matching logic works really well, but the linkage to recovering a name from memory is a bit broken?

Aspie Hints and Tips

AS Get a smart mobile phone that puts a little avatar picture of the person next to the phone number that is ringing you. The relationship between number, name and picture will eventually strengthen.

F

Faking It

You may often wonder how you got into this predicament in the first place. How did you not recognise or realise he was so different? That is because you married a master of disguise; a chameleon. An actor who has been observing normal human behaviour all his life. He has seen what other people do. He doesn't necessarily understand it and he sometimes gets it wrong, but he will pride himself on getting it right and carrying it off.

Many an AS man has gone undiagnosed by professionals. Even when their partner, wife or parent has taken them to see a specialist and described how they are, the professional will say that he seems perfectly fine to them.

They will ask the AS person to fill in a psychological questionnaire and he will come out perfectly normal. There is your proof. Nothing wrong with him. The family are sent away.

The professional however, has been duped. The family know this and the AS person knows this. He will be so proud of what he has achieved. Today was his big day and he has proved to the world that he is normal.

There are very few professionals out there who really understand what it is to be an intelligent man on the autism spectrum. They underestimate their patients. They do not realise that a half hour conversation and filling a form in is nowhere near enough to diagnose someone who is so good at pretending to be normal.

Even if the AS man does want to be diagnosed, quite often he cannot avoid the challenge of proving that he is good at what he does. It is extremely hard to open up about your feelings. To admit that sometimes you get it wrong. That you upset your family. That you are 'lesser' than everyone else. One session is not going to do it.

The loving family will come away mystified, confused by what has happened. They may even start to wonder if it is them that has it wrong. Perhaps he is fine after all?

The Husband Says:

 Time for some plain talking, Aspie to Aspie.

Karen talks a lot of sense here. If you know, like me, that you are well along the spectrum, what have you got to lose by admitting this? Keep faking it to the outside world by all means, but perhaps if you let your guard down with your spouse, things might actually start getting better faster? Try turning what you think the world has as negatives to being your positives. Look at some of my other comments for our Aspie strengths that are in demand from our partners. She married you didn't she? That's a big dollop of approval right there.

Faking it all the time is exhausting. Give yourself a break with your partner.

Family and Friends

Family Perception of ASD

I had no idea how relieved and delighted David's parents were when they discovered he had a girlfriend. I don't know who was more shocked, me or his mother, when I walked down the stairs in David's little house to find his mother there doing the ironing. He hadn't told me she was likely to visit and she was completely unaware of my existence.

Neither of his parents had any inkling that David had Asperger's. Indeed they had never heard of the condition back in 1995. However, looking back, they did often drop hints about David and his peculiarities especially regarding him as a small boy. He apparently had a penchant for drilling holes in the sitting room walls to 'see what was behind there'. This was said with humour some twenty years after he had grown out of the habit but I suspect there was less humour at the time as he ruined the wallpaper. It was put down to having a curious mind, and what was wrong with that?

They also dropped hints about him being less than patient with other people, something I didn't witness until he had to help out at the family business. They told me that he didn't "suffer fools gladly". Well that is certainly true.

When our oldest child was eventually diagnosed at the age of 10 with AS, David's mother was not at all surprised. She had worked with autistic children many years before and admitted that she had suspected he might have been. I had interviewed my mother-in-law for my dissertation about Asperger Marriage as I had posthumously diagnosed my father in law as having AS. She had no recognition that her husband was possibly autistic and had put his bad temper and unsociable ways down to the fact he had Type 1 Diabetes.

It is hard for any mother to come to terms with the fact her child might be autistic, even if he is in his forties but my mother-in-law was very much aware of how David could be so unreasonable and verbally abusive at times. She did not argue with me when I suggested it. She has in fact been very grateful that I have stayed.

How to Explain ASD to Family and Friends

The first thing you need to do is your research. If his family are genuinely interested in helping they will have a lot of questions. To get a diagnosis, the clinician will often ask for a close family member to go along and answer questions about the (suspected) AS person's childhood as the answers are often revealing. If his mother is willing, she would be the perfect person to take along as she would provide good first-hand information and also feel involved - and thereby more open to her child's diagnosis.

F

Some family will never accept the fact that your husband has a diagnosis. They will see nothing wrong in his behaviour and may even resent your intervening. It is best to choose which of your battles to fight and there are some people whose minds you will not change.

Fear of Rejection

This is mostly regarding the AS individual but there are relationships where the Husband can reject his partner because he gets overwhelmed by her actions.

The Husband Says:

This one runs deep.

It is the fear of rejection that, a few hours after that big blow up argument, makes me want to make up and come back to Karen. She could walk out the door any minute and she might be better off by doing so. Or at least one of my inner voices says so.

But she hasn't yet. Perhaps my fear of rejection is unfounded and just adding further to my stress levels?

Feeling Overwhelmed

This can apply to both of you, NT and AS.

Neurotypical Without Support

As the Executive Secretary in this relationship most of the everyday responsibilities fall to you. From getting yourself up, making sure the kids get off to school, household chores and going out to work. You will have found there is no time for you to take time out for yourself. You will also have realised that you are not getting the reciprocal support you need from your other half. As time goes on, not only do you have the responsibilities of daily life on your shoulders but you have to shoulder everyone else's troubles and emotions, by yourself. No back up.

NT It is hard to step off the carousel and take time for yourself but this is what you need to do. You also need to make clear to your Aspie husband that you are struggling and cannot do it all alone.

Have you considered joining any support groups? Sometimes it just helps to vent your frustrations to other people who understand even if there is no solution. Look up local autism support groups in your area or look into counselling. If the counselling is just for yourself they do not need to be an ASD specialist, though it helps.

There is a website specifically to support Asperger wives. They have discussions in relevant topics, arrange Meet Ups around the country and they all provide useful information such as ASD counsellors in your area.

Try not to fall into the trap of medication or self-medication. It seems like an easy solution at the time but it can often add to your burden when you realise that you rely on these too much.

Look at other article on here on how to communicate better with your partner.

On the Spectrum and Overwhelmed

AS
Signs that you are overwhelmed:

- Anger and irritation at people and inanimate objects
- Not wanting to get out of bed
- Severe procrastination
- Drinking too much
- Staying away from home
- Working too many hours
- Tiredness and possible depression
- Meltdowns and shut-downs

If you recognise these signs in yourself then you need to ask for help.

Your first port of call is your partner. You need to be honest and communicate with them to tell them you are not coping. All your partner can see is that you are angry at them. Your partner will be confused and hurt and will become defensive making the situation worse for both of you:

Tell them how you feel. If you cannot verbalise if then write a letter or an email that you know they will read.

- Ask them for understanding and patience
- Ask for help and support
- Don't place all the burden on them.

Try and work as a team to solve your problems. You will be surprised at how willing your partner is to help you. Their happiness is intertwined with your happiness.

F

Feelings

People with AS have been unfairly described as "not having any feelings" when this could not be further from the truth.

They do, however, find their feelings hard to describe and are often not aware of them building up until they erupt. In this way they could be seen as being unfeeling, but only because they are not aware of the subtleties of their emotions.

Fiction

If you haven't yet had enough of autism and Asperger's, then here are some fiction books I highly recommend that you read. These authors have worked hard to portray autistic characters in a non-patronising and informative light:

- The Curious Incident of the Dog in the Night-time
- House Rules
- The Rosie Project
- A Different Kettle of Fish

Fidelity

This is generally a very positive side to your AS partner. You know that you can trust him and he will never stray. This is true for the majority of your Aspie men.

However, there are exceptions and generally these exceptions are true to Aspie form of being extreme. There are some men with Asperger's who will never be faithful and can never be trusted.

There are also some men on the autistic spectrum who will leave their wife and children and never give them another thought. Their new partner is their new "obsession" or "special interest" and they cannot focus on anything else.

Fight or Flight

When stressed the body goes into a fight or flight reaction. This releases adrenaline, making the heart work faster but also reduces the intelligence of the person temporarily. This will make them less reasonable whilst they have an increased heart rate.

Finding Things

I hold my hands up. I'm not organised, or at least on the surface it looks like I'm not. I put things down and sometimes can't remember where I've put them, but they eventually turn up. I've never lost my mobile phone or purse though I have had my purse stolen.

I still make the mistake of asking David if he knows where an item is. Instead of saying "No" he will start pulling the house apart in a frenzied and angry fashion until it is found. If it is not found, he takes it quite personally.

Therefore, I try really hard not to ask him as it isn't worth the stress. I generally find my car keys or whatever I was looking for when I retrace my steps.

When I was a child my father was a pipe smoker and he would constantly lose his pipe or matches. I think he discovered early on that the best way to find it was to ask me. I would be able to use common sense to track it down successfully whereas my dad just couldn't.

I notice this with my children that they find it hard to find things. Every morning they ask me where their shoes are and every morning I point out that I have tidied them up and put them in the porch.

The Husband Says:

Several meaty topics all rolled into one.

Let's start with the "confession" from Karen that she moves things and tidies them up. The whole theory of mind thing means that I'm unlikely to figure out that Karen has been on a tidying spree and that there is some external mechanism that has caused my stuff to move. I didn't move my stuff; I didn't see my stuff move so my stuff must still be where I left it.

Aspies often have phenomenal memory, but memory that works in an unusual way. It's not a computer database that you can query using a fixed syntax. You need a trigger to make the recall happen, and that trigger is likely to be very "sensory" for an Aspie rather than written or spoken - so a picture or a smell is more likely to trigger a recall of where I have left something than a list or inventory for me. It sounds perverse, but I go to the place where I think I may have lost the thing to try to get a trigger to find it again. If that doesn't work, well the brute-force search of every possible location is the only thing left to do.

For me, finding stuff depends on the habit of putting stuff in logical and habitual places. Logic can go horribly wrong. Like being on holiday recently in France and thinking I had lost my mobile phone. In a water park more than an hours drive away. I tried using Karen's phone to ring my 'phone but I just got a French tone that says unobtainable. I panicked. Only eventually did Karen point out to me that we were in an underground car-park with no signal - we went above ground and my phone started to ring - it had slipped down behind a piece of plastic in the dreadful hire car we had been given. Never again will we hire an Opel Meriva.

F

Aspie Hints & Tips

Put a cabinet or table close to the normal exit door for the house. Put keys, money, 'phone, watch - all that day to day "pocket luggage" in that location - pick it all up when you leave, put it all back when you return.

Fixations

Your Aspie has a single track mind. He will become fixated on hobbies, worries, anticipations and (especially) negative thoughts.

It is easy to recognise a fixation as, generally, it is all he will talk about. It is hard to derail them when they are fixated on a topic.

Sometimes it is worth letting them get their feelings out. Make them feel listened to and then try and move on. If they insist on constantly regurgitating the same issue with no end or solution in sight you need to be firm and tell them that you have listened and that you would like to move on.

It is worth giving them a time limit/parameters and rules, on occasion, so they know what is expected of them - and for the sake of your sanity and temper.

"Fixer Upper"

A friend of mine has been trying out online dating but has rather high expectations. She is dating someone who really likes her but, even though I can see she likes him a lot, he does not meet her high expectations in certain areas.

I was telling David this and said that she needs to realise that finding a man is like buying a house; you can't get everything you want and have to compromise somewhere. He replied that what she has is a "fixer upper". I laughed and agreed but said "no woman looks for a fixer upper". David, the man when I first met him, showed me a "show home" and I fell for all the obvious perfections he had to show me, but he had hidden behind new paint! The dry rot and the mine workings didn't show up on the survey.... so I ended up with a fixer upper with collapsing foundations.

The Husband Says:

Take away from that a positive message! Whilst Karen thinks I might have deceived her before marriage by hiding my faults, she considers that I am a fixer-upper; my faults can be

repaired or tolerated and she doesn't need to move out either physically or metaphorically. I'll be even more valuable once Karen finishes the repairs.

Flapping

Flapping is not so obvious in the adult Aspie. I have noted that some Aspies, whether excited or nervous, cannot help do it to some extent, but it is subtle, constrained and controlled. I think I have a finely tuned radar for noticing it these days. In women and girls, flapping is a little more obvious but, at least when they get older and excited it can still be acceptable for a female. But your male Aspie is aware enough to know that it makes him look odd. It can be brought down to subtle finger tapping within the lap where most people wouldn't see or notice.

What is Flapping?

Why do they do it? What do they get out of it and is it something that is like a nervous tic that they cannot help?

The Husband Says:

When I was younger, I didn't overtly flap, but I had a behaviour that was in the class of "flapping" - when I was bored in school assembly and forced to sit cross legged I would close my eyes and rock back and forth. So I guess that all of these "flapping" behaviours fall into the stimming (conscious but habit) and tics (unconscious behaviour) categories.

Another physical action related to flapping is seeing an Aspie up on the balls of their feet like they are about to start a sprint race. I guess this is because you are less stable and this results in stimulus to the sense of equilibrioception (balance). There may also be a link to Proprioception (the sense of where you are in space) and the apparent needs of Aspies to link information from multiple senses together, possibly for confirmation and reinforcement.

Forewarned is Fore Armed

I was really proud of David recently. We had been to a meeting about our daughter's recent diagnosis and it had been very positive. I think it had given David time to reflect on himself and recognise a lot of his daughter's traits as his own.

After we left the meeting he turned to me and said that he'd just like to warn me that he was going to be in a foul mood this coming weekend. A little startled, I asked why and he informed me he had to do his tax return. He hates anything related to tax and resents the time he has to spend doing the government's work for them - as he sees it. I immediately understood and thanked him for warning me.

F

Previously he would be in an absolutely foul mood and take it out on me and I wouldn't know why. I would react negatively to his treatment of me and our antagonism towards each other would spiral. Now, forewarned is fore armed. I know not to take it personally. He is able to understand himself enough now to predict the kind of mood he is going to be in and he has learned, through conversation with me, that I find upsetting when he is horrible to me because he is having to do something he doesn't like.

Just the fact that he knows that I know what the problem is will most likely reduce the problem! I will be more understanding and supportive and he should respond in kind to my positive measures. It may not be a particularly enjoyable weekend but we should come out of it with our marriage intact.

The Husband Says:

See, I'm learning. Another coping strategy.

AS *Explain what is going to drive forthcoming behaviour because you as an Aspie are the arch-planner and know that this set of circumstances is going to happen. Turn that to your advantage.*

Forgiveness

You can't have a successful marriage without being able to forgive. Once you have gone past seeing your partner's point of view and, more specifically, not wanting to see it, there is probably no hope for the marriage.

NT **AS** It also has to come from both sides.

NT To find forgiveness for abominable behaviour (I'm not referring to violence or abuse here) doesn't have to be difficult. Perhaps the first thing you have to do is remind yourself why you married him in the first place. What are his good points? Then you have to work out exactly what was behind the behaviour. What were the triggers. What was his intention?

Did he actually mean to embarrass you by telling you off in public or had his anxieties become so much for him that he wasn't even aware of where he was? Perhaps he doesn't actually understand that you would mind being berated by your husband in view and earshot of other people? Perhaps he has no concept of neurotypical embarrassment and social decorum?

F

If you can see what lead up to the behaviour, it is possible to forgive the behaviour. Yes, there will be the fear that he can and will do it again, but there are steps you can take to reduce these triggers and head the unwanted behaviour off at the pass.

The Husband Says:

It's unfortunate, even ironic, that us Apies really struggle with forgiveness. I bear grudges lasting months and years. Karen seems to take a little time, but almost always seems to forgive my errant behaviour by the end of the day.

Friends

As a Support Network

It is good to have friends. I find I have two types of friends. Those who are involved in the autistic world and those who aren't. I need these people at different times and for different things. Of course, it isn't 'never the twain shall meet' but it is good to have friends who understand your situation and it is also good, in a way, to have other friends who don't. The less-autism-aware set talk about other things, and you realise there is a life outside of autism and anxiety. It is nice to be able to talk about other interests with people.

The Husband Says:

I don't have such "deep" friendships as Karen does. It's probably because I have difficulty judging emotion and how much emotional investment a prototype-friend might be making in me and how much I should reciprocate back. My long standing colleagues have the same sort of status as my friends.

"Proper" friends is rather tricky for us Aspies - that way leads to more emotional angst. I'm very happy with my relationship with Karen as partner and "special-friend"; making the emotional investment in Karen is worthwhile, and Karen will forgive me if I get something wrong. "Ordinary" friends might not be that forgiving.

An awful mess ensues when I say something inappropriate with "ordinary" friends. They don't seem to realise it was an accident and that I wasn't deliberately trying to insult them.

I really struggle to apply logic to friendship to understand its nuances. NTs promote this ideal that friendship should be unconditional - that defies logic and analysis.

Further Reading

Books I Recommend

- Tony Attwood, Complete Guide to Asperger Syndrome

Forums on Facebook to Follow

- Aspergated Wives (A closed group, you need to request membership)

- Different Together (Also a closed group)

F

G

- ✧ Gait
- ✧ Gaslighting
- ✧ Genius
- ✧ Gift Ideas
- ✧ Girls
- ✧ Gluten
- ✧ Going Mad
- ✧ Grief
- ✧ Gross Motor Skills
- ✧ Growing Out of It
- ✧ Guest in the House
- ✧ Guests in the House for Special Occasions

G

Gait

Once you know what to look for, it is one of the more obvious physical signs of having an ASD. Toe walking is mentioned in the diagnosis of children with Asperger's and ASD. What isn't mentioned is that this continues throughout their life. It becomes less pronounced, especially if you are 6 foot 2 and twenty stone but the bouncing walk is still there.

Gaslighting

This is a term used when one partner makes the other think that they are 'going mad' by twisting their words or denying that something had happened. It is named after the old black and white movie Gaslight where the husband hid items from his wife and then accused her of moving them. He was intentionally driving her 'mad' in order to get her certified and institutionalised for financial gain.

It is fairly common for wives whose partners are on (or suspected of being on) the autistic spectrum to accuse their husbands of 'Gaslighting'. The wives feel that their words and actions are being misrepresented in order to make them look and feel less.

This has happened to David and I, especially in our earlier marriage when he would accuse me of having intentions I did not have. He would misunderstand my words and my actions and be paranoid that I was angry with him or against him in some way, when I was not. Or at least I wasn't angry with him until he started accusing me of behaving in a negative way.

This behaviour from the man you love really does, after a while, make you start to wonder whether you really are going insane. Being accused of something you didn't do or ever intend to do is confusing and soul destroying. Having the person that you love and rely on most in the world be angry with you is devastating and very lonely. You have no one to turn to when this happens. How can you explain to your friends about your husband's paranoia? Even when you try and write it down it seems almost trivial, but it is not trivial to experience time and time again.

Is Gaslighting Abuse?

This kind of behaviour form the man you love feels very much like abuse. It often comes out of the blue and makes you feel diminished.

NT However, you need to realise that if your husband does have Asperger's Syndrome, this behaviour of his is not intentional. Yes, I agree it does have the same effect as a psychopath or a narcissistic meeting out sadistic ways to his partner, but he does not mean to hurt you and that is the difference.

Making Your Husband Aware of His Behaviour

NT You need to be honest with your husband. Every time he inflicts this belittling behaviour you must inform him of what he is doing. Tell him that you understand that he is upset but what he is saying is not true. Also inform him that he has hurt your feelings by doing this.

How to Avoid these Situations from Occurring

NT You need to make note of when this happens and what the triggers are. It may be something as simple as lack of sleep making him irritable or that his social cup is full as you have had unexpected visitors who have overstayed their welcome. Once you recognise a pattern that affects his behaviour you need to take avoiding steps.

Supplementation

The above advice is valid and I do try and use it myself but David's behaviour can be unpredictable at times like this. What has vastly improved his overall behaviour over the last two years of our marriage is providing him with healthier meals full of nutrients and supplementation to his diet. Though I try to get more fruit and vegetables into him, unless they are fermented he really isn't that keen.

Certain vitamins, such as Vitamin D3 (which is actually a hormone) and vitamin B complex, do not make overnight improvements but they are worth persisting with for overall physical and mental health, especially if your partner is like mine and not keen on sunshine and exercise.

On days I forget to give David his supplements at breakfast he is not nice to know by tea time. He is tired, irritable, paranoid and uninterested in us as a family. He lacks a sense of humour and likes to comfort eat food full of carbohydrates and gluten and drink alcohol. None of these things make him agreeable. I curse myself for my lack of organisation on these days. He does not seem to be able to motivate himself to take the pills himself.

NT What has made an essential difference to his behaviour is 5-HTP which can be brought from health food shops. It raises his mood very quickly as it contains both serotonin and melatonin. He is a much nicer and even mannered person when he takes 5-HTP. Be aware, this does not cure his autism. David is Aspie through and through but once you reduce his anxieties he is a lovely person to know.

Behind all his bad behaviour is lurking his (and your) nemesis, Anxiety. Get rid of that and you will want to stay married to your husband.

G

Genius

Back in 1944, Hans Asperger himself described the quirky children he observed as "little professors".

If you are talking about autism being on a spectrum, then there is also a wide spectrum of intelligence from Learning Difficulties (an approximate IQ of under 80) to the Einstein's of this world. Actually, it is suspected that Einstein did not have Asperger's but high functioning autism (HFA) as he was mute for the first five years of his life. In fact, though Einstein's IQ was high, there are many children with Asperger's and HFA who would have a higher IQ than Einstein's 150. David was tested as a child and it was certainly higher than that. I believe it is actually less common to test a child's IQ these days. David and I certainly don't know what our own children's are but they are certainly bright kids, though in very different ways.

There are many kinds of genius and some 'Geniuses' have actually had to put in a lot of hard work to get there.

My idea of a Genius is someone who just knows without having to put the work in. This is often the case with many Aspies who have their own kind of intuition, compared to NT intuition. They look upon us as wonders of social and emotional communication and we look upon them as the innovators and great logical thinkers of our world.

The Husband Says:

Let's tread carefully on this subject. You kind of want to find some positives about all this Aspie "thinking differently" stuff. Assigning genius to an above average memory and a logical approach to logical subjects like the sciences might just be trying to make the best of a bad job.

Gift Ideas

The TV Series "The Big Bang Theory" has a story on this subject: Season 2 Episode 11: "The Bath Item Gift Hypothesis".

Aspie Hints and Tips

Listen carefully. Large hints will be being given. But do try to add a controlled element of surprise. Buy a card, wrapping paper and a bow - it feels like a waste of money, but NTs like this frippery.

- *Do not buy a "practical present" like a vacuum cleaner or a dishwasher*
- *Don't buy the technology that you want as a present for yourself*

- *Avoid clothes, especially underwear, despite the adverts at Christmas and Valentine's Day: getting the right size is tricky, you probably don't have enough taste to choose something fashionable and that fits with her existing wardrobe.*

- *Flowers are good, but avoid lilies - they traditionally signal a death and they smell and might give you sensory overload*

- *A voucher is versatile, but not a very thoughtful present*

- *Jewellery can be good for a partner, but check carefully that the recipient uses that particular kind - e.g. does she have pierced ears? Rings can be quite subjective (and difficult to size). Watches and pendants are good. Understated silver might be better than gaudy gold*

- *A night out on the town at a good restaurant? But beware the hazards of eating out*

- *Concert or show tickets for a favourite type of music, comedy or play. Do your research - e.g. opera would be a very unusual and unlikely choice*

- *A spa day with transport there and back. Don't choose the treatments though*

- *Chocolates and alcohol are tricky - they might take you to a debate on body image and dieting*

- *Roller-coasters, funfairs, activity days - but only if you are prepared to join in and go on all the rides too*

- *Vases, ornaments and the like. But be careful to choose things that fit with the existing household decor. Don't rely on your sense of style - go to a small shop and ask the assistants for help.*

- ***NO PETS!***

- *It doesn't have to be expensive - very definitely it will be the thoughtfulness put into the gift that will count.*

- *But don't talk about the selection process - it needs to look effortless.*

Girls

From the time autism and Asperger's Syndrome was first mooted, the attention has been on boys and the men they have grown into. For some reason the girls were ignored. Statistically the current thinking is that the ratio of boys to girls on the autistic spectrum is 4:1 but some professionals suspect it is not so skewed. It is just that the girls have not been diagnosed or, perhaps worse, have been misdiagnosed with another condition.

G

As a mother of an Aspie girl, I myself spent years wondering about and observing my daughter. It wasn't until I went to an NAS conference about women and girls on the autistic spectrum that I knew for sure my daughter had Asperger's. I confess I did a lot of crying that day but came away determined to help my daughter.

It took a lot longer to get her diagnosed but through my stubbornness and persistence this has eventually happened. My daughter is quietly pleased. She knew she was different from her peers and now she has a reason why. In fact, when I told her she had got an official diagnosis, she threw her arms in the air and cried, "Where's my certificate?"

So though this App is aimed mainly at the wives of autistic men, I am aware that I should be aiming it at both sexes. I am even aware that there are quite a few same sex relationships where one partner is on the spectrum.

Yet, as this help guide is being written from my perspective as the Asperger Wife, with input from the Asperger husband, we have decided to refer to the majority of NT women/AS men relationships for now. I hope no one feels excluded.

The Husband Says:

I have the wrong mix of chromosomes to give any insight into this.

That might not be the flippant answer you think it is at first sight. There is a school of thought that thinks that autism and Asperger's is a result of lots of similar gene mutations scattered across many chromosomes. A theory of why girls may be less affected than boys is that girls have two X chromosomes to go at, so the tolerance to error in genetic material is naturally higher - there are plenty of "good" genes to outweigh the "bad". Boys, with X-Y, have half as many "good" chances to begin with so might be more susceptible.

Gluten

What is Gluten?

Gluten is found in many products such as wheat, rye, oats and barley. It is a composite protein, acting as a glue and helping foods keep their shape.

Gluten Intolerance

Gluten Intolerance has been dismissed by the NHS as 'fashionable' and some doctors just believe this is a new health fad and actually think that people are depriving themselves of certain foods. The NHS however, do admit that Coeliac disease is a serious problem.

My Gluten Journey

I myself was seriously ill ten years ago and was losing my eyesight. The ophthalmologists after many tests and examinations could not find a cause and referred me to the neurologist. The neurologist did many tests (none of which he explained) which I later discovered related to his concerns about Multiple Sclerosis. I was sent for MRI scans, CT scans, EEG's, lumbar punctures and muscle biopsy tests. I must have cost the NHS a fortune but I was not at all well and it wasn't just my eye sight. I was lethargic, suffering from severe migraines and generally felt very ill.

In the end they washed their hands of me as they did not know what the problem was. Not once did anyone ask me about my diet. Sometime later over a casual coffee with a friend she mentioned she might be gluten intolerant and that she was going to get tested. I didn't believe in that kind of quackery but after my friend was tested she cut out gluten and felt much better. I wondered if I had any intolerances. I went along to a local clinic and, though I told him I wasn't generally feeling well, I didn't talk about any of my food likes or dislikes and he didn't ask.

We did a double blind test which took about half an hour. He told me that I was intolerant to parsnips, leeks, milk and wheat.

I have to say I was astounded as I had always hated parsnips with a passion (inherited from my father) to the point I would refuse to have any potatoes on my plate that had been roasted next to a parsnip. My mother would get infuriated with me (she loved parsnips) but my father completely understood. My body was trying to tell me something.

I immediately cut back on all wheat and tried different types of milk. I didn't really get on with any of the alternative milks such as rice, almond and soya, but I know plenty of people who swear by them. I wanted something that wasn't milk that I could just use as milk. Thankfully, I found lacto free milk and changed all our milk to this with little protest from my family. What a difference it made.

It was difficult at first to give up gluten. Giving up the breads and pastries I loved was hard enough but also having to check for hidden ingredients. Who knew that the flavours on crisps that I loved so much were full of gluten?

My life changed very quickly for the better. I lost weight, was less puffy, less irritable and less tired. My gut no longer acted like a washing machine after lunch, my headaches and migraines disappeared and my eyesight became clearer. Occasionally I would become complacent and convince myself I would be fine if I ate that slice of pizza or gave in to the cajoling from well-meaning friends. I never was fine. There was always a price to pay. It may be ten minutes later with the loudest gurgling tummy the world has ever heard or several prolonged trips to the toilet later that evening. It was never worth it.

G

Gluten and Autism

At the time I became aware of my gluten intolerance, my son was eight years old and still at first school. He had been getting upset at school and the teachers were worried about him. I had put it down to anxiety about his imminent move up to middle school. The teachers took me aside and suggested he wasn't getting enough sleep. He wasn't a great sleeper but he had a strict bed time routine. However, I could see why they were concerned: he had dark circles under his eyes and was regularly upset. He had also been suffering from bad tummy problems for a while. He hated going to the toilet and I would often find him lying on his bedroom floor in pain and sweating, constipated. He was sometimes in a terrible state. Eventually I put two and two together and wondered if I was gluten intolerant then he might be too. Looking back now I don't know why the lightbulb didn't go on sooner.

He was in such an awful state, not only was he constipated but he had diarrhoea as well and basically didn't have much control over his bowels. I sat him down and discussed seriously with him my idea. Considering his age he listened attentively and agreed it was a good idea. This put into perspective how desperately miserable he was.

The plan was to take him off all gluten for a week and see if anything changed. Well it was little short of miraculous. We cut out the pizzas and cookies he loved and all the little snacks in between. He made an effort to eat a bit more fruit but mainly I was careful in planning meals and not giving him the pizza and pasta he and his sister basically lived on. He started to sleep better, he was less anxious, the circles went form under his eyes, his teachers reported he was no longer crying at school. The most noticeable thing was that he hadn't been to the toilet all week and I was worried I may have done the wrong thing. But at the weekend he went off to the toilet and called me in after. There in the toilet was the biggest most solid poo he had ever done in his life and for once he was proud of it. I knew then we were on the right track.

When he went to middle school his behaviour became worse and he was eventually diagnosed with Asperger's Syndrome, which has since explained an awful lot. The school were only prepared to give him gluten free food if he had a letter from the doctor so, even though we knew one hundred per cent that he had this problem, we went along to the GP and he was referred to a paediatrician specialist. To our horror this Consultant insisted that he be put back on gluten for three months before he had his bloods taken. We decided to do as we were told and also I kept a food and behaviour diary. Morgan was suddenly allowed to eat all the things he loved with abandon. Within days he became ill, tired and moody again. We decided not to keep up the gluten filled regime it just was not worth it. Shortly before he was due to have his bloods tested, I let him eat some gluten foods in moderation. He passed his test with flying colours and was pronounced officially gluten intolerant. I felt a great deal of satisfaction about being proved right but I didn't confess to the Doctor that we had not kept him on the gluten for three months.

G

Even now I regularly hear Consultant's and GP's say there is no harm in gluten and that it does not affect autistic behaviour at all.

The Husband Says:

One more voice promoting gluten in moderation. Mine. I don't go for quackery, but in blind testing I have found that bread at lunch time makes me sleepy in the afternoon. I still eat bread but it has to be the best sourdough rye to make the expected dent in my performance worth the taste sensation.

In addition, the more "commercial" the bread (with flour improver and the like) the worse the symptoms of my mild intolerance. So it's not just the gluten to blame.

Going Mad

If you have had this feeling in your marriage, then you are not alone. You are also not going mad. Believe in yourself and your instincts.

There really were times early on in our marriage when I started to wonder if I was going mad. His reactions to everyday situations were over the top. He managed to alienate us from our neighbours and friends. I couldn't understand why people were being so mean to us. It turned out they weren't, but the way David related back conversations from his autistic perspective made me think other people were unreasonable and uncaring. I was naive and in love and I looked up to my husband as he was so clever and talented. I had managed to stamp on my doubts and insecurities, whilst wearing my rose tinted glasses, in order to marry a man I knew loved me unconditionally.

His paranoia and unforgiving nature influenced me at first until he started not just being unreasonable about the people around us, but with things I had said and done too. I started to realise that he would overreact to situations and not see things the way I saw them. I still wasn't sure who was right. My under reaction or his over reaction?

This wasn't something I could talk about to anyone. What could I say? How would it sound? On the face of it he was a loving, hardworking husband. I was confused and dispirited.

NT Let me tell you now, you are not going mad. Believe in your instincts. If you feel he is overreacting about a situation, do not mentally follow him down that path. Realise that he is in an unknown situation and he doesn't know how to react to it. Don't let him be forceful with his opinions or actions. Stay calm and, when he has calmed down and become more rational, gently talk him through it. Get him to see sense.

G

Grief

Are you grieving for the loss of your marriage? See Stages of Grief.

The Husband Says:

Grief represents a collision in the Aspie world. We care, we just don't show it like you. Social norms dictate that we attend funerals when asked (we won't volunteer). Expect us to be quiet and withdrawn, showing little empathy, but practical and accommodating. Funerals have a set timetable and expectation which we can plan for. We are attending because you want us to.

We will bottle it up and be quietly sad for ourselves later. We don't really want to reminisce and we certainly don't want to relive this again.

My dad said: "The only funeral I need to attend is my own."

Gross Motor Skills

Surprisingly, Gross Motor Skills (i.e. walking, running, throwing, catching, jumping etc.) are usually nowhere near as affected as fine motor skills by autism and Asperger's.

Growing Out of it

The Husband Says:

I don't think you ever "grow out of it"; this is a condition for life. Your act - your coping strategies may become so sophisticated that less and less people notice - they might think that you are "growing out of it".

The energy required to keep up the act may lead to a fake relapse. How many older people do you know that you label eccentric or cantankerous; could these be Aspies who have run out of energy to conform to your social norms?

Guests in the House

This is such a major issue for us. Because we do not have a spare room, it is difficult to accommodate people to stay. When the children were younger they were happy to share either with each other for a few nights or with the guest depending who it was.

Our son, at the age of twelve, suddenly demanded to know why he had to move out of his room every time grandad came to stay. I didn't have a good enough answer for him as I could see it upset him. He was not able to access all the things he needed whenever he wanted to and, as he also has Asperger's, he was not able to deal with it as well as a neurotypical child would.

The next time my father visited we set him up in the study on the sofa bed, but this had even more dire consequences. Even though David had access to the bedrooms, bathrooms, kitchen and living areas, the only place he wanted to be (and the only place he couldn't be) was his study, his man-cave. He threw an enormous tantrum which, for me at the time, came completely out of the blue. It was a terrible atmosphere to live in until my father left. I have had to ask my dad to stay in a hotel now if he wants to visit, which is expensive and inconvenient for him.

The Husband Says:

I like Karen's dad. But with autism and Asperger's conditions with a significant genetic linkage, it comes as no surprise that gatherings of relatives where the children also have a diagnosis will be hot beds of further Aspie bad behaviour.

Social norms dictate that you should respect your elders. But there are so many aspects of our elder's belief systems on science, politics, the weather, sport, you name it, that are just plain wrong. It is very difficult to ignore these matters when they are being preached to you and your own children under your own roof.

In the particular series of incidents that Karen recounts, we had no shared topics of conversation that we could consider "safe" - free from inherent conflict. Karen's dad had invaded my territory - my office with my television, so I couldn't escape to relax with a beer and a dose of crappy TV. We just rubbed each other up the wrong way.

We are renting a house at the moment; deliberately chosen with a guest room and enough television and computer points that guests can live a self-sufficient experience, and I don't have to give up what I consider "mine" when they are here. I don't feel like I should have to adjust my normality when guests are here - they should change their behaviour when staying under my roof.

I also need to learn the NT trick of saying "stay as long as you want, no hurry" whilst sending a body language "vibe" - please go now we want our lives back.

Guests in the House on Special Occasions

This is actually more tolerable for David. There is generally a certain amount of structure, depending on the occasion, and I have learned to give him responsibilities which get him out of the main social melee and also give him a

G

purpose. He will happily cook food and serve drinks and will chat to the people he comes across, but he is able to have a "get out clause" at any moment which gives him more control of the situation.

NT We tend to invite good friends over and not strangers, and we have structured occasions such as a Games or Quiz Nights. This is fun for everyone as they like to be challenged and show off their knowledge in a fun and safe environment. Also, the fact that the occasion starts at a certain time and ends at a certain time is easier to cope with.

The Husband Says:

Agree with this completely. It's Karen's friends visiting of course, because these are "close" friends, and it is Karen's social circle that is neurotypically in a neat hierarchy to allow that distinction and choice.

The right amount of self-administered medication (alcohol) and taxis on call helps to lubricate the situation. There is also a "point" to the evening - the game or quiz. You might think this could lead to a tantrum on losing, but who minds coming third in such exalted company!

G

- ✧ Hans Asperger
- ✧ Happy Facade
- ✧ Harm
- ✧ Having a Purpose
- ✧ Head in the Sand
- ✧ Health
- ✧ High Expectations
- ✧ High IQ
- ✧ Hobbies
- ✧ Holidays
- ✧ Holidays with other People
- ✧ Hope
- ✧ How to Initiate Sex
- ✧ Hugs
- ✧ Humour
- ✧ Hygiene
- ✧ Hypermobility
- ✧ Hyper/Hypo

Hans Asperger

Hans Asperger was an Austrian paediatrician and wrote his paper "Autistic Psychopaths in Childhood" in 1944. However, due to the war and his nationality it was not well received and was not translated into English until the 1980's by Uta Frith.

Lorna Wing and Judith Gould who worked on the translated paper coined the term for the 'little professors' that Hans Asperger had written about as Asperger's Syndrome.

Happy Facade

I suspect this is one most likely to be for the female with ASD, but with all subjects on the autistic spectrum this is not exclusive to the fairer sex.

Many girls on the spectrum surround themselves physically and immerse themselves mentally in a world that makes them happy and comfortable. For many this world is full of rainbows, unicorns and princesses with pretty dresses and magic powers. Others latch on to a particular period in history and adopt a period style and even speak in a certain way. These things are their special interests and make them happy.

However, much in their life causes them stress and anxiety and they use their special interests to divert their thoughts away from this, almost to the point of convincing themselves that it is just a hobby/plaything and not a tool to take them away from other people and their fears.

They create this facade so well that they convince themselves they are fine. That everything is fine. If you ask them how they are they will smile and say everything is good because in their head, in their world, everything is good. That's why they created it. Any disasters that befall the residents of their secret world can be controlled and fixed by them. Often with the flourish of a pen.

It doesn't take much to scratch the surface of this facade. It may be cruel to point out to someone who is living in denial of their own anxiety, but sometimes this has to be done, to face up to the reality of an avoided situation. Facing their fears doesn't mean they destroy their comforting world, just put it to one side whilst help can make the happiness real.

Harm

Staying in an abusive marriage long term can do you untold harm.

It can also harm your partner.

NT **AS** Have you considered that you are doing each other harm?

You are both being defensive. Both believe you are right and never giving in. Where has the love and the compromise gone?

The Husband Says:

I've never contemplated physical harm. But that doesn't make up for all the mental harm I've caused over the years.

Having a Purpose

David finds it hard to define his identity. The problem is in many ways he doesn't know who he is. He is therefore not even confident about going into a supermarket and doing the weekly shop. He might get it wrong. Though I tend to do most of the shopping myself, he occasionally comes with me. I have noticed over the years that he is very uncomfortable wandering aimlessly around a shop.

NT The first thing I do is to make sure he has the trolley as, firstly, it defends him from all the other people with trolleys and second, it gives him a purpose. This purpose may only be 'trolley pusher' but he is happy with that. It also helps if we have a shopping list so he knows what aisle to aim for. He hates me meandering up and down aisles 'without purpose' as he sees it.

I am confident enough in my own self and ability to wander into a place without purpose and see what surprises me.

The Husband Says:

Being assigned tasks to do means that you have given me a purpose. This might be a double edged sword, since you might have been able to achieve that task more easily on your own, and now I'm asking endless questions about the specification of the deliverables and the timescale and budget for completion. But at least I'm busy and not directly making mischief.

Head in the Sand

NT This is often brought up in discussion with other Aspie wives. Their husband rarely asked about their day or after important events. It comes across as so very uncaring and uninterested. The wife feels very unloved and insignificant.

H

There are two main reasons for his behaviour

1. He very much compartmentalises his life into areas which 'never the twain shall meet'. Or as my husband puts it in Ghost Busters terms 'crossing the streams'. Despite the fact that life is not neat and tidy and able to be put into separate, labelled boxes, this is what they try to do to organise their life and their mind. If he is at work; naturally he thinks about work. If his phone rings from a personal number at work he will not answer it. That is crossing the streams. It takes too much mental energy to extricate his mind out of one box and work out what is happening in another.

2. This is the main reason he ignores the problems occurring in your life. Unless he is directly faced with a crisis he will do his best to avoid it. If you think back he is much more likely to ask you about happy and positive events that were due to happen than the ones you were dreading. He can deal with those emotionally.

It is a common and poor Aspie strategy to literally block out anything bad that they cannot handle. If you were going to the doctors to get a lump investigated it is quite possible he will not ask you for the result as he is too scared to find out. Yes this is cowardly but despite how it looks it is because he cares too much and not because he doesn't care at all. If he doesn't find out the answer, then he won't have to deal with the consequences. His low emotional intelligence just cannot cope.

He is hoping that by living in denial that someone else will fix it and the problem will go away. He also knows that you are likely to be the one to fix the problem and this is one of the attributes he finds attractive about you.

Health

There will be some Aspies who have healthy obsessions such as running but my Aspie is a desk jockey. His obsessions from a very young age have been sedentary and mostly computer based in some shape or form. Exercise is very low on his list of priorities.

Thankfully (for me) David is rarely ill. He is a terrible patient. He often thinks he is going to be ill because he mirrors other people around him and assumed because I have a headache that he has one too.

The Husband Says:

Karen has a difficult task - to remind me of my health but without nagging.

Do us Aspies make a conscious decision about health - that health is all about later years, so we don't need to worry about it now? Perhaps that's the reason Karen points out that it is low down my agenda and something that can be "put off" since it has no immediate deadline; no overt here and now impact.

But I do care what people think. I am obese, stir in a bit of dyspraxia and I can guess what NT people are thinking - clumsy oaf draining our NHS.

I am determined to do something about it, but it will be after my priorities of doing enough work to deliver the lifestyle my family deserves. There's an elliptical and treadmill just down the hall nagging me to get back to them. Better they do the nagging than Karen.

High Expectations

This probably comes under one of the extremes umbrellas but many of our Aspies have very high expectations for themselves. There is nothing wrong with having high expectations per se, as they are great motivators and many Aspies have gone on to great achievements in many areas of life.

The problem arises whilst coping with, and implementing the hard work that goes into these great expectations and also coping with the crushing disappointment when the expectations have not been met.

Why do people with Asperger's Syndrome have High Expectations?

Many of our Aspies have above average intelligence, good memories and an eye for detail and in school were able to prove themselves to teachers and their peers by doing well in exams. This will have raised their self-esteem and they would have received praise and other positive signs of admiration. Therefore, they would have wanted to repeat this to achieve the happiness that came with high achievement. Often, if they do not do well at something it is not worth doing as they do not achieve that high again. They do not understand the (very British) concept of "It's the taking part that counts." Indeed, my little AS family have poo-pooed this statements and said in no uncertain terms, "It's the winning that counts."

Implementing High Expectations

It very much depends on the circumstances and often within a structured environment such as a school or office, there are strict rules and regulations which your Aspie can adhere to, in order to structure their time well. Often without this structure, their deficit in Executive Functioning, can cause problems in being organised enough to achieve their aims.

In a less structured environment, unless the aim in question is also their special interest, anxiety and procrastination can get severely in the way of progress.

Fear can be a great motivator for them to do well and in some cases, if your Aspie can find some resilience to beat their anxieties this helps them to work hard and finish what they started. The fear is often fuelled by someone in authority who also

H

has high expectations of our Aspie. Often if they have delivered good work before, they are expected to repeat this or even improve on it.

Reducing Anxiety

Sometimes your Aspie can feel overwhelmed by the size of the task they have set themselves or have been set. They may have started off enthusiastically but the more work they have done, the more they have realised they had to do. This is often because they cannot see the bigger picture and find it hard to judge the scale of a task.

They may become depressed if they feel it is outside their control or decide to ignore it in the hope that it just goes away.

On the other hand, and this is the opposite to the 'head in the sand approach', they keep working on it day and night, not knowing when they have done enough. Not knowing when to stop. I have had people say to me that they just keep going in the hope that they have covered everything. This behaviour can be quite frantic.

Coping with Disappointment

Whether it just be an Expectation Violation or a major blow, I'm afraid our Aspies don't cope well with disappointment. They feel it so deeply. They have difficulty reacting appropriately to the different levels of disappointment in life.

NT Sometimes it is best just to let them wallow in their own misery and pity. Because they are not so in touch with their own feelings it takes them longer to process their thoughts and bounce back.

They do have coping mechanisms to deal with disappointment which they have nurtured over the years and the most common one is the Special Interest.

Let them indulge some in this as it takes their mind of their disappointment and gives them the serotonin they need to cope. Give them space, patience and encouragement and understanding.

Perhaps at a later date discuss with them what went wrong and if appropriate help them decide whether they should attempt to do it again. Some may lose all interest in the subject but others when they have reviewed the situation will see that they did achieve what was needed or that they were not far off their original goal and that it may be worth having another attempt.

High IQ

Many people with Asperger's Syndrome do have a high IQ but it is not necessary to reach the dizzy heights of Einstein in order to qualify.

I recently found out that genius level is from 130. Reports of Einstein's IQ vary from 152 to 160.

David informs me that when he was tested by a educational psychologist at age eleven, that he had an IQ of 160. He may have remembered this wrongly.

A high intellectual IQ does not mean have you have a high Emotional Quotient nor any common sense. Most 'normal' people have a good mix of all three.

Hobbies

A hobby for an Aspie can quickly turn into an all-consuming obsession. Most people like to have a hobby to enable them to relax and think of something less serious that isn't work.

An Aspie takes this to the extreme and may indeed extend the hobby to unreasonable lengths, letting it interfere with his work or stopping him from working at all.

The reason they do this is the same as everyone else, to relax and to let their brain do something it enjoys that is not stressful. The difference is that they use it to shield them from the rest of the world. They know they have problems and jobs that need doing, but it gives them an excuse not to do it. It is their way of burying their head in the sand, often in the hope that if they do so for long enough, the problem will go away or someone else will fix it for them.

The Husband Says:

Hobbies turn out to be a bit obsessional for us Aspies. If (like me) you have a hobby of watching pulp-TV, then you can't just watch the one episode - no, it has to be the whole season, then the season after that, then the last season where the show really "jumped the shark" and everyone acknowledges is awful. Like Pokémon, you just have to collect them all.

Hobbies, to me, seem to be about sorting, sifting, cataloguing and curating. Like putting the music collection in alphabetical order on the shelf (when we used CDs) or trying to persuade Microsoft Media Player that albums by "The Beatles" should be grouped beside albums by "Beatles" on the PC.

Now this obsessional behaviour can be a power for good - if a hobby coincides with something that is actually needed - like if your job in IT coincides with a hobby of computing, then all might be well. Likewise, DIY - the compulsion will be a force to complete and finish the activity - the danger is that us Aspies see every flaw so nearly finished or nearly good enough is not actually fully complete.

On that last completer-finisher note, us Aspies often go looking for NT "approval" that the job is done. We can see the flaws and the things that aren't complete but, if you NTs can't see the mistakes, this might give us comfort to stop.

H

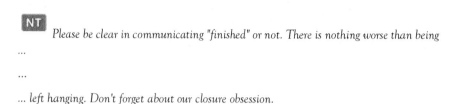

Please be clear in communicating "finished" or not. There is nothing worse than being

...

...

... left hanging. Don't forget about our closure obsession.

Holidays

Until recently family holidays have been a complete nightmare. On the surface, two weeks in Europe with a villa and a pool sounds idyllic. During those holidays there have been moments of calm, excitement and joy, but the overwhelming memories were the stress, the blame, the tension and the silences. Sitting by the pool with my head in my hands wishing I was anywhere else. Knowing that I had to stay cheerful and calm for the children and get through the next few days until we could get home.

On return I was reluctant to have another family holiday (the children were no problem). I didn't want to put myself through that again.

In the new year, the traditional time to plan our summer holiday I set some rules down. I had never done this before. I thought it would be badly received and yet I think there was relief on his face. Possibly he thought, "At last! Structure and planning!"

The Husband Says:

Got it in one! I like structure and planning. I don't like "holidays" that are spontaneous and exciting and unplanned where I have to be on best behaviour all of the time.

It's bad enough for you NTs if you don't know the language, but bear in mind for me I'm having to work on the "social language" (body language differences) as well as the spoken language.

As an example, we were in France a couple of years ago and went to a tiny restaurant - not a word of English spoken. We thought we had communicated quite well; we were the only diners and we chose the fixed price menu, but none of us realised that we had to serve ourselves with salad as the first course to trigger the rest of the lunch serving process. I would have sat there for hours waiting for service, but Karen had the presence of mind (after quite a while) to go into the kitchen and enquire. That would not have occurred to me - we had followed all the "visible" rules.

Last time, in Rome, was much better than any holiday before. Karen gave me time to figure out how things like metro-line ticket machines worked. And technology has moved on - the city centre mapping in my 'phone was reliable so I felt more "in control" of what was going on around me.

I think I'm probably a bit like other Aspies on holiday. I don't want to sit around a pool doing nothing; but I'm not active and sporty. Going to a museum or reading a book are more my "thing". Just not doing my day-job is holiday enough.

Oh, and I'm in charge of the barbecue.

Holidays with other People

This is like in the "having guests in the house" situation but so many times worse.

We went to Italy a few years ago and my dad came with us. It was possibly the worst week of my married life. David could not relax at all, he blamed me for every little thing that went wrong and he even made up things to go wrong. I couldn't understand why he was like that but in the end he confessed it was because my dad was there. He felt he had to be on his best behaviour all the time and he just couldn't cope with it. In the end he showed my dad his worst and rudest behaviour. I was mortified and very upset. Yet I still had to carry on and help the kids have a great holiday. I came back from that holiday swearing we would never go away again.

 Advice: Don't do it.

The Husband Says:

I'm trying (and failing) to forget two horrible holiday incidents. The first is as Karen recounts above with Karen's dad in Italy. I felt like not only did I have to protect my immediate family, but that I had some duty towards Karen's dad too. Matters really came to a head for me over the Diesel incident: I like using the self-service pumps because I don't have to speak any Italian - just shove card or cash in and off you go. The hire car was running low on fuel and for several days I'd been trying to fill up; the only card I had that reliably worked to pay for holiday meals just didn't work in the fuel pumps. I tried cash, but the pump wouldn't start and it just kept my money. My confidence in buying stuff in Italy just crashed - including buying stuff for us, as an extended family, to eat. I was totally miserable until I plucked up the courage to use a few carefully rehearsed words of Italian to get an attendant to fill up the car and use his credit card machine to complete the transaction. It went through! Relief! I wasn't locked up for trying to steal Diesel!

The other incident continues to embarrass me. We went on holiday with close family friends sharing a villa in Florida. The first week was fine, the second week OK, but then an Icelandic volcano exploded stranding us in Florida with no estimates of when we could fly home. It was the not knowing that drove me bonkers. What better place to get stranded than in Florida? But there's only so much Mickey-Mouse one Aspie can take! And we were running out of money and space on credit cards - this wasn't a package deal. And since it wasn't a package deal, the airline had us at the back of the queue for repatriation flights. I'm self-employed and all this unplanned time away from clients was costing us a fortune - if I'm on holiday, I'm

H

not earning. To top it, all our close friends got a flight home before us. It felt so unfair - I felt like they were almost bragging that they were going home because I couldn't read their facial expressions properly - I was mistaking a relieved expression for something more smug which caused me to flip. In the end though we wound up on the same relief flight, but our friendships were very strained by my behaviour.

So, pleasant as a shared holiday might be for you NTs, Aspies don't share the unexpected nicely, so shared family trips abroad full of surprises and an element of competition are a no-no. Serendipity is fine - like the last night take off of the Space Shuttle whilst we were in Florida, or finding the Haribo museum in France.

Hope

I am aware that by being completely honest on here, at times I can come across as being very negative. I also want you to know there is hope for your marriage.

I have struggled with how much negatively I am writing about at times but, in order for you to understand and relate your situation to my own, I have to be completely honest. I would not be writing this help guide if I had not been to the pits of despair and managed to claw my way back again.

I want you to come away with growing empathy, understanding and hope for your marriage and your husband's situation.

By taking on board many of my tips you CAN, with time and patience, improve your marriage and maybe even rediscover the man you loved and married in the first place.

I lost "My David" for a while but he is coming back to me now.

The Husband Says:

It's hard to write these articles in such a short space of time. They involve delving into a murky past; hardly pleasant. But Karen is one hundred percent right - all this introverted analysis is having the effect of making me review my behaviour (innate, learned and self-taught). There is, indeed, hope. And lots of it.

I wonder if it would be good for Aspies to keep a diary or journal and review it from time to time. That way you can see how the coping strategies develop with honest feedback from a partner, and how life just gets better and better. After all, this project was spawned by Karen's insight from her reflective journal. Keeping it modern - why not write a blog - private or, if you are brave, public? I'm finding this cathartic; you might too.

H

How to Initiate Sex

If you want to have an intimate and enjoyable time with your wife after the initial excitement of new love has worn off and you have settled down into the everyday humdrum of work, household chores and kids, it can be difficult to find the time and the right moment.

You need to take into account that everyone has a different libido which means that though they enjoy sex, the frequency of how much people need varies very much from person to person. It also depends upon how healthy, stressed or what responsibilities are on that person at that time.

For example, after the birth of a baby your wife will naturally put the needs of your helpless infant first and in order to do this she also needs to put her own needs second. These are mainly to eat and sleep until the baby is older and into a routine. The fact your wife is paying you less attention is only natural and is not to be taken personally. Your wife will also most likely be conscious of her less than toned body after having given birth recently and she may not feel confident enough about herself to want or to initiate sex. Try and be sensitive towards her body conscious feelings. You may still she is as sexy as ever in which case it would do not harm to remind her of this.

Tips on Attracting your Wife

- Hygiene is very important here. Make sure you brush your teeth regularly and shower every day. If your wife is not keen on stubble you should try for a smooth shave. You will be surprised at what puts a woman off.

- Make sure you will not be disturbed. Your wife will not relax if she thinks the neighbours will hear or the kids are about to wake up.

- Appearance is also important to your wife. She won't mind you putting on a little weight but an overhanging beer belly is not attractive and cannot be hidden just by buying larger clothes. A man who looks after himself is attractive in more ways than one. In the same way, make sure you get your hair cut regularly and washed.

- Compliment her.

- Tell her you love her. They like to be told more than once in a marriage even if your feelings haven't changed.

- Choose your words carefully and in advance. Make sure you are not issuing a back handed compliment.

- Arrange a break away with jut the two of you with the kids looked after by someone your wife trusts if they are still young. She will appreciate the time you have spent organising it for her. Do not go beyond your budget.

What Not to Do

- Do not just stare at your wife in the vain hope that she will notice and take pity on you. Women don't actually enjoy pity sex. They want their man to take the initiative. If she is ignoring you doing this it is not because she hasn't noticed. She knows what you want but either she is too busy, to tired or just not turned on by your helplessness.

- Just because she is your wife you should never take her for granted.

- Don't come home drunk and demand sex.

- Do not try and initiate sex when she is preparing a meal with a sharp knife. This is dangerous.

- If you suggest a nice massage for her do not assume this will turn into sex. Let her know this is what you want. Don't surprise her. If she initiates it than great.

- Never assume that just because you want sex that she will.

Hugs

NT
There is good evidence and plenty of research that tells us that hugs are good for us. They raise our serotonin levels, make us feel wanted and happy. Of course, being Aspie men, our husbands like to take things to extremes. They are either very keen on something or completely avoid it.

If your husband is a hugger, make the most of it. Try not to reject him when he offers a hug. He may well take it to heart, even if you are really busy. Remember they think in black and white and not in grey areas. They won't necessarily understand about 'the right time'.

What is mostly complained about in Asperger marriages is a lack of physical contact.

In this case, it is worth explaining to your partner that you would really appreciate a hug every now and then. If you let him know that the physical contact makes you feel wanted and connected with him, and that it makes you like him more, he may well be willing to do this for you. Try and leave the emotion out of it. Ask him for regular hug contact, depending on how he feels about it, once a day or once a week. He may even start to enjoy it himself.

The Husband Says:

Hugs are a tricky area on (at least) two counts. There's the whole sensory thing, and for me, hugs are good - but not every Aspie's hot beverage of choice. But the other thing is the social acceptability and social norms thing. I don't think any Aspie likes public displays of affection - the "rules" are really complicated here with even NTs finding it difficult to measure what level of near-intimacy is allowed in public.

Now perhaps the way to break open any Aspie-hug-stigma is to get some Italian blooded friends. The expected social norm here is big hugs, not shaking hands. Thanks Paulo, Maria and Gwyn.

Humour

There is a very common misconception that people on the spectrum do not have a sense of humour. They can sometimes have a different sense of humour, or a very dry, witty humour but I have not come across someone who has no sense of humour at all. One of the reasons I married David was because we could make each other laugh and we still do. It is difficult to have a marriage without being able to laugh at life. What marriage can survive without a shared sense of humour?

Perhaps the reason for the misconception is that when one is feeling anxious it is very difficult to see the funny side of things. Thinking back to when I have felt particularly anxious, just before singing a solo at a concert for example, I pretty much have a sense of humour failure.

I have noted he is not generally a fan of shows where he has to work hard to recognise more subtle humour such as impressionists or everyday sitcoms which are often setup around unspoken social rules. These are neither relaxing or amusing for him to watch.

Our daughter, who is a chip off the old block, is a very literal thinker. I don't know if David was like this when he was younger, but her grasp of comedy is very slowly evolving. She has to explain her jokes to me and I often have to explain jokes to her. She loves puns though. They are very punny.

Favourite Humour

- We have a shared love of the American sitcom, The Big Bang Theory though I think for very different reasons. David describes it as a documentary and empathise very much with Sheldon.

- The Last Leg

- Word play; puns; Sorry I Haven't Got a Clue; Tim Vine; Ronnie Barker

- Observational humour: Jason Manford, Michael McIntyre, Alan Davies

- Quirky Humour: Bill Bailey, Eddie Izzard, Monty Python - David is, of course, word perfect on Python and even holds the scripts of all the sketches.

- High Brow Humour: We also enjoy topical and satirical shows such as Have I Got News for you where the panellists are highly intelligent and quick witted, and Stephen Fry as host of QI.

Q: What's brown and sticky?

A: A stick.

However, their humour isn't always funny or intentional.

The Husband Says:

They call impressionists "comedy" or "entertainment". I don't agree. All I can see is that they get the impression wrong; the things they have the characters say are trite; the entertainment is meant to be in the performance, but I like the real thing with real words to say.

Some situational comedy works for me, but very little of it. The humour has to be quite refined or extremely dark for it to chime. Thus "Father Ted" or "Mrs. Brown's Boys" falls flat, but the pinnacle of that art for me is "Black Books".

Hygiene

This is one of those ASD areas where they are either "Hypo" or "Hyper". As in they have no interest in their appearance and cleanliness or they are completely obsessed with it to the point where it can affect their daily lives. This often leads to the Co-morbidity of OCD.

There is a general stereotype of geeks and nerds with unwashed hair and bad clothes. Well there is some truth in this. With their social difficulties it does not occur to them that it is offensive to others if you do not wash.

The Husband Says:

Another delicate subject. As an Aspie, I have a general failing to prioritise hygiene highly enough. Work and clients require me to be clean and tidy but at home this seems less relevant - I prioritise, and there is a level of avoidance.

Why is hygiene avoided? Well there are some deep sensory impacts in performing one's ablutions. There's lots of hypersensitivity issues related to tooth-brushing (it REALLY tickles my gums, and I'm convinced all my teeth wobble and are always on the point of falling out) and hair-cutting (the tugging of my hair and pressing on my scalp). Everywhere you look on the human body where hygiene is important, it's a bit intimate and squelchy.

But having a partner is a long way towards a cure for these problems. Karen is careful to encourage day to day husbandly hygiene, suggesting when I need a haircut and reminding on the keeping of dentists appointments. Karen has even taken the lead and explained my sensory issues to our dentist which has in itself gone a long way to relieving my anxiety. I have become more well-drilled on the social conventions of getting a haircut and dental inspection.

Hyper/Hypo

This is in relation to the extremes of sensory issues. Hyper is when you are over-sensitive to stimuli. Hypo is when you are under-sensitive to stimuli. This is often connected to the dysfunction of the vestibular system.

Hypermobility

Hypermobility Syndrome or HMS is occasionally comorbid with autism and Asperger's Syndrome. Most people with AS can use this to their advantage but others can end up in a lot of pain from it.

I suspect that supplementing with Vitamin D3 will help considerably.

The Husband Says:

Weird.

This must be some kind of freaky coincidence - I can see no reason why my "different" brain processing should result in being more bendy than most people. But I am - my fingers bend backwards more than most NTs and my ankle joints are prone to twisting in unintended directions and sprains. I may be mildly dyspraxic, but I'm also ambidextrous. What a jigsaw puzzle of symptoms!

H

- ✦ Identity
- ✦ If he's Happy, I'm Happy
- ✦ If it's any Consolation...
- ✦ Illness
- ✦ Inanimate Objects
- ✦ Indirect Influence
- ✦ Infidelity
- ✦ Inflammation
- ✦ Injustice
- ✦ Insensitive
- ✦ Instincts
- ✦ Intent
- ✦ Interruptions
- ✦ Intimacy
- ✦ Intolerances
- ✦ Intolerance of Uncertainty

- ✦ Intonation
- ✦ Intuition
- ✦ Invisible
- ✦ Invisible Disability
- ✦ Invitations
- ✦ In touch with Feelings
- ✦ Irrationality
- ✦ Irrelevancies
- ✦ Is There a Cure?
- ✦ It only has to happen once to become the norm
- ✦ It's not all Rainbows and Unicorns
- ✦ It's the Little Things
- ✦ I am only Human
- ✦ I didn't Sign up for This

I am only Human

Even though I am armed with years of experience of being an Asperger wife, mother and daughter, and have this experience reinforced educationally by my Master's degree in Autism, there are days when I get it completely wrong or I get to the end of my tether.

I am only human.

On occasion, I will lose my temper with him. On occasion, I am tired and feel that I just don't care. On occasion, I have had enough. On occasion, I just have to get away.

I am not infallible. I make mistakes. I often have these mistakes pointed out to me by my Aspie family. Sometimes, depending what mood I am in, I shall laugh it off and other times I just have to grit my teeth. I am able to forgive myself my weaknesses. I know I am strong most of the time but I am not superhuman. I get tired, overworked and hormonal. Some weeks are easier to handle than others. I do not beat myself up over my failures. I just pick myself up, learn from my mistakes and carry on.

I Didn't Sign up for This

It isn't all bad or I wouldn't be here writing this self help guide. I could have gone and found a different type of life (I can't say it would have been "better" as life is full of unpredictable trials and tribulations).

I have a picture of my mum and dad signing the register on their wedding day. In 1967, they made a beautiful couple. My mum was 21 and had just finished her degree and my dad was 24 and had just started on his doctorate.

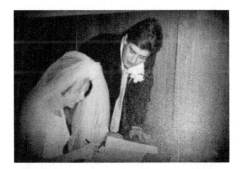

I'm sure they had a very similar marriage to David and I. There they are signing the register. He had her. He had a piece of paper to prove it. I sent my dad that picture and another one of them standing outside the church. He sent me a text back saying 'Just looking at the photos you sent me. Pretty little thing your mum wasn't she. Perhaps I can be forgiven for looking smug!'

I think he can too.

However, that ritual signing of the register, whether consciously or unconsciously, signalled to my dad that he had got his prize, he had won and maybe he didn't have to work quite so hard at wooing her any more. He could slip into his true personality. Become the curmudgeon he naturally was when he wanted to be.

So actually, my mum and I did sign up for it. We have witnesses and pieces of legal documents to prove it. We made our vows in churches full of friends and family. Not only did we declare our love for our men, we signed ourselves over and we just thought it was a ritual - one that the meaning had been lost in the mists of tradition. Not to our husband's it hadn't.

The Husband Says:

It's interesting that you get onto the subject of a marriage contract. As part of my profession I do a lot of contract management. One of the key things you do before entering into a contract is a due diligence activity where you check that the promises made by the other party are true. You might even go as far as to get written warranties.

So I suppose that courtship allows partners to do their due diligence. Perhaps it's just a shame that the traditional and standard marriage contract doesn't include clauses for warranties. Pre-nuptial anybody?

Identity

Many people with autism struggle to know who they are. They struggle to recognise their emotions and they struggle to make choices and decisions. Therefore, when you think about it, it is not surprising that many of them struggle with their own identity.

As NT's we often develop strong personalities early on and, as young children, often decided what career we would like to have as an adult. This normally changes and develops with experience which we use to help us develop a sense of identity as well as learning to understand and like ourselves.

Our Aspies swing from self-hate (often the source of meltdowns) to complete arrogance. There is little in between. It is hard to know exactly who you are when you are constantly going through those extreme emotions.

When asked to make decisions they find it difficult because they feel they have to analyse everything in fine detail before they give an answer. We NTs may find them slow to respond to a question and thus assume they don't have an answer; this can often result in us answering for them. Sometimes they don't answer because they are too shy or they really just don't know.

Our son recently signed up for sixth form college and we went along with him for a computer 'health check' where he had to meet the course tutor and show an initial understanding of what he was getting into. Our son was very quiet and, though he was listening avidly, did not really show any outward sign of this. Everything was so new and daunting to him.

The tutor tried to engage with him and asked him which area of computing he would like to specialise in at university. Morgan again kept quiet. I wasn't sure of the exact reason why but eventually as the silence stretched I felt the NT urge to answer for him. I hate doing this as I really want him to answer for himself but he often looks to me for answers. I don't want the teachers thinking I am putting ideas in his head. I hope what I am doing is interpreting for him. So I spoke up and said that I knew he had a particular interest in Ethical Hacking. This seemed to be a good answer for the tutor and also for Morgan as, if he didn't like my answer, I'm sure he would have let me know somehow.

I know once he settles into college and starts enjoying his course and builds up a relationship with his tutor, that he will come out of his shell and vocalise his own ideas, and hopefully produce some excellent work. In the meantime, as his mother and the person who understands him most in the world, I am there to help him shape his identity.

Having said all that, I know my son has a very strong online presence. He has a good understanding of all things gaming, resulting in him currently having more of a virtual identity! This is where he and millions of other Aspies are most comfortable.

The Husband Says:

It's not that we don't have a strong identity, it's just that what you consider to be conventional identity traits are spread over our multiple personalities where we choose which one we are using for what purpose. It's too much work to have each of these personalities fully populated with a complete set of identity, so we put in only enough for each personality to function.

Our identity is the sum of each of those personalities and the logic we use to choose among them.

If he's Happy, I'm Happy

David's moods can affect the whole household. There is no escaping it, whether he is on a high or a low. When things are good, they are very, very good and when they are not, they are terrible.

The happy, positive side of his personality is very attractive and the reason I fell for him. He can't do enough for me or for anyone else he cares about. He is charming and witty and chatty and fun. I get sucked into his "high" and life seems good.

The Down Side

The moment his mood changes though, it is all pervasive and again the whole house feels it. There is no getting away from it. Everything that can go wrong, goes wrong. Every person has something against him and nothing is ever going to be right again.

These days I try not to get sucked into this maelstrom of emotion but it is still hard. If I walk away he thinks that I am cross with him as he cannot understand that I am just trying to preserve my own sanity.

These extremes in moods have caused problems when psychologists who are not experts in autism and Asperger's Syndrome have misdiagnosed Aspie mood swings as Bi-Polar Disorder.

If it's any Consolation...

His behaviour is truthful and consistent:

- He wouldn't have married you if he didn't love you.

- He trusts you enough to stop faking it and show you his real self.

- He is probably madder with himself right now than you are.

- When he is charming to others and not to you, it is because he is scared what others think of him, whereas he knows you love him because you have told him.

Illness

We've all heard of man flu but Aspies tend to either be hypochondriacs or will ignore any pain and carry on, often in denial.

Low Pain Tolerance

Like most things with your Aspie, there is no moderation; hyper or hypo. Pain is either excruciating or non-existent. Either way it is hard to know how to treat them.

When my son was little he would regularly fall over and he would scream. Usually it was just a graze that I would deal with easily and lots of cuddles calmed him down. With a small child, you tolerate these instances and don't think they are unusual.

One day he fell out of my sight but I heard the screams and it sounded like he was being murdered. He came running towards me with his face covered in blood and I was horrified thinking that he had broken his nose. The screaming went on for ever and I was scared. Once I had cleaned him up, I realised it was just a nosebleed and he was fine. They cannot gauge how badly they have hurt themselves and all "bad" is bad and unbearable. Our son gets this from his dad. The amount of times David has stubbed his toe but acted as though he was crippled for life. At first I was sympathetic, but over the years I have found myself walking away. No sympathy I can offer helps and he can be very hard to handle and abusive. It is distressing for me too.

High Pain Tolerance

Our daughter on the other hand must be hypo-sensitive to pain. She does feel it but she really plays it down. This is just as dangerous as it is hard to judge how badly she is actually hurt. She ended up in hospital as a baby as she did not cry even though she had an obstructed bowel and must have been in a lot of pain. It was wrongly diagnosed and we nearly lost her.

I have heard of instances of children on the spectrum who complain about a "bit of tummy ache" but end up in hospital with a burst appendix! Such a scenario would be even more likely if the mother was away and the father, also on the spectrum, had no empathy.

Hypochondria

I'm pretty sure I'm not a hypochondriac. The only time in my life I've enjoyed being ill was to get time off school. Since then it's usually quite an inconvenience. I'm not one for taking pills for everything either. If I have a headache I see it as a sign that something is wrong and I should do something about it. Generally, it will mean I'm tired or dehydrated or hungry or tense. My body is telling me to stop and take care of it. Only when I feel a migraine approach with the flashing lights do I immediately take some ibuprofen and go and have a lie down in a darkened room if I can. Sometimes it isn't possible and I get some water from somewhere and sit quietly in the car with my eyes closed until it has gone.

I don't particularly consider myself to be stoical or have a high pain threshold, and I am a complete wuss about touching hot things (though this mainly stems back to a bad burn injury when I was eight and I screamed the waiting room of Cardiff Royal Infirmary down for an hour or more).

David, on the other hand, carries around a vast supply of throat soothing sweets, Paracetamol, Ibuprofen and sinus treatments. He will pop any of these at the first sign of a headache, ache or cough. He will tell me all about it in great detail and give me regular updates on how he is doing. He will stop work and hide if at all possible. He is best left alone for both our sakes.

Coping with your illness

Unless he can hear me vomiting, or sneezing and constantly blowing my nose, he has no idea that I might be ill. Early in our marriage, I just assumed he knew I was ill but that he wasn't bothered / didn't care.

Even now, if I tell him that I feel ill he will immediately tell me that he feels poorly, even if he showed no signs or symptoms before.

I don't think he is doing it for attention, I genuinely think he believes he is ill or that he is empathising with me. However, like in the reciprocation chapter, expecting much sympathy is like getting a hug from a brick wall.

There are a couple of possible reasons for this:

Like with his inability to know when he needs the toilet, he cannot tell whether he is feeling poorly or not. He finds it hard to assess how he feels. Perhaps he is just a little tired or grumpy (pretty normal for an Aspie) but, since you are his barometer in so many ways, perhaps if you are ill then he may have it too?

Of course, if you have a broken arm or, God forbid, breast cancer, then of course he cannot feel like that. In fact, it is probably easier for him to deal with in some ways as it is clear cut. He does not have a broken arm. He does not have breast cancer.

Will this make him more sympathetic and look after you more?

Well, I broke my elbow out on a dog walk one morning. I hadn't realised what I had done at first but when my friend came around to visit and saw how pale I was looking she took me to casualty. Once I had been x-rayed and the break was confirmed, I texted my husband. When he arrived home from work that evening we discussed what had happened and how inconvenient it was. I don't remember getting any hugs or him asking what he could do for me. I do distinctly remember he made me a cup of coffee. Why do I remember that? Because it was the only cup of coffee I got in the whole six weeks of healing time.

I am a resilient independent person, perhaps this is my downfall, but I don't like to just sit and be waited on, (perhaps this makes me the perfect wife for an Aspie?) so I quickly made myself a cup of coffee with just one arm. It isn't too difficult it just takes a little longer, and of course, I didn't just make one for myself. He got his usual cup. In retrospect, this was a big mistake as I proved to him to that nothing had changed. Situation normal. He didn't offer to walk the dog for me. I knew that, even if he did it for the first few days to help out, I couldn't expect him to stay off work to look after me. The dog still had to be walked and the children still had to be fed and sent off to school. I got on and did it.

I wonder what would have happened if I had taken it easy and just left him to it?

I

NT

So, how should a person with a more open personality deal with being ill in an Asperger Marriage? I believe you should gear it something like this:

- Tell them you are ill

- Tell them exactly what is wrong with you

- Tell them what you can't do

- Ask them for help in doing the things you can't do

- Tell them how to do the things you need help with

- Tell them they need to keep helping until you consider that you are better

In hindsight, I probably only told David the first two of those points. I didn't really ask him for help after that, so why was I surprised that I got little or no help?

We NT wives have a particular type of disease which our husbands do not. It is called Assumption. We make the natural mistake of assuming he will know what to do or that he knows what you are thinking. He doesn't.

At the time this freak event occurred in our marriage (though it was only four years ago) I did not have my mantra of 'never assume'. Never assume that he knows what you want. Never assume that he can see the obvious. To an AS man the obvious is not obvious. He does not have your perspective.

The Husband Says:

NT

Can I echo the bullet points above. Make it absolutely clear by means of command that you are not well and must be not only helped, but replaced in the household function for the time period it takes for you to get better. NO AMBIGUITY.

These will be stressful times since your Aspie is ill equipped to look after everyone's needs - after all he can barely manage his own without your help. Take heart though that you will get better and a disaster area of a house is transient. The family is resilient and will survive on one-pan-meals or takeaways for a few days.

Inanimate Objects

Most Asperger men are not violent but you may have been disturbed when seeing them fly into a physical rage with an inanimate object.

If something goes wrong with the object they never fail to take it personally. David tells me the printer is peril sensitive. It always fails when he has a tight deadline.

This failure may just be lack of paper which is easily resolved, even if it takes a fair amount of swearing to put it right.

I have witnessed pieces fly off the computer when he has been in a rage. To David this is not an object without thoughts and feelings but one that despite it supposedly being there to help him, its whole existence is to spite him and cause him distress. The PC, or particularly the new Apple Mac know when he is stressed and delight in making things worse for him by deleting files or just crashing.

I always used to think it was just a running joke and despite Aspies being logical thinkers they can at times be extremely superstitious.

I believe David is reflecting his negative thoughts onto the offending object. We all need to get our frustrations out. I do tend to shout at the dog a little bit, rather than at anyone else and I think David probably feels it is safe to take his anger out on the computer or printer as it can't' retaliate and he would never be violent with me. It's also easier to blame something else for making things go wrong rather than your own fallible humanity.

In Touch with Feelings

As a NT you are most likely aware of your feelings even if you are not always in control of them. Desire and fear are literally gut feelings and emanate from the same place in your 'second brain'. You can tell the difference between these two diverse emotions, yet many on the spectrum cannot.

Often times their feelings come as a great surprise to them. Many are so curious about these feelings they will educate themselves to top psychologists.

Indirect Influence

David has occasionally admitted over the years that meeting me was a good thing. I encouraged and supported him and talked him through his fears and decisions when he was not brave enough to take the leap. My faith in his ability gave him confidence. I would describe that as direct influence.

Sometimes when I try to directly influence him (or nag as it has been called) he resists and fights back. These days I try more to discuss options with him and let him come to his own decisions, using me as a sounding board.

Indirect influence is a little more complex but actually can be much more affective.

For example, I was experimenting by writing out a Social Story and I created a scenario of a genuine issue in our relationship that I have not been able to fix. It was about the little things in life, the small gestures that makes a reciprocal relationship work. I drew some stick figures and a kettle and some mugs and made up a simple story about how making two cups of coffee, instead of one, makes your wife happy. The point of the actual exercise was to see whether I could with my very limited artistic skills draw something that would work. I showed David what I had produced. He seemed to think it was passable.

However, this scenario must have played on his mind.... in the morning I received an unsolicited cup of coffee in bed. It was a nice surprise. It was a one off situation, but I enjoyed it for what it was.

One of the interesting issues that arises here is that the way an Aspie is given directions and instructions can impact on their response. They like to be in control and make up their own mind about when they are going to do things. Being told what to do is not attractive to them but, when asked nicely if they could do something, they generally don't mind. Take that a step further and they will actually enjoy surprising someone by showing them they can do something well without being asked. However, don't expect a repeat of this any time soon. Proving he can do something once doesn't mean he will do it on a regular basis (or ever again).

Infidelity

What happens in a marriage to make people unfaithful or to just look elsewhere?

An Asperger Marriage can be a very lonely place to be. Some women have turned elsewhere just for some love and attention, whilst still staying in the confines of their marriage.

I can't see how that is healthy but perhaps, if both partners were in agreement, it could work.

For my part, I would not accept any form of infidelity from David and I wouldn't expect him to either. Trust is very important and, though we have been in despair at times, the one light has been that he has not been unfaithful to me. He knows I wouldn't put up with it and that would be the end of the marriage.

After all what would be left? Why would I put in all this hard work if there was no firm foundation?

The Husband Says:

I wouldn't even dream about being unfaithful to Karen. I might lose her. Not even the so-called "window shopping".

This can lead to tricky conversations - the type where everyone comes out unhappy and unfulfilled - for example: We can be watching TV and Karen might ask "Do you like Davina McColl?". Now I find Davina extremely attractive, and she comes across as witty and intelligent, so the straightforward and truthful answer is "Yes". But my Aspie mind has the conversation going into the direction of "Would you be unfaithful to me for Davina?" The answer is of course "No", but this territory is full of traps. I'm clearly attracted to this public figure. Our paths would never cross so the opportunity would never arise that I could actually be unfaithful to Karen with Davina. Nonetheless, even the thought that Karen might consider I could be unfaithful, is scary to the point that a simple and innocent conversation has to be closed down as soon as practical, preferably without alerting Karen to the fact that I am uncomfortable! Her examination of the reasons for my anxiety could lead directly to the one thing I'm trying to avoid - the discussion of infidelity.

What a tangled life us Aspies lead.

Inflammation

Research is very much ongoing in this area but it is thought that people on the autistic spectrum are more susceptible to food allergies.

Inflammation is an auto immune response that is meant to protect your body from attack by toxins. This causes swelling and pain in joints, migraines, IBS and mood swings.

Injustice

Your Aspie partner will most likely have strong feelings about injustice, especially if it is aimed at themselves. They may be very vocal about it or withdraw into themselves entirely, not knowing what to do about it. Someone wasn't following the rules and this has upset their equilibrium.

The Husband Says:

Here's another example of how us Aspies are black-and-white type people with no shades of grey. Justice and injustice go hand in hand; justice is meant to be moral and unambiguous - so injustice is exactly the opposite - illogical and improper.

I wonder if many in the legal profession are closet Aspies. Especially the high court judges that have to rule one way or another on a complex case.

Insensitive

My Aspie family likes its routines, Chinese takeaway on a Friday night and Scotch pancakes on the griddle on a Saturday morning always go down well.

Recently, my twelve-year-old daughter was seeing an Occupational Therapist and one of the topics that came up was "helping out around the house". My daughter admitted she didn't do much to help me and that perhaps she should. So the following Saturday morning I asked her if she wanted to help me with the pancakes. She loves my pancakes, and she does like cooking, so she jumped up and said she would. I had to do a little bit of supervision but mostly let her get on with it whilst I set the table, made the coffee and hot chocolate, sorted out the vitamins and juices to wash them down and so on. After several attempts I managed to get my sixteen-year-old out of bed and dragged David from his computer screen to come and sit at the table.

Our daughter was complimented on her pancakes and how evenly cooked they were. I commented that she only had the pancakes to concentrate on whilst I normally did everything at once, resulting in my pancakes coming out rather random and occasionally burned.

David then turned to me and said "I don't know why you bother multi-tasking as you are so bad at it."

I was left there open-mouthed and hurt while he giggled at how amusing he had been. He has no concept of how hard I work behind the scenes. His philosophy seems to be, if you can't do it perfectly, don't do it at all.

My defence, which I didn't bother to vocalise, is that if I didn't anything multi-task, nothing would get done and no one would get anything to eat!

However, I decided to take a deep breath and let it go. Look on the bright side it has given me more material for this App.

NT The thing is, in days gone by I would have retaliated as I am not a personality to be trampled on. I would have got cross and shouted but then it would have ruined everyone's day. It is better for me to smile sweetly sometimes and let it go.

Why? You may ask. Because I know that he isn't being malicious. He thought it was humorous. It wasn't big and it wasn't clever, but it was really nasty. Not worth getting het up about. He's just naturally insensitive.

Instincts

As neurotypicals, we are generally intuitive and trust our instincts. We don't even have to think about it when we meet someone in the street. We immediately size up whether we recognise them, what social class they are from, whether we like them, what mood they are in and whether they are happy to see us.

How do we do this? We use our wealth of knowledge stored in our brain - that which has been gathered as we have grown and learned about the world around us.

As babies we quickly learn to smile back at our parents, knowing it makes them happy and that therefore smiling is an indication of happiness.

We are not aware of these thought processes when we greet an acquaintance, we just think, "Oh no, it's that annoying neighbour again and he looks grumpy", for example.

Our partners, however, do not have this ability. They have learned over time to look out for information that signals whether they recognise someone, but they have to go through the thought processes one by one before coming to a conclusion and even then they are not sure whether they are right.

For example, recently, David encountered our local female vicar whilst getting into the car. She doesn't live in our street so he wasn't expecting to see her there. He doesn't go to church but I do, so he knows who she is whilst not being familiar enough with her to talk easily. As convention dictates, he said "Hello" (as it would be rude to ignore your vicar) but after that he was completely stumped. This was to the extent that, when I got into the car, he was notably flustered and it affected his driving for quite some time. I'm not sure if he was cross with himself or just flummoxed by a simple social situation. The main problem was that it was unexpected.

The Husband Says:

Just because I'm a bit "blind" to emotions and facial expression doesn't mean that all of what you NTs consider to be instincts are broken. I still have a "gut feel" for right and wrong, especially in technical and creative fields - I have never learned music but I instinctively know if an in instrument is out of tune. So instincts must fall into several classes and I'm just wired up a bit wrongly for some of them.

Intent

To intend to do something, you have to plan and be aware of the consequences of your actions and how these will affect other people.

Autism is a condition which causes a deficit in Theory of Mind or Empathy. This means you are less aware how your actions will impact on others as you assume they share the same perspective as you.

Therefore, if your husband lashes out verbally at you it may seem that his intent was to hurt your feelings but it may be he was reacting to other circumstances beyond his control.

I

Interruptions

I hate having to interrupt him. I try and time it exactly right and wait for a natural pause in his work or a glance to see whether he's on Facebook or not. Usually he is deep in thought and absolutely hates having his train of thought broken. Is it harder for Aspies to recollect their thoughts?

Either way, regardless of what it, is I am not in favour when I interrupt him. I quite often place his food in front of him or otherwise he would not eat. Sometimes that is ignored as well. I hate it as it makes me feel inferior, as if I'm the little 1950's wife wearing a pinny and making sure her lipstick is on right. Keeping the peace can be demeaning and it does not put me in a good mood.

The Husband Says:

Quite a number of times we have joked about the idea of a little flag-pole on the corner of my desk so that I can run up a little flag saying "Available" or "Busy". I have this excuse that I often work from home, so some of my time is automatically designated "busy, working, productive, earning". But this is often an excuse for what I think is a common Aspie male thinking pattern:

Us Aspies like to put things in order so that there is a clear beginning, middle and end, with a clear single path passing through them all. We are single task focussed and terrible multi-taskers. We hate the context switch time necessary to swap from task to task. We like to see things closed and finished. We can be self-absorbed ignoring the passage of time and neglecting basic human functions like drinking, eating and hygiene.

It is actually good for me to be interrupted; to take a break. On customer's premises it is good to be interrupted to ask if I want a cup of coffee, otherwise I would remain glued to the computer screen.

So interrupt, it is the right and proper thing to do, but perhaps ask for a summary of what I'm working on or thinking about whilst offering coffee and biscuits. Be prepared for the first few seconds to be gruff and unthankful, but I'll get over it. It might also take up to perhaps half a minute for me to acknowledge your well-meaning interruption, whilst I "park" what I'm thinking about in a state that I can return to it easily. I'm juggling lots of things in my head so this takes time.

Here's a metaphor. My thought processes are like the circus act with the plates on top of the slender rods. In time, the spinning plates slow down and fall off, but a quick flick of the rod can speed the plate back up again. I've got lots of thoughts in my head at any time - all plates on sticks. When you interrupt me, I need to dash around all of the plates, give them all a quick spin up to full speed and then I know that I can listen to your "interruption" and when I come back to my plates they will all still be spinning - perhaps slowly, but will not have fallen off their sticks.

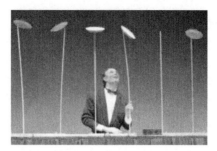

Intimacy

Intimacy is about letting someone in to your life. It is about trust and not just about letting someone touch you or having sex with them. Intimacy is about so much more.

Not every AS/NT couple have problems with this, but I have come across quite a few that do.

Part of the problem is that the AS man is happy with the status quo and the level of intimacy, which might just be sharing a house or a bedroom, is enough for them. Some do not even have the need for sex and view it, quite literally, as a way of mating and having children, though these men are in the minority.

What is missing in their marriage is reciprocation. The woman craves it desperately. David is fairly accepting of my hugs for example but I do have to time them right. He doesn't appreciate them if they distract him from a vital piece of work. He has complained, when I have kissed him on the cheek whilst walking past, that my kiss was "too noisy".

When these things first start to happen, as a young wife, you cannot help but see it as rejection. Even though they are tiny instances, they are like little paper cuts to the heart.

Not knowing or not having a firm diagnosis can be so damaging to a relationship. These days, knowing helps. I can sometimes laugh such instances off as I know it isn't personal, even when it feels personal. Of course, it is not allowed to go the other way. Any rejection from me is taken very personally on David's part. I have to be so careful in what I say and what I do.

Suggested Strategies

  Some suggestions for both of you:

- Talk about needs
- Talk about limits

- Massage
- Set aside clear time for intimacy

The Husband Says:

I think that intimacy on NT terms requires a level of spontaneity, and spontaneity is the one thing that doesn't fit well with coping strategies based around planning.

I'm beginning to wonder if, as part of our Aspie social blindness (manifested in me as difficulty with detecting mood in my partner), that perhaps we don't communicate our own mood state outwardly in the way that NTs would expect to "receive" subconsciously. With intimacy so dependent on mood, perhaps that's why it might be difficult to kindle intimacy - neither of us is clear that the other is "in the mood"? So we give it a go and sometimes it works and sometimes it doesn't.

Intolerance of Uncertainty

Though everyone, NT or AS, suffers from varying levels of anxiety, the intolerance of uncertainty is owned by our loved ones with ASD.

If allowed to get out of hand it can rule or even ruin their life and can be quite disabling.

Uncertainty is something we all experience from time to time, and this lack of knowledge of what is about to happen makes us nervous. We feel reluctant to do something or we get butterflies in our tummy.

Yet we know from experience as adults, the best way to deal with uncertainty is to face it head on.

Now your Aspie partner may agree with you here in principle, but they find uncertainty extremely hard to cope with and will do their best to avoid unknown situations.

Uncertainty makes them grumpy and tired and can eventually lead to a meltdown. But why does it affect them like this?

It is often said that those on the autistic spectrum do not learn from their mistakes, and to a certain extent this is true. It can seem like they do not learn from past experience. Generally, they do not make the same mistake twice if the situations to avoid are very similar but, what they cannot do, is situational transference. Which means that, unlike us NTs, they have difficulty using past knowledge and experience to apply to a new situation. They are unable to predict what is going to happen. This is something that we do naturally with barely a thought.

It is quite scary going to new unpredictable situations on a regular basis. The Aspie will decide it is better to avoid the social gathering or job interview as they cannot cope with the anxiety brought on by the uncertainty.

Intolerances

Nobody quite knows why intolerances are becoming more prevalent these days. Some claim it is pesticides or a lack of nutrients. Others claim it is vitamin D3 deficiency.

All I know is that for some years now the ASD society have been talking about the difference that diet makes to autistic health and behaviour.

There are many food substances which people are intolerant to but the main ones are Gluten, Lactose and Yeast.

Gluten

There is a common misconception that gluten is just found in wheat and bread products. It is found in so many more places which you thought were 'safe', such as oats though the amount of gluten present in oats is less than in wheat.

The Husband Says:

It is very easy to dismiss the idea of food intolerances as quackery. Especially if you are an Aspie-logician. But being a stubborn Aspie-logician scientist, the one sure way to expose quackery is to do the experiment and show that it doesn't work. Well that back-fired on me. Some simple diet change does beneficially work.

If I consume too much gluten, I feel sleepy starting about an hour after I eat the bread or pizza or whatever. Taken to excess and I will be running for the toilet. The same goes for the corn starch found in American soft drinks "at the fountain". I can eat more rye bread or high quality organic bread before feeling sleepy. So now I can choose - pleasure of the taste of bread and pasta versus loss of efficiency in the afternoon if I have them for lunch.

Now to lactose. Upset stomach and lots of gas with ordinary milk and no such symptoms if I use lactose free milk in my coffee. Cut and dried.

Yeast? Well the jury is out. I tend to have a banging hangover the morning after drinking beers and ciders and less so if I drink some wines and spirits to the same number of units. I like a bit or marmite on toast, but is it the bread or the yeast extract that is not good for me?

As an Aspie, am I more prone to full blown allergies and intolerances? Probably so. On top of my food intolerances, I'm severely allergic to Penicillin (anaphylactic shock levels of allergy). I get hay-fever - although this has improved recently - has diet change and vitamin supplement helped? - the jury is out. I'm also intolerant of some naturally occurring resins from wood - I get a pain under my fingernails that subsides if I thoroughly scrub my hands. Penicillin and resins are sufficiently unusual to hint that as an Aspie I'm different. But one data point does not a correlation make!

Intonation

The subtleties of language can often escape an Aspie - and I don't mean the vocabulary. Intonation seems to be a difficult one for them to pick up. It is not just the actual language, but the way we voice it, that can make all the difference. They understand whispering and they understand shouting, anything in between is lost on them. I have for example, often been accused of being miserable when I have answered a question, when in fact I am just tired, or perhaps I am trying to concentrate on something else, and not giving him my full attention.

Many a time as a teenager, when I staggered downstairs after tired and was sitting with a coffee contemplating the day, my father would walk into the room, take one look at me and say, 'What's the matter with you?' Well this never went down very well with me. Teenagers are touchy at the best of times. I usually hadn't even decided what kind of mood I was in by the time my father appeared, but he always managed to make me feel miserable after that comment and I learned to reply 'Nothing until you came in.' This probably wasn't the nicest thing to say but was at least honest. It's perhaps a good thing that I went off to university as my parents and I needed a break from each other. I was allowed to grow up and they were allowed to miss me.

NT When I remember to, I will be especially cheerful when greeting David in the morning, so that he knows I am in a good mood. It feels almost a bit 'Disneyfied' but he gets those exaggerated expressions and then he doesn't have to try and figure me out. It is hard work though when you haven't quite woken up and are busy making a cup of coffee and rushing around getting everyone their breakfast! Remembering to slap a cheesy grin on your face and sweetly greet your rumpled husband doesn't come naturally to most. He is allowed to look miserable in the morning but I am not. Life just isn't fair.

The Husband Says:

Like all things "Aspie", intonation (or more properly called prosody) can be either hyper or hypo as either given or received. As a child, my conversation was at first considered monotonic and monosyllabic by my teachers. I was encouraged to consciously have a sing-song delivery. Perhaps I over do this now?

As I have studied languages to a basic level, I now understand that lots of contextual information comes from the prosody of the person talking. In French, for example, making a statement with a rising tone at the end of the sentence turns that statement into a question -

I

like a bit of self-doubt - the rising tone says without words "I think so, I'm not sure, can you confirm?"

So prosody and intonation is important to full understanding of the spoken word and can be lost on Aspies in the same ways as spoken and written puns and metaphors. If hypo, the intonation may be stripped away depriving meaning. If hyper, then meaning may be assigned to even a sigh when none was meant by the NT.

Intuition

Intuition describes the ability of the mind to acquire knowledge without inference or the use of reason.

In other words, in certain situations we NT's 'just know' what is happening without having to go all Sherlock Holmes and look at the fine details to give a verdict.

This is something that our AS partner's lack and are probably quite jealous of our innate ability. We can't even describe to them how it is done. It is very hard to describe something to someone that just comes naturally. My daughter asked me to describe to her how I manage to whistle the other day and I couldn't get much further than purse your lips and blow. She did this and no musical tones were made. She was most frustrated.

I should think we would have the same conversation about how I know she is sad yet she doesn't know that I am.

The Husband Says:

Karen's article talks about intuition being a social and emotional think devoid of reason. I don't fully agree. Intuition has a broader technical and scientific sense. It refers to innate ability to recognise pattern. I believe that many Aspies, whilst not wired for emotion, are wired for logic. Instead of following every step of a logical or mathematical argument, we can innately "see" what is the correct answer. The number has the right "feel" about it.

There are patterns in the natural world. If there are patterns, then they can be described mathematically or with logic. Many Aspies resonate with and innately understand these natural patterns. Social expectation, with an absence of pattern and at times a defiance of superficial logic just does not chime.

Invisible

NT As the wife of an Aspie man you can often feel invisible. He is busy with his obsessions or in another room keeping his own space. He doesn't greet you when you come home or notice when you place a coffee on his desk.

He takes for granted all the everyday tasks you do around the house and never appreciates them or thanks you for doing these repetitive, mundane tasks.

You wonder what would happen if you just stopped doing them. Would he notice?

Solution

To be fair I have never been a domestic goddess but when we first started living together we both did the chores. We both worked during the week and relaxed on a weekend after having spent a small amount of time sorting out the washing and cleaning the one bathroom. It didn't take long.

These days we have a much bigger house, kids, a dog, far more responsibilities and a lot more stuff. I can't remember the last time we had a relaxing weekend. There is always stuff to do. Therefore, I do have a bit of an excuse to not keep everything tidy and perfect. I think if I did he wouldn't notice all the effort I put in.

Bizarrely, he is much more appreciative of my efforts when I have let the chores build up. I think part of it is that it's a visual representation. It had got so bad he could see there was a problem that needed fixing, even if he wasn't going to be the one to fix it. Therefore, once I eventually found the time to get around to sorting out the pile of clean washing into people's rooms, he could see it was a task that had been done and he could appreciate the effort (and the clean shirts hanging in his wardrobe).

Invisible Disability

An invisible disability is one that is not immediately apparent. I have had many people tell me that my husband "does not look autistic". This is a strange thing to say, after all what does autistic look like?

In my head, when I think of someone autistic I think of someone with a special interest and how they put it to good use, so they may be a scientist wearing a white coat and safety goggles or an engineer wearing a hard hat and holding a clipboard on a construction site.

Of course, to those in the know, they only have to watch a person's gait to see if they are toe walking or notice the little Stimming movements the adult Aspie tries to discreetly hide when they are nervous or excited but that is not what the person in the street means.

I am loathe to use the word disability towards autism, because as a family unit we do not feel disabled. In fact, we quite often feel "enabled" by the way David and the children are able to think outside of the box. Where we come unstuck is through the onset of anxiety, usually caused by the catalyst of other people's actions and expectations and doing new, unknown things. Is anxiety a disability? Well, it comes and goes - but it is there a good deal of the time at differing levels for our Aspies.

Sometimes it stops them from doing things and other times it forces them to work harder to succeed, often resulting in something amazing. So to use the label Disability is a tricky one and I think it depends on that particular person on that particular day and how they feel.

Mostly, anxiety is invisible, especially if it keeps you indoors.

Children with an ASD are less likely to be able to (or want to) cover up the fact that they are anxious, but by the time they get to adulthood, when most want to just appear "normal", they may be an expert at pretending to be.

What happens behind closed doors is another matter. If your child or your husband has been working so hard at keeping their disability hidden all day, they will be shattered when they return home. The moment they step through the front door they know they are safe and they will shed their cloak of invisibility.

This is the point where their differences become most visible.

The Husband Says:

A simple and crass answer: I don't think I'm disabled - I don't need a blue badge on the car.

More sensitively though, Disney recognise autism and Asperger's as a disability and allow you to skip the queues at their theme parks. They recognise that anxiety (over the wait, the apprehension in the queue) can be disabling to enjoyment.

Invitations

Does your heart sink when you receive a joint invitation to a party or event? Mine used to for several reasons. I knew he wouldn't want to go and I knew it would be stressful for both him and me. Neither of us would enjoy it. We would spend the time leading up to the event dreading going.

NT These days I am clear from the start. I will tell the person who is inviting us whether to expect one or both of us. I would much rather go on my own to most events. I am relaxed socially and can enjoy myself. I don't mind meeting new people, even if I may be a little nervous before turning up somewhere new by myself. It is much better than having to deal with his discomfort which makes life miserable for both of us.

Some events, he is happy to attend. These are ones where he generally knows what is going to happen, he knows the people and he has a purpose in being there. Hanging around chatting and drinking is not his idea of fun, especially in a noisy crowded room.

NT Give him a task, be an Usher or server of drinks and he will be the best Usher or server you have ever had. He will feel wanted and useful. I even often volunteer him for such events and people are always grateful for his help and ask him to come again.

The Husband Says:

In this day and age, it shouldn't be the social norm that all invitations are accepted unconditionally; but sadly that does seem to be the case. Karen flouts these social norms (very carefully), and perhaps I should learn to do the same independently rather than relying on Karen as "social secretary" for our household.

So if I could change the "rules", what would I do? Well for starters, I'd want some indication with the invitation of how big a social receptacle I will need to take along. Experts talk about how Aspies "social cups" fill up more quickly than NTs and how sociability then slops on the floor and the Aspie has to "escape" the embarrassment. So in this invitation - is a cup going to be big enough? Fancy dress party - that's going to need a social skip. Dancing involved? - that's at least two social bucket-fulls. Supper and a board game with two other couples - well that's my social cup just nicely filled.

Does this invitation have a "get out" clause? Can we just drop in for an hour and, if we like it, stay? Or is the course of the evening timetabled and fixed and, having attended, would we be expected/forced to stay to the bitter end? Is there a quiet room other than the disco? Will there be surprises?

Irrationality

There is always a reason behind this behaviour. However, it is hard to judge whether it is worth delving into it at the time. Often it can only be discovered and looked over in hindsight and in a calm situation.

Example: The other day we found ourselves with only one car for the day. David had forgotten that I had committed myself to an 8-week research course every Thursday morning, this being the fourth one, and he had forgotten that he had a doctor's appointment. He was in quite a bad mood when he realised this as he believed he had thought it through when arranging for one car to be taken away and the new one arriving 2 days later. As he had planned to work from home for two days, he didn't think it would be a problem.

He decided that if I dropped him off at the doctors that he would walk home. I was surprised as it is a good three mile walk through the countryside. It is a walk I regularly do half of (I turn around about half way) with the dog and sometimes I do all of it. David is not a walker. As we were leaving the house I saw him put on his everyday shoes, basically the plain black ones he wears to work. I suggested he would be better off putting his walking boots on. He carried on putting his shoes on and insisted he would be fine wearing them. I asked him if he would be walking along the road path and pointed out it would take longer. I said the riverside path was shorter but would be muddy due to recent heavy rain. He said he would be fine and by the tone of his voice he did not want to be told what to do. I stopped as I know when I am fighting a losing battle but I didn't really know why he insisted on wearing his smart shoes.

When I was at my research group, he sent me a text me to say he had done the walk and was hot and sweaty and that he had met lots of people on the way. He said he would have done the walk in 60 minutes if he had not. Was this a reference to the fact that he could walk it faster than me? I hadn't realised we were in competition. However, I ignored that and praised him for doing the walk. I had half expected him to get the bus especially as it was still raining.

Later that day when I got home and after having seen the muddy state of his shoes, I asked him why exactly he hadn't worn his walking boots. After some thought he explained that he wanted to be smart for his appointment and didn't think it was appropriate to wear his walking boots there. I pointed out that the nurse or doctor would have been over the moon if he had told them he was going to walk the three miles home and would have applauded his choice of foot wear. He did not know how to explain this to me. Of course if he had, I would have suggested that perhaps he change his shoes but I suspect this also would have caused him consternation.

The Husband Says:

Just the one point on the story before I generalise. I wasn't in competition on the time taken to walk back. I was more trying to recount how I'd met the great and the good of the village on the walk, and they, rather surprised to see me at all, just had to engage in pointless social conversation, with me all dishevelled and sweaty (I'm not a walker remember!). My social cup was overflowing and I wanted to tell you how I'd coped and not behaved badly in front of the village glitterati.

This article should really be called Rational-Irrationality. For Aspies and NTs, for every given situation or puzzle there are a myriad of solutions. You NTs automatically factor in the social and the practical. I depend more on logic. What is the doctor expecting? I expect a professional to professional discussion. Is there a "uniform" for a doctor's appointment - yes there must be - smart casual with easy access to arms for blood pressure, blood samples etcetera. Does it matter about taking a muddy path home in smart-ish shoes - no they will clean up when I get home. Will it matter that I'm muddy and dishevelled on the walk home? No, it is unlikely that anyone will see me.

BZZZZTTT! Wrong assumption and answer on that last point. That was the only flaw in the logic. But I coped. Sort of. I didn't appear as the headline in the Parish News so I must have got away with it.

1

Irrelevancies

Some markers in our NT lives are highly important to us, like our age but to many Aspies it is just an irrelevant number that plays little part in their lives.

So I came across David having one of his regular shouts at the bank for causing him inconvenience and embarrassment, only he couldn't get through the security protocol. I heard him shout that he was 48 at the call handler and then again and then he told the call handler how he came to his conclusion. He had subtracted this year's date from his year of birth. I knew he wasn't 48 until later this year and had to remind him that he was 47. I wonder how many other autistics have trouble getting through security protocols because of what they consider irrelevancies which everyone else assumes that you will immediately know.

It makes me feel a little better that my dad still can't remember my birthday.

The Husband Says:

...And the really odd thing about all this was that the bank DID want the answer 48 even though I am only 47 at the moment because they clearly stated that I had to answer with my age at my next birthday.

47, 48, what's the difference?

Is there a Cure?

The short answer is No.

The longer answer is more hopeful but requires a lot of work from both of you.

Autism is a difference in the way the person's brain is wired. They think differently from you and I. There is nothing 'wrong' with them per se. Our husbands and our diagnosed children look at the world differently from us. Because we are wired differently to them we perceive their reaction as being 'wrong'.

NT First of all you need to accept this.

AS Secondly, it would really help if your husband could accept and even be proud of this. There are many plus points about being an Aspie.

Thirdly, you and your husband, indeed the whole family, should try and be at optimum health through a healthy diet which will help with your own resilience and your husbands' differences.

It only has to Happen once to Become the norm

You may have noticed that something that you did once, long ago and never again since, will be looked upon as your default behaviour. This will usually be something that they regard as negative behaviour from you. They will fixate on this and not take into account any of your positive behaviour since.

The Husband Says:

I'm pattern matching. I'm trying to group similar events together to establish what the social norm might be. This can be dangerous.

If all I have in any given category is one experience, then this MUST be the norm that us Aspies should abide by - even if your NT social sense tells you otherwise.

If I have several examples of similar behaviour pattern with one that differs, I might not have "processed" that category to out-vote the outlier to properly establish the norm for that category. It takes time to consciously think and edit out the noise of behaviours that don't fit an emerging pattern.

Aspies can seem to get "stuck in a groove" like this. It's also very tempting to dwell on the negative and allow the negative to define a pattern rather than seeing a new positive experience as breaking a pattern.

It's not all Rainbows and Unicorns

Being in an Asperger marriage isn't so unique...

It's in our vows on the day we get married, "For richer, for poorer, in sickness and in health". For centuries starry eyed brides and bridegroom's have spoken these words and all have assumed the bad stuff will never happen to them.

Of course, if we didn't think like that, we would never make the commitment in the first place. It's natural to start off your married life with optimism and joy.

Look around you and you will see the 'normal' marriages struggle too. The reality of babies, work, health and finance, always put a strain on any marriage. It's how you deal with it that matters.

It's the Little Things

It is probable that this marriage is not your first serious relationship, and you will have some positive memories of previous NT/NT relationships. These may not have ended well eventually, but it is likely you have fond memories of reciprocal behaviour from previous partners - such behaviours that are sorely lacking in your marriage now.

Little romantic gestures like offering to pick you up from work after a late night shift or finding spontaneous little presents on your pillow. Those are nice gestures but you probably also received the ones we don't even think about in a NT/NT relationship, someone bringing you a cup of tea and a biscuit when they make one for themselves or reaching over to hold your hand in the cinema when you are scared. These things rarely happen in an AS/NT relationship as it requires your partner to imagine that you would like these things.

At first it may not be obvious, as you will provide many of these gestures yourself and your new AS partner will mimic them for a while (without you recognising this is "copying" rather than instinctive). However, it will take great thought on his part to carry these out and, once he has ensnared you into marriage, it will rarely occur to him that these little gestures are still wanted, let alone needed, to keep the relationship alive.

It's the little things, the tiny caring nuances in a relationship that gets missed by your AS partner but is desperately wanted and increasingly so by the NT as years go by.

The Husband Says:

AS
   BIG HINT for Aspies: planned spontaneity. Look it up. Now go and do some for her.

- ✧   Jealousy
- ✧   Jekyll and Hyde
- ✧   Jobs
- ✧   Judgement
- ✧   Judgement of Character
- ✧   Jumping to Conclusions
- ✧   Justice

Jealousy

I have never viewed David as a jealous man. I have never given him any cause to be, so it may be that he just doesn't have any experience in this area. Though I cannot speak for every man in every Aspie marriage, I feel the majority are very faithful men. They have chosen their woman and do not feel the need to go elsewhere unless their partner has given them real cause.

David works away a lot and I have never worried that he will stray. He works too hard and he knows that I understand him. I'm not saying I am a rare being but someone as understanding and tolerant as myself would be hard for him to find again!

Yet, there is a jealous side to him. This stems from his feelings of inadequacy. He is the only one who feels this way about his abilities. But, it is from his 'lack of ability' that his jealousies stem. For some time after I had graduated with my Masters in Autism, he kept talking about how he should be going for a Masters or a Doctorate. He has never felt the need to before as he has a good first degree and has had a very successful engineering career. Some of his colleagues have PhD's but he is not considered any lesser than them and, in many cases, he is the more practical part of the team, the one who has not just theorised but actually carried out the work successfully.

I know he was proud of me when I graduated but at the same time, my achievement made him feel inadequate, which of course was never my intention.

With some couples I have counselled, jealousy and inadequacy have been a major bone of contention, even to the extent that the husband has refused to attend his wife's' graduation. I have even come across cases where the AS father has been jealous if his child gets praise for schoolwork.

The Husband Says:

I'm glad I give such a good impression to Karen. Sometimes I can get a bit jealous of the attention that Karen occasionally gives to an ex-boyfriend. I struggle to tell the difference between a platonic friendship (which this relationship with the ex must be) and any form of infidelity. There's an element of jealousy in any time Karen gives to others that she could be giving to me.

I also have jealousy towards those that have gained advantage through what I perceive to be injustice. I'm also jealous of people who gain advantage through luck, but I'm not tempted (e.g. to gambling) which others might be. Logic dictates that gambling or reliance on luck is a mug's game.

J

Jekyll and Hyde

Do you feel that you live with this fictional character by Robert Louis Stevenson?

The author was intrigued by his character's split personality, where Dr Jekyll was the good character and Mr Hyde the evil.

Dr Jekyll was a meek, mild and kind man, whereas Mr Hyde was portrayed as quite a psychopath. The narration in the story follows them initially as two separate men and it is discovered eventually that they are one and the same.

Using the term Jekyll and Hyde provides an instant image of someone turning from good to bad and back again with hardly an explanation for it. This is often what it feels like to be living with a man with Asperger's Syndrome.

As the wife, and thus the one not aware of all the little nuances affecting his mood, it seems that his sudden eruption of temper has come out of nowhere. In fact, there will be a reason for it, an email from work or a driver tailgating him that you are not aware of. He will unleash his frustration on the nearest person.

Now Mr Hyde was a violent and uncaring character, so it is a little unfair really to compare the AS man with him in reality. It is rare for an adult with AS to lash out physically at someone they love. I would not advocate staying with such a person. I certainly would not be with David if he had ever raised a hand to me.

Where the situation compares is how his character reverts back to the meek Dr Jekyll once he has got his frustration out of the way. Unfortunately, as his partner who has had to absorb his abusive outburst, you are left reeling from the onslaught while he is quite relaxed about it.

Jobs

In days gone by workers had much more job security and often a 'job for life' especially in large companies and academia.

Our Asperger men in the past had less anxiety in their life due to routines, lack of change, respect and less competition. They had a role as breadwinner in their household and were happy with their role and place in society.

During the last 30 years, in the UK and in other developed countries, has come constant change in the name of progress. This brought about redundancies due to global recessions and cost cutting.

Imagine the stress this has caused in families over the decades where the man of the house has had the rug pulled out from under his feet, control and certainty wrested away and he no longer has an identity or the means to provide for his family.

This happened to my undiagnosed father who, in his early forties, was forced to take 'voluntary' redundancy from his university post due to a merger and cost cutting. I witnessed first-hand his breakdown. Though he found a new job very quickly, we had to move country and he was on a contract that was renewed yearly. He never had job security again. He ended up taking early retirement as he couldn't cope with his life teetering on the brink and the constant change. He was never the same again.

Judgement

There are no grey areas in the mind of the AS man. It is either right or it is wrong. It is black or it is white. This is why so many make fine policemen and members of the armed forces (but don't tell the MoD or they will have to sack half of their staff!).

My family members are very moralistic, which is not a bad thing, but because they only see the right or wrong in the situation, they do come across as judgemental and not very forgiving. For example, if I had been a smoker I would not be writing this now as David would never have asked me out. That was a definite no-no for his life partner. For me, I have never smoked and would not have been keen on dating a smoker but if that was their only failing, I would have been prepared to look past it or help them to give up.

I have always been a fence sitter and able to see both people's perspectives, the pros and cons of both situations. At times I have been jealous of people who have very firm convictions about major issues and never regret their decisions, there is a certain advantage in it, but not necessarily if you want to make or keep friends.

The Husband Says:

I'm definitely very judgemental, but I think we need to be very careful suggesting that all Aspies in relationships are also judgemental. Let's also be careful what we mean by judgemental; if you are thinking about Myers Briggs "judging" versus "perceiving" then you are conflating two separate discussions. Judgemental here relates to justice - the pursuit of right and wrong.

Judgement of Character

I don't purport to be a particularly good judge of character as I have made severe mistakes in the past. On the whole I like to take people at face value and believe the best in them.

David on the other hand prefers to think the worst of people until otherwise proved. However, who is the happier person with more friends? He also doesn't believe in forgiving people for their sins and foibles which may be another reason why I have a fairly large circle of friends and he doesn't. I know I am not perfect and I can't really expect my friends to be so all the time. Besides, it always gives us something to talk about.

The Husband Says:

Compared with Karen, I like to think I'm a good "first impressions" judge of character. As Karen says, I dwell on the negatives, and it can take me a long time to forgive someone of their perceived wrong-doing or foibles. There are certain subjects, with certain people that it is just best not to talk about.

Jumping to Conclusions

You are married to a literal thinker. It is quite possible that he interprets your words in a completely different way from the way you intended them.

This can go badly wrong when you are making a joke or using sarcasm as they will sometimes think you are being rude or just not funny.

It is easier to see literal thinking in children as the adult Aspie brain has usually learned by now that you speak in code and metaphors and when we NT's say one thing, we actually mean another. What a minefield our language is!

I was shopping with our daughter and as a treat I suggested she choose some sweets. She chose some fizzy jelly sweets which had a very sour taste to them. I wasn't sure it was a good choice for her and said "They'll blow your head off." She looked at me very concerned and said "Really?" and then was a little upset that I burst out laughing.

We have all found humour in books for Aspies explaining metaphors and our son in particular was in a fit of giggles for a whole car journey after reading "toasting the bride" and imagining the literal connotations.

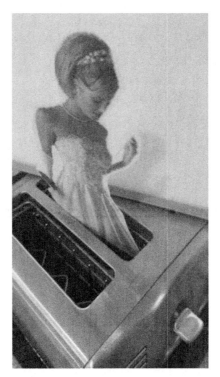

There is a good book on this subject complete with humorous illustrations: 'It's Raining Cats and Dogs: An Autism Spectrum Guide to the Confusing World of Idioms, Metaphors and Everyday Expressions'.

The Husband Says:

I take a different slant on 'jumping to conclusions'. The way my mind is wired up, for many maths and logic puzzles, I seem to be able to jump directly to the answer - the conclusion. Even if I can't jump to the correct answer straight away, I have an innate "feel" for what the answer should be and in multiple choice questions, which the red-herrings are and why.

I also try to jump to conclusions on matters that you NTs have an innate ability on, to try to act like you. Quite often I get this wrong, so I'm learning to slow down and trust my analysis of the situation rather than try to use an NT's "social sense" that it turns out I just don't have.

Justice

Our men have a strong moral compass. They think very much in terms of right and wrong and black and white. They are not so good at looking at the grey areas of life (see Meh). There are no rules there.

J

You will find that people with AS make very fine lawyers and policemen. They get great satisfaction from rules and regulations and carrying them out.

However, their rigid thinking does sometimes go against them and they may not be able to see that sometimes justice should not be carried out on minor indiscretions. Rules are there for a reason and need to be carried out to the letter.

They therefore have strong feelings and even fear of injustice. To the point that they will get involved in campaigns or become very emotional about something that is very unfair or tragic that they have seen on the television.

The Husband Says:

Again I'm agreeing with Karen. I wonder if our abilities as Aspies to spot nuances of emotion in people's faces makes us blind to the depth of emotion that a person is suffering as a victim of injustice? Can our responses ever be properly proportionate when 'an eye for an eye and a tooth for a tooth' is an emotional response to being wronged emotionally? Us Aspies are poor at measuring the depth of emotion and the depth of hurt. You really, really don't want me on a jury if there is the remotest chance you might be guilty.

Could this 'hang-em, flog-em' right wing attitude have a significant genetic component linked to my Asperger's? Very probably.

- ✧   Keeping the Love Flowing
- ✧   Kids
- ✧   Killjoy
- ✧   Kindness
- ✧   Knock-On Effect
- ✧   Knowing Everything

Keeping the Love Flowing

 It's the little things that count.

To a man with Asperger's, showing his appreciation of you does not come verbally but in his actions. Putting up a shelf or mowing the lawn. Remembering to pick the kids up for you. In his head this is all for you. It probably adds up in his head in an internal quota. He probably gets to a point in the day when he feels he has done enough for you to show his love. That is when if asked, he will be reluctant or just ignore your request or do it with bad grace. Hasn't he already shown you how much he loves you and NOW you are also asking him to empty the bin?

For us NTs our love is pretty much limitless. When we truly love someone we will do anything for them. We don't count our actions. We just instinctively get up when the baby is crying or make our husband a cup of coffee when he comes in. Not so for the AS man.

NT Likewise though, perhaps you could turn this to your advantage? Make a visual list for him to see all the tasks that you automatically carry out for him during the day. He may not need you to do this as he probably does note that you do them for him but he will also to an extent take them for granted.

Sometimes when I am annoyed with being taken for granted I will be rebellious and just make a coffee for myself!

Does a Relationship need Romance to Survive?

From the very outset David refused to be coerced into romance. What he meant was going to a restaurant on Valentine's Day and being forced to pay inflated prices amongst a room of soppy eyed couples. He just wanted it to be natural and not because some advertising agency had told us we had to.

In fact, I had no problem with this as I felt the same way myself. David had been very thoughtful from the beginning of our relationship and so a soppy card or an enormous teddy bear I didn't want, was not going to do it for me. Besides, I had had all that in my previous relationship, the flowers, the six-foot panda the three-foot card. What I didn't have was fidelity, trust and reassurance. What is more precious?

Every now and then David will say "I nearly bought you flowers" which makes me laugh but I think he now thinks it's too late to start bringing me flowers after all these years. I suspect he is worried that I'll think he is being unfaithful. As previously mentioned, I have no worries in that area at all.

K

Kids

No matter how much preparation you and your partner do, the arrival of a new born baby will still be a surprise.

There is no manual for each individual baby and the moment you think you've got them sussed, they change.

Not all Aspie men will be helpless, unwilling fathers but the majority I have met have floundered in this area. They don't have the natural skills to work out what their child needs or the ability to adapt to ever changing situations.

NT Be patient with them and give them clear, concise directions. If you have to leave the baby with him make sure he knows exactly when and how often the baby needs to be changed or fed. Don't be vague and say to check the nappy. Tell him to change the nappy at a certain time or he will wriggle out of that nasty task. It isn't that he can't do it (as I was led to believe) but that he won't do it.

Killjoy

Aspies get a bad press where having fun is concerned. They really don't like having surprises sprung on them but if you give time to plan they can psyche themselves up for almost anything.

Kindness

Surprisingly, my husband can be very kind.

When I first met him I was told he was a lovely, generous man and it turned out to be true. He still is. He is very generous with his time for other people. It is helpful if he knows in advance what people would like him to do but once he has decided to help out he will give it his all.

This can sometimes, unfortunately, be to the detriment of his family. He used to be Chair of the Parish Council and it took up so much of his time that his work began to suffer as did his moods. He became very stressed because of very difficult local politics. At times we hardly saw him. In some ways it was a very good experience for him and it helped his people skills no end. People in the village still have a lot of respect for him but I was glad when he resigned.

K

Every Day Kindnesses

I'm not sure he always notices my everyday kindnesses. For example, I think it is simple courtesy to make coffee for him when I am making one for myself. He very rarely returns this gesture. It is very irritating. He will actually stand and chat to me while he boils the kettle and makes himself a pot of coffee and all the while I'm waiting to be asked and watching to see how many mugs he gets out of the cupboard. What really gets me is that he knows this annoys me and yet he still does it. I may sometimes say "No, thank you", which is possibly why he doesn't ask as perhaps he thinks I never want one? As women, we put great store into simple gestures and even if I don't want a coffee I would just like him to ask. It makes me feel wanted.

The Husband Says:

Cups of coffee and tea are a peculiar example. I don't think every Aspie will act like I do over refreshment. Lots of this stems back to my early career in Engineering where making the teas for the whole team was a rite of passage for the young Engineering trainee. Eventually you develop new skills and tea-making is put behind you; the new apprentice has to make the tea from there on in.

Karen, you might be reassured or horrified that at work I seldom "get the teas in". It's such an inter-personal battleground; at my current client they even have otherwise identical company mugs with their names printed on. It would have been so much more useful to print their "recipe" on the bottom - 'White tea, strong, two sugars' or 'Black decaff coffee, one sweetener'. My current client even notes in his diary, as a joke, each time I get the coffees in.

Instead I go for the planned spontaneity strategy - during Wimbledon fortnight I brought in strawberries and cream for the team. At Christmas, on 'Black Eye Friday', I get bacon sandwiches for everyone. You probably wonder why I don't do this at home? It's all a careful strategy to project a particular 'work persona' to clients and colleagues. You are justified in saying "If you can do it at work, why not at home?"

Knock-On Effect

Unfortunately, life rarely happens in a predictable way. Even for an adult Aspie there is a very narrow margin of error in the way the day falls. Most of the little annoyances, such as running out of coffee, can be overcome without too much trauma but having your train cancelled last minute can have a serious knock-on effect for the rest of the day.

Well surely that is true for everyone? If your train is cancelled, you end up late for your appointment and so on. Indeed, but we Neurotypicals manage to claw back incrementally from the day, little bits of time and effort here and there. We might just take half an hour for lunch instead of an hour, by grabbing a sandwich rather than a hot meal. We may postpone a less important meeting in order to make sure we get to the crucial one of the day. But most importantly, though we are disgruntled and inconvenienced by the fact our train was late, we quickly and mentally get over it, perhaps by having a little moan on Facebook or to our boss, and then we move on.

Our Aspie on the other hand lets this one, early morning inconvenience affect their mood and their behaviour for the rest of the day. They feel inclined to tell whoever they meet about the poor service and perhaps even have to compose a letter of complaint, rather than shrug it off as one of those things.

Their agitation and anxiety caused by knowing their train is late does not diminish once the situation has been resolved and they arrive at their destination. They feel rushed, unsettled, aggrieved and anxious. They can't settle to what they intended to do and cannot give anything their full attention. They still try and carry out their day in the order that they had planned without making any time concessions. They are not mentally prepared for the changes and do not perform well when normally they would.

They are also distracted by their concern that the train home may well be delayed again. They may have to constantly check updates online to see if the cause of the problem has been cleared or reoccurred.

They carry their mood outwardly, especially when they get home. They are worried that it might happen again tomorrow and the anxiety does not recede until normality resumes the following morning.

Knowing Everything

David has a phenomenal amount of knowledge and a phenomenal memory but he doesn't know everything. Yet, he is very good at giving the impression that he does. I think he sees it as a weakness to admit to not knowing something. People refer to him as The Oracle. They are not far wrong I suppose, if only because he can manage to fool them.

Part of it is that he uses his extensive knowledge and experience to quickly work things out and, by adding some of his superior vocabulary, can at least sound like he has an informed opinion. What is extremely annoying however, and it took me years to work out that he does this (as he does it so well), is that the moment you tell him something, before you have closed your lips on the last word, he nods wisely and says "Yes" confidently, as if he knew that all along and just hadn't bothered to say it to you. I had to test this theory out a few times and, though not deliberately making things up, when I told him snippets of newly learned information or gossip he couldn't possibly know he would still do it!

K

I don't know if he sees it as a weakness in myself when I admit that I do not know something. I think it is a weakness not to admit you don't know something, as experience has taught me it is easier to ask. Most people are always willing to impart helpful or useful information and it is so much easier, especially if they offer to do it for you.

The Husband Says:

You are right. Again this "knowing everything" stems from what I do at work. My signature, and I think one of the reasons people hire me, is that in my subject of energy technology, I have a very broad base of knowledge - I know a little bit about everything, so I can jump about from topic to topic and give management a "helicopter view" of the whole situation. When deep knowledge is required, I know who to ask or what standard text book to refer to. When nobody knows, I'm willing to apply Occam's Razor and eliminate the impossible to leave the probable and guess which of the probables to follow - often so many around me have the same intellectual capability, but they won't gamble and simply must know the full and complete answer before giving an opinion. Clients hire me because I don't suffer from paralysis in technical decision making.

I'm guilty of bringing this tactic home. But you also know I have a phenomenal memory for trivia which is only ever some use on Quiz Nights. I'm also (and this only comes with age) more willing to say "I don't know", pause and then add "...but I know a woman who does."

K

L

- ✧ Lactose
- ✧ Language
- ✧ Lashing Out
- ✧ Laziness
- ✧ LCHF
- ✧ Lead by Example
- ✧ Leaky Gut Syndrome
- ✧ Leaping to Conclusions
- ✧ Leo Kanner
- ✧ Letting things Go
- ✧ Letting you Down
- ✧ Libido
- ✧ Light at the end of the Tunnel
- ✧ Listening
- ✧ Lists
- ✧ Literal Thinking
- ✧ Loneliness
- ✧ Lorna Wing
- ✧ Love
- ✧ Lowering your Expectations
- ✧ Low Emotional Intelligence
- ✧ Lying

L

Lactose

It took me years to realise that I was lactose intolerant. I don't think it is something that just happened. As a child I didn't like milk but we were forced to drink it at school. I think my body was trying to tell me something back then.

Some people do not produce the enzyme lactase which helps you to digest milk.

Lactose Intolerance

This should not be confused with a milk allergy which is an auto immune response to food and can be dangerous.

Lactose Intolerance is the inability of adults and children to digest milk. Lactose is a sugar found in milk and, to a lesser extent, other dairy products.

Symptoms of lactose intolerance include: bloating, flatulence, stomach cramps, diarrhoea, rumbling stomach or even vomiting.

There is still a lot of research to be done around a healthy gut and its effect on autistic behaviour.

Since I gave up milk with lactose and stopped having gastro problems I have been mentally happier, healthier and stronger. It has literally helped me cope with the day to day of being an Asperger wife and mother.

As a family we only buy lactose free milk. This milk tastes the same and can be used exactly the same as normal milk. The only difference is that it doesn't make me ill and, on the down side, it is more expensive in the supermarket - but that is a small price to pay.

Language

I was on the train with my daughter the other day, and we could not help by overhear a young man's conversation on his phone. I was not impressed by his use of language which mainly consisted of giving the other person his poor opinion of a mutual friend and what "body part" this friend represented. This is not the kind of language I wanted my daughter subjected to on public transport, and I would have appreciated it if this young man had cared to consider his language for his audience and not just his friend.

As parents we learn to use a different language around our children than we do with our partners and close friends. I remember one of my mum's friends, when I was a teenager, telling me that my mother swore like a trooper. I still don't believe it. I have no evidence of my own to base it on.

L

So why do we not consider what we are saying more carefully to the person we vowed to spend the rest of our lives with? Don't they also need consideration and a tactful use of language on our part?

In our early married life when I assumed I was married to a 'normal' man, I would just say whatever I felt was right at the time. I didn't really temper what I was saying or worry about how he would react to my words. As time went on and I realised I had to be careful with what I said, I would think things through before speaking to him. After David's unofficial diagnosis of AS, I would give even greater thought as to how my conversations would affect him. I would find myself loading the dishwasher whilst, in my head, I was going over conversation starters and even intonation to try and get it right and not to upset him.

NT What I found was that it was very important not to use negative language as he would fixate on that. I had to try and find ways that he would feel positive about a situation or at least know that he had control over a situation. Or if I had to tell him bad news I would try to give it a positive spin. However, he isn't daft and can see through these things.

I don't want to sound patronising and say you should talk to your husband like he is a child, but you wouldn't come out and tell your unsuspecting child straight away that their dog had been run over, you would temper it. You would lead up to it, give them a little bit of warning.

The Husband Says:

As a contrary Aspie, I'm going to comment on a different aspect of language to that being discussed by Karen. Picking up on the swearing point: I think I might be the same as a lot of Aspies in that we are keeping up an act so we tend to mirror, reflect or mimic those around us. When working in a shipyard, I'll be swearing along with the labourers - I do this to fit in and it's not a conscious decision anymore.

I pick up and adopt other people's accents, idioms and patterns of speech very easily and adopt them into my own. In a teleconference with a French native, who is working hard to speak fluent English, I tend to pick up on the noun-verb reversals (like "post-box red" instead of the English "red post-box") that come from the French speaker and start to repeat them, even after the phone call. I know my daughter often "parrots" in this sort of way too.

If I like the sound of a particular piece of language, I'll subconsciously steal it and incorporate that sound bite into my language, both spoken and written.

Lashing Out

This happens when their levels of anxiety are so high that they are overwhelmed with their feelings and they lash out. I am speaking in the verbal sense. David has

L

never been physical or violent with me. I would not stand for that and I would not forgive that.

Observing young children on the spectrum you can see, particularly when they are tired after a long day of school, that their poor mother's get all their bad behaviour. The mothers are bewildered by this especially when the school say their child is a model pupil.

There is a time limit to being good.

Also the child instinctively knows that their parents love them unconditionally and will forgive them and protect them. I think that this is how David feels in his home environment. He knows I love him and will forgive him.

However, a warning to all Aspie men from your women: We do love you and we will forgive you but this is not an unlimited offer. It is very traumatic to have to deal with your outbursts which are very unfair and irrational and sometimes unpredictable, especially when we are blamed for something we did not do.

As we did not give birth to you, our love is not necessarily unconditional. A time will come when we may stop loving you, or if we don't stop loving you, we will end the relationship to save our own sanity. You cannot take us for granted forever. You know yourselves that having your skills taken for granted at work may be flattering at first but quickly becomes very tiresome. You may dream of having another job where you are appreciated. Don't blame your wife for thinking the same thing.

The Husband Says:

Heed the above!

Laziness

My opinion of this one has come full circle. I used to just think he was lazy and didn't want to do certain things and would try anything to get out of it. Then I discovered he had Asperger's and realised after some time that there was a reason for his reluctance.

However, having now learned the subtleties of his behaviour, and also realising that he does have Asperger's but is foremost human (and a man), I now know sometimes he is, in fact, plain lazy!

The Husband Says:

See my comments on the article on avoidance for my thoughts between anxiety induced avoidance and laziness-avoidance.

Aspie Engineers are quite deliberately some of the laziest people I know (I am one). Our job is to find the best way to fulfil a need in, usually, the cheapest and simplest way to achieve the desired result - and that can come across as lazy. So now we have another "tension"; not just avoidance compared with laziness but efficiency compared with laziness.

LCHF

Low Carbohydrate and High (or Healthy) Fat Way of Eating

Thirty years ago our eating habits changed as we were told by our governments we needed to be eating more healthily to avoid heart disease and cholesterol. We were all meant to live longer. Instead, diabetes, has become an epidemic as we eat the high carbohydrate foods and low fat, sugary foods that were recommended to us.

I remember, years ago, my mother and her friends became obsessed with the F Plan Diet which seemed to mostly consist of baked potato and baked beans. I'm not even sure why we did it as none of us were overweight at the time.

Now governments (to some extent) are holding their hands up and telling us that they got it wrong after all. Sugar is bad for us (who knew!) and fat is not bad for us. We don't actually have to eat five a day to be healthy.

It turns out that eating too many carbohydrates is actually unhealthy for us and causes inflammation in our bodies. Inflammation causes us to be bloated and tired and have "brain fog". We ache and we fart and we consider these all normal signs of life. It turns out they are not.

If you cut out of your diet grains, rice and sugars you will start to feel energised and rejuvenated. Your body will stop aching, you will sleep better, lose weight, be less bloated, and less moody.

David and I have just started doing this and we feel so much better, losing several pounds each within a week. Yes, it can be hard to cut out processed foods and sugars at first, but the benefit is well worth it.

Books I recommend from experts:

- Eat Bacon, Don't Jog
- The Real Meal Revolution

The Husband Says:

These books seem to contain some science. Which is more than can be said for Government advice.

L

Lead by Example

NT If you want your husband to do something for you, you should probably check first that he knows how to do it. Now that might sound like an odd thing to say but there are a few reasons for this:

- They don't care to admit they have a gap in their knowledge, especially if it's is considered simple and obvious.

- As young boys and men they will have often skilfully avoided any household chores and are still unaware that woollens should not be tumble dried or that bins don't magically empty themselves.

They genuinely do not see the world as we do, so do not have the 'common sense' that we have always taken for granted.

However, if you want him to do something for himself and he still won't do it, the best way to get him to do it is to lead by example.

For instance, David is really not into his exercise. He can see the point of it and he likes the results but actually getting around to it, well there's always something more pressing that needs doing.

I go through phases of trying to get fit and I can generally be self-motivated, unless I have too much on and then fitness is the first thing to go. When I am motivated I will go to the gym and start feeling better about myself. This is when David starts making noises about "perhaps" he should start going again.

NT Obviously, all men hate to be nagged, so the best way to get them to do something is not to nag them. You will get the blame regardless.

It's hard to pinpoint whether I inspire him to go to the gym by my obvious glow and changing body shape, or whether I just shame him into it. Either way, my going (and the subsequent positive results) can get him off the sofa and on to a treadmill.

Conversely, the moment I get overwhelmed with stress again and can't find the time to fit a run into my day, he starts slacking off as well. Does he see this as silent permission to stop?

He never says to me, "Oh you haven't been in the gym for a while." He never even tells me that I'm putting on weight. I don't know if that is a good thing? No one likes to be told they are putting on weight but, on the other hand, if someone points it out to you, you are probably more likely to do something about it.

This means that I am the instigator of pretty much everything that goes on in my house, be it good or bad. I would love the support from a partner who would tactfully and supportively point out when things are going wrong. Instead I have to be my own moral compass and guide. It is very wearing and, at times, I flounder without the mental support.

The Husband Says:

Taking the lead, for an Aspie, can be dangerous territory. Unless the direction in which to move is absolutely clear then sooner or later some social decision making, rather than technical decision making, will come into play and then we fall down.

Karen is right with the gym thing - I need to see leadership to encourage me. I know that when Karen has set aside time for exercise, then I can have that time too because there is nothing else (perhaps social) planned that will clash.

On the "you're putting on weight thing", that's a minefield for an NT to NT conversation, never mind for a blunt, opinionated, none-too-subtle Aspie with NT discussion. It's only one step divorced from giving an honest answer to the dreaded "does my bum look big in this?" and only one more step to marriage-divorce!

Leaky Gut Syndrome

This list was put together by Dr Amy Myers. This is not necessarily related to autism and indeed is not even acknowledge by the NHS as, to them, it is too vague and would cost them too much money if acknowledged. However, I believe most people with autism and AS should at least consider whether they have this and whether they could do something about it.

If you are in good health you will have a healthy gut. If you are not in good health the chances are you do not;

Signs you may have a Leaky Gut

1. Digestive issues such as gas, bloating, diarrhoea or irritable bowel syndrome (IBS).

2. Seasonal allergies or asthma.

3. Hormonal imbalances such as PMS or PCOS.

4. Diagnosis of an autoimmune disease such as rheumatoid arthritis, Hashimoto's thyroiditis, lupus, psoriasis, or celiac disease.

5. Diagnosis of chronic fatigue or fibromyalgia.

6. Mood and mind issues such as depression, anxiety, ADD or ADHD.

7. Skin issues such as acne, rosacea, or eczema.

8. Diagnosis of candida overgrowth.

9. Food allergies or food intolerances.

How to Avoid a Leaky Gut

The main culprits are foods, infections, and toxins. Gluten is the number one cause of leaky gut. Other inflammatory foods like dairy or toxic foods, such as sugar and excessive alcohol, are suspected as well. The most common infectious causes are candida overgrowth, intestinal parasites, and small intestine bacterial overgrowth (SIBO). Toxins come in the form of medications, like Motrin, Advil, (American trade-names for painkillers) steroids, antibiotics, and acid-reducing drugs, as well as environmental toxins like mercury, pesticides and BPA from plastics. Stress and age also contribute to a leaky gut.

The Husband Says:

As I've said in other articles, I don't hold to quackery and faddism, but again I've got to acknowledge a grain of truth in the leaky gut theories. By scientific abstinence and substitution, I can show a direct link between what I eat, how clearly I think, and my response to minor ailments.

The full blown "leaky gut as a cause of autism" theories stem back to Paul Shattock around 1998; the now discredited Andrew Wakefield (of autism and MMR infamy) adopted some of Shattock's ideas. I don't subscribe to those theories at all. But it is unescapable that having reduced levels of yeast in my diet (and yeast is known to damage the intestinal tract), and reduced casein and lactose from milk, and reduced gluten (some of those difficult to digest components of a modern Western diet), I do feel physically better. Add them back in and I feel worse: sleepy, sluggish of thought, and shall we be polite and say "gassy".

It's hard to argue with fact.

Leaping to Conclusions

We NT's are good at this, particularly when you know a person well, there is often no need to mention certain things that are obvious. We therefore leap to conclusions that our husband actually understands our thought processes better than they do. So when he 'lets us down' by failing to do the 'obvious' we get cross, thinking that he either didn't listen, is lazy or worse, just doesn't care.

It is confusing because, when you first meet and you share your every thought and deed so closely and discover what you have in common, it often seems like he does really know you. The difference is that often you are bonding over a similar interest and therefore he can relate. Knowing that you wanted him to vacuum the stairs because you were going to be late from work and the plumber was coming to fix a tap in the bathroom does not compute with him.

He may even have been in the room when you mentioned that the stairs would need hoovering but he would not have realised that it meant he had to do it. Unless he has the comorbidity of OCD, putting a vacuum to the stairs is not on his radar.

Leaping to His own Conclusions

David and I were discussing the other day about intuition and whether he had it or not. After some thought he said he did have intuition but it was different to the NT version of intuition.

For example, when a NT sees someone they know approaching them down the street, within a nanosecond they make the decision whether they want to speak to that person or not and quite possibly whether that person wants to speak to them. If you do stop to talk and pass the time of day, two NT's conversing will each assess the other's mood quickly. Often the conversation is quick and to both person's "social interaction satisfaction" allowing them to move on.

For you typical Aspie this everyday occurrence is actually one that causes great anxiety and best to be avoided if possible. They have no intuition that they can use to evaluate in a moment the mood of their 'opponent' and conversation may become adversarial.

They leap to conclusions in other areas too, and in a way we cannot understand and which is actually hard for them, themselves to describe.

For example, our son never made it into the top maths stream in school. We knew he had a natural ability with maths so we could not understand why. On conversation with his maths teacher we found out that he was not answering the questions in the way that she liked. Was he getting the answers wrong? No, he was getting the answers completely right. However, in her eyes this was not good enough. She needed to know how he came to the conclusion. She insisted that he write out the methodology to explain how he got to the conclusion.

Well, to our son and to my husband, this seems like a complete waste of time. Once they have read the question, their mind (depending on the type of question) leaps to the answer without having to 'work it out', therefore when Morgan's teacher asks him to write down the methodology, he finds this difficult and pointless.

Leaping to the Wrong Conclusions

Unfortunately, David using his logic and experience of worldly matters, will often leap to the wrong conclusions where social situations are concerned. He will use previous situations to try to help explain current situations but not notice subtle and different nuances from the time before. This is where he gets socially unstuck and can easily offend or annoy.

The Husband Says:

The above is quite accurate. I'll expand a little:

With a near absence of social information in a decision making process, Aspie's eventually become accustomed to "making do" without that information. This leads to social mistakes. But in business, I turn this to my advantage. I have become accustomed to decision making without the full information available; I'll make a decision based on what scant information I do have and I'm prepared to set out on that course of action. That makes me different from many NTs who can't make an important decision without all the facts, triple checked and certified. It looks like I'm gambling, and there is an element of that, but I'm relying on an adapted form of intuition.

Leo Kanner

Leo Kanner was an American psychiatrist who was born in Austria. He wrote the seminal paper regarding autism in 1943 'Autistic disturbances of affective contact'.

Though Hans Asperger, a fellow Austrian published first, Kanner never made reference to his work.

Letting Things Go

Your Aspie has a one-track mind. This is one of the reasons why he finds it hard to drop a subject.

Yet, if someone has upset him and he doesn't understand why, it could take him months to get over it. It may be something as simple as not understanding why someone doesn't obey the rules to being upset about events on the evening news.

Until he has some kind of resolution e.g. reporting illegal parking to the police, or researching every detail he can find online about a certain subject, he will not be able to relax or even sleep. His mind won't let him. It won't matter if his obsession inconveniences others. This takes priority,

NT Understanding is the key. Helping him make sense of the world around him. Sometimes it helps to join in with them if you have the patience. It will validate his thoughts and hopefully resolve them quicker.

Letting you Down

He would never knowingly let me down. He wants to be supportive and be seen to do the right thing, yet it is difficult for him to know what the right thing is when no one has told him.

Of course, an intelligent man in his forties should know what the right thing is by now, surely? Well the answer to that is "Yes" and "No".

Certain situations come up time and time again, and he has learned along the way how to behave, but new and uncertain settings come up almost daily which you and I just 'wing' without a care. This laid back attitude we have for certain situations is something that our husbands are very jealous of. They wish that they had this magic ability to "read" a room or a situation with a glance or just by hearing the tone of someone's voice.

They don't mean to let us down, they either just don't understand the demands placed on them, or they get so emotionally overloaded by a situation, they switch off and react by disappearing and leaving you to it.

Don't forget, although this is a secret that they probably haven't confessed to you, they married you because of your magical ability in social situations. The company, cookery, and sex are just added bonuses.

One of the many reasons I took to David was his unswerving love and support for me. Yes he has let me down in certain unpredictable situations, but when it comes to the big stuff he has been there for me. When I most needed him, such as the day my mum died, or the day I graduated and I was a nervous wreck, he took control and calmed me down. I don't know anyone else who could or would do that for me.

The Husband Says:

I don't set out to knowingly let you down. Happenstance may be such that events conspire to affect my decision making. This may lead to me behaving in an unexpected and non-NT way - that looks to you like "letting you down". I had no intent, no pre-meditation to do that.

Libido

I have read and heard very mixed stories regarding an Aspie man's libido. Some are perfectly "normal", a few very high, but most of what I have come across is complaints from the wives about their husbands lack of libido and of her feeling neglected.

It isn't necessarily something that goes hand in hand with ASD at all but can be a side effect of it. Certain medications for depression for example are known to affect libido.

There is also gathering research about the effect of Vitamin D deficiency. In the northern hemisphere and especially in Britain we suffer from a lack of sunshine and therefore many people do not get sufficient sun exposure to enable them to make their own vitamin D. Vitamin D is crucial to good health and many people who have supplemented with it believe that it has helped motivate them in all areas of life including their sex life.

L

The Husband Says:

There are lots of things under this topic to discuss. Aspies like me have a reputation for being blunt, but we are also quite shy so forgive me if now that I'm "put on the spot" to comment on libido that I blurt out what most people might only hold as private thoughts in their own head.

First of all, since getting married and our children arriving on the scene (and no, I won't do a birds and bees piece!), I will say that opportunities to exercise my libido are greatly reduced. I don't think my libido is any lower (other than old-age kicking in), but it has fewer outlets for the time being. NTs indicate to me that love and sex are best when spontaneous, so in depth planning to take time off work or have the children looked after for a weekend of husband-wife time rather spoils the moment. The only surprises can be what happens during that time you have made to be together. But don't be too surprising or extreme - for our NT partners - all things in moderation.

And then there is the filtering of expectation that has to take place. NTs can spot a joke or a leg-pull and comments on libido by NTs, especially males, can be quite ribald. As an Aspie I have to work harder to filter out truthful information from bawdy lad-talk hyperbole. Am I average in the libido department? Probably, but there is so much "noise" that I can't tell for sure. It's a difficult enough subject for an NT to talk about seriously, never mind for a shy Aspie to strike up the courage to even talk about the subject. Us Aspies trust few people and the conversation on libido requires the very highest level of trust. On that tack, it would be near impossible to get me to talk openly and honestly with a third party counsellor (a popular agony aunt answer to libido problems) - how could I build up enough trust?

In a cold and clinical examination (what else do you expect from an Aspie?), husband and wife would probably seem to get the most out of the sexual parts of their relationship when their libidos and expectations are somewhat matched. As an Aspie though, I'm "blind" to many of the signs of success in a sexual relationship - one area of human behaviour where communication is much less on what is being said and much more on what is being done and particularly facial expression. I want an example to follow, but Karen is my first, only and hopefully last sexual partner? Do I come up to standard; can I claim to be at least average? There are some anxieties here through lack of hard-to-come-by-experience.

Light at the end of the Tunnel

There was a time, a few years ago, where I could see no end to the darkness of my marriage. There was no light at the end of the tunnel. In my mind, it just stretched on and on with no respite from his moods and behaviour. I even started to think I was depressed but was assured by my GP that I was 'just under a lot of stress'. He was right of course, but I couldn't see how to reduce the stress.

So how did I turn the corner in our relationship?

It was a slow process and, though we have come a long way, we are perhaps not there yet.

NT What made the differences were a series of instances I would not have put together initially. His psoriasis and my gluten intolerance. I was looking for a solution to his terrible skin condition. I came across some interesting research regarding Vitamin D3 and it sounded convincing. David, though cynical, was happy to start taking 4000 iu a day of Vitamin D3 and also Omega 3. Slowly his skin condition started to improve. There was no other change in his lifestyle other than this. Bizarrely, however, after a few months I realised that he had been a lot calmer and more motivated than usual.

Further investigation regarding Vitamin D3 and autism revealed research regarding the improvement of behaviour of children who were accidentally given high doses of Vitamin D3 by their parents. This made me realise I was on the right track and I started to investigate further. It was such a relief to see there might be a light at the end of the tunnel for us. This was a significant step forward for our marriage.

The Husband Says:

AS *I wouldn't want to rather unscientifically suggest that taking vitamins is the only thing that saved our marriage and helped me, in particular, to appear more normal. Can I start a list?*

- *Sorting out an embarrassing skin condition certainly helped. For any condition at all - eat more healthily, get a medical check-up, and get anything that is broken, fixed.*

- *Accepting, and then beginning to promote a label for myself as an Aspie that is able to cope, succeed and flourish is important to me. I've sort of "Come out of the Autism Closet"*

- *Talking very openly with Karen has given me a lot more coping strategies to add to the twin acts of David at home and David at work.*

- *Telling a few selected friends and colleagues why, from time to time, I might behave differently to their expectations.*

- *Writing my response to Karen's thoughts for this book and App has been beneficial - perhaps keeping a diary or a blog and analysing your situation might help?*

- *Realising that outside of my small circle of friends, family and colleagues, that I'm never going to see that person again, so why should I care about what they think.*

L

Listening

Do you ever get the feeling that your conversations are rather one sided? Most Aspie wives tend to be very good listeners. It is one of our men's' most obvious traits that they love to talk about their special interests irrespective of whether their captive audience is interested or not.

We end up in that Asperger Marriage Paradox while he is spouting about his work or his hobby. We Aspie wives want to see them happy and interested in something and much prefer an atmosphere where he can talk about his favourite subject, than one where he is silent and ignoring us or, worse, getting irrationally angry with us about something that happened that was beyond his control.

Yet, especially when you are in the car on a long journey and he is telling you for the 96th time about some intricate tax law that he is having to explain to his stupid work colleagues, you do feel like ripping your own ears off! You know that if you disagreed, with him or tried to change the subject when he is on a roll, that he will inform you in many ways how you are completely wrong, or will just get back onto his favourite subject.

Remember the days when you first met and you found this endearing? Maybe it was because you had work or a hobby (probably where you met) in common? He seemed to be clever and interesting back then and he would listen to your opinion too?

I suspect he doesn't do much listening anymore.

The Husband Says:

I'll start my comments on this subject with the opposite of listening: talking. You see that's what gets us Aspies into the most trouble. Our social awkwardness has restricted the number of topics on which we feel we can hold a conversation. We like to be expert in what we talk about. We hate it when we are stopped with a rightful call of "bullshit" and will work to avoid this by becoming ever more expert on an ever narrower range of topics. Now add in the fact that Homo Sapiens are social creatures - we all feel like we must keep communicating in order to be human, so we fill silences. We get tense when there is a silence. Aspies even more so. You know the bit on X Factor where they announce the most recent loser and, to build tension, they make you wait exactly ten point zero, zero seconds for the answer - that feels like an eternity, yes? For Aspies even more so.

Karen gets annoyed when we are in the car and there is silence and I ask her why she is so quiet, me assuming something is wrong because I've miss-read her facial expressions again - deep thought looks so much like stubbed toe.

L

Karen Says:

Okay I have to interject here. Those silences in the car you mention? Those are meant to be companionable silences when we are listening to music or watching the scenery go by. Just because I am not saying anything, doesn't mean I'm cross.

Back to the Husband:

Now look at the flip-side: listening. Chit-chat is boring; can I re-purpose those neurons processing listening for something else? Why yes - "polite" listening where you don't listen at all but try to give the impression that you are. NTs and Aspies both do this and both get caught, but NTs can be brazen whereas Aspies can be apologetic. It's a shame there is no socially acceptable way, other than in comedy, to interject in someone's conversation and say "you are really boring, you've banged on about this for 20 minutes, and on top of all that, you are wrong". Perhaps we need a new social convention - a small flag you can wave perhaps? Or perhaps we all need to learn the value of silence - that means you, NT-person, too.

Lists

 Your partner may be obsessed with lists. This might be beneficial.

My (suspected) ASD father, for example, regularly makes lists of things that he needs to do. Sometimes he even starts to do the tasks on his lists but very quickly he loses his list and can't go any further. On another day he will start again by writing a new list. It is a family joke, but also a reality, that he will start the second list with this:

1. Find List

I have come across many wives who complain bitterly about their husband's lack of organisation. They tell me that they have tried to organise him to the point of syncing up their digital diaries, putting tasks on whiteboards in the hallway, sending them long texts with detailed shopping lists on and so on.

They cannot understand and have no sympathy when their partner ignores their requests or comes back with the wrong item. They get frustrated and cross with them, berate them and then write them another long list of things to do.

What these women are not doing is trying to find out why their partner has not managed to do what, at first glance, seems like a very simple task. After all, what is difficult about looking at your phone on the way home from work and reading and sticking to the shopping list sent by your wife?

Well first of all, as an Aspie who has had an extremely long and difficult day at work having to deal with the neurotypical disorganised way of working, they will be mentally and physically exhausted as they leave the office. All they will be thinking about is putting on their favourite music in the car as loudly as they can to enable them to relax. They will be focussing on the long drive home but they may also be finding it very hard to switch off from some technical detail they are having difficulty with at work: as they have a one track mind, they will be concentrating on that. It may be that they will drive all the way home ruminating on this fact and, despite your reminders, will have completely forgotten to go to the supermarket. As they get home and walk into the house, they will suddenly remember that they have failed to complete the one task you have given them that day. This will most likely make them feel like a failure and angry with themselves.

Of course, what is the first thing that you say to him when he gets home? 'Did you get the shopping?' You are immediately pointing out his failure. He will react badly to this and blame you for giving him the task in the first place when he is overworked and tired. He may well resent the fact that you have been in the house all day "just" looking after the children, whilst he has had to go out and deal with unpredictable people and situations all day long. He will resent the fact that you have the (seemingly) easier task of childcare or your own (less important) work. He will be jealous of the fact that you find these tasks so much easier to deal with than he does, and then you pile more tasks on him instead of doing them yourself. This is where resentment and arguments build up. He needs time to decompress.

However, he may have had a good day, or you may have sent him a timely reminder to go to the supermarket, and he has actually got there. He hates supermarkets! - they are bright and loud, full of people aiming trolleys at him, there is too much choice and the staff ask him ridiculous questions at the tills. He is already stressed about the experience before he gets there...and before he takes out the list you have given him.

Whilst avoiding all the maniacs with their ankle bruising trolleys, he tries to remember where items are kept. Supermarkets have a very annoying habit or changing their aisles around just when you think you have learned them.

Then there is the list; have you just sent him a list that says milk, rice, baby wipes and bread? Or have you sent him a more detailed list that lists exactly what brand of item you need? Giving him the exact item is a good idea but he can come unstuck if the item is not there. Quite often they will get overwhelmed by the choice of similar looking products and worry that they will get the wrong one. In some cases they will not get any type of product for fear of getting it wrong, not realising that ultimately, if you need baby wipes urgently, any brand will do (as opposed to no wipes at all).

It would be worth giving him second and even third options here - or put a reminder on the list: 'Ring me if you are not sure'.

Some Aspies actually enjoy the freedom and choice of a supermarket especially when they don't have to go very often. They get sucked in to the clever marketing and believe the large signs and dazzling offers that are on display. There was many a time my dad would be sent to the local Sainsbury's by my Mum to get a loaf of bread, and he would come home laden with reduced price goods because they were a 'bargain'. I still remember the confused look on my mother's face as my dad presented her with a pint of single cream that had been reduced. He was very proud of himself but could not actually give her a reason why he bought it other than it was a good price.

Some Aspies stick rigidly to the list while others enjoy going off piste. The more spontaneous, like my dad, might need a little bit of training to make them stick to the list and give consideration to whether they actually need any other items they see that are not on the list.

NT

Pointers to making a good effective list:

- Do not make the list too long

- If it is a list of tasks rather, than a shopping list, try and keep it to a maximum of 3 tasks for the day (otherwise he will get overwhelmed and end up doing none of them or feel like he is being burdened with the whole world's problems and do them all with bad grace).

- If it is a joint list of tasks make sure that the tasks are clearly marked with people's names so that he does not feel he has to do all of them. However, this does not work in my household, regardless! Even if I write a list for myself and name it "Karen's List of Things To Do", in his mind, he still sees it as "David's List of Things That Karen Wants Him To Do". These days I tend to stick to mental or hidden lists for myself to avoid him seeing them and getting cross about them. If he believes there is a job to do, he thoroughly believes that he is the only person who can do it right.

He also believes that if I start a job, I never finish it. This is annoying for both of us and we have different ways of going about tasks. I do indeed like to get things started but I am not as single-minded as him and will generally do a job in stages. I get bored easily and like to alternate tedious tasks with something else or a rewarding cup of coffee. Also, as a mother, I am at the beck and call of the children (and indeed as his wife) hence I have to stop and make the tea, do some cleaning and put the bins out on time. Whilst I see this as multi-tasking, he sees this as lack of commitment to a task.

Frustratingly, I will often get back to a task to find out he is finishing it for me. Sometimes I am secretly glad but, mostly, I find this very annoying. I wouldn't have started it if I didn't think I could do it. David also has very different techniques from me - some that I don't always approve of.

L

Tip: if you are writing a list of named tasks, you may want to specify how long it will take you do it and whether or not you believe you may want help. Perhaps colour code in red if you do not want help at all. Hands Off!

The Husband Says:

On shopping lists: What flipping type of wipes? Am I psychic? Are you cleaning the baby, your shoes or the toilet? How many? What scent? Any particular brand? I'm the one who is supposed to have the communication disability!

There. Got that out of my system. Normal service can be resumed.

I make lists for several reasons (I can feel a list coming on...):

- *To make sure I do everything that people seem to be expecting of me - to gain closure.*

- *To put the list of tasks in some sort of priority order; I can only do one thing at a time so I'll put the most important one at the top.*

- *As a signal that I'm looking to take on tasks and that I'm brought into a planned event, e.g. preparations for visitors at Christmas.*

- *My memory is great, but sometimes not that great (see avoidance). I will write down nasty chores that I must do, rather than feel particularly willing to do. This is a form of martyrdom.*

- *Last, but not least, so I can get the satisfaction of crossing things off the list when they are finished! A big red felt tipped pen is best. I'll secretly put some easy to achieve stuff at the top of the list so that I can cross that off quickly - it makes it look like I'm making progress.*

I am Master of the Lists! Gantt charts are the ultimate in Aspie list writing - they are list writing disguised as business.

Literal Thinking

Aspies are literal thinkers. If you say you will do something in a minute they will keep an eye on the clock and inform you that you took longer than a minute. They may consider that you were lying, whilst you were in fact just being vague.

The Husband Says:

Over the years, I have been exposed to many of the metaphors and phrases that tempt Aspies into thinking the worst. So I think I'm almost immune to the faux-pas that this can generate. One place where I still get stuck on literal thinking (which can lead to social gaffes) is in the

double meaning of sexual innuendo. I either see innuendo where none was meant, or miss the innuendo that I've accidentally uttered with brain on auto-pilot, that all the NTs pick up on with it being out of social context.

Loneliness

There you are in a marriage with children, a busy life, perhaps work and a good social life, yet you feel alone.

It's hard to put your finger on at first, but it slowly dawns on you that you are the only one who knows what it is like to be you. On the outside things look rosy, but underneath your smiles you might be dying inside from lack of love and understanding.

Worse, the person you married with the intention of spending the rest of your life with him, is cold, thoughtless, and often angry with you for no reason. In fact, you can't reason with him and you can't explain to your parents or your close friends what is going on, because you don't really understand the situation yourself.

Later you may suspect or even have a diagnosis of Asperger Syndrome for your husband. This however, does not magically cure loneliness and the lack of reciprocation in your life.

NT Don't let me make you think it is all doom and gloom but it does take a lot of hard work on your part and also, to a certain extent, your husband's.

Finding an understanding counsellor is a good start. Someone who will listen to you without judgement and who knows what it is like to have a husband on the spectrum. At the moment they are few and far between but I know there is training going on out there.

Join a support group. There are several on Facebook and a particularly good one, run for NT partners, called Different Together. Look it up. There are forums of people exactly in your situation. They even have Meetups organised locally where you can have a coffee and a chat with like-minded people.

Talk to your husband. Get him to read this App. See if he will pick up some of the tips. Even being offered a cup of coffee once a week by him is a good start and shows that he cares. I'm still working on that by the way.

Lorna Wing

Lorna Wing trained as a medical doctor but specialised in psychiatry. In 1981 Wing was the author of a number of books and papers on autism, her most significant being 'Asperger Syndrome a Clinical Account' which made known Hans Asperger's translated work and coined the term 'Asperger Syndrome'.

Much of her pioneering research work was carried out with Judith Gould and, together, they set up the National Autistic Society.

Love

NT
How often do you tell your partner that you love him? How does he react when you do? If he is pleased you should keep telling him.

The Husband Says:

AS
FELLOW ASPIES: *Keep telling your partners you love them. The NTs can't get enough of this. To you it is boring and repetitious - "I told you yesterday I loved you, and I still feel the same way, nothing has changed overnight, so why should I repeat myself?". Well just humour me, do it, and see the reaction.*

Here endeth the sermon.

Karen Says:

For me it depends how much you snored during the night.

Low Emotional Intelligence

The medical term for this is Alexithymia.

The Husband Says:

I was recently talking about being an Aspie with a colleague whilst in the car. We got onto the subject of intelligence, and he commented that he thought I was very intelligent. A nice compliment to get. I had to remind him, though, that "intelligence" comes in many forms. Intellectual intelligence can be measured through testing, but emotional intelligence (about perceptions of feelings, mood and emotion in others) is much harder to test, but no less important than out and out intellectual brain-power. My Aspie brain is probably no "better" than his, but my brain is wired for pattern and logic where his is wired for recognising emotion and appropriate social behaviour.

L

Lowering your Expectations

NT

Every marriage starts with high expectations and, eventually, reality hits when the humdrum of household chores, long working days, and the negatives of sharing a bathroom kicks in. It perhaps happens sooner in an AS/NT marriage.

To make a marriage successful, both partners need to understand where the problems lie and be prepared to do something about them. However, if you are the one who is most unhappy, but still want to save the marriage, and you are the one with the high emotional intelligence, the first steps should come from you.

First of all, as he will not change overnight, you need to lower your expectations of what your idea of marriage is. This does not mean that you can't have a happy and balanced marriage, but you need to be pragmatic: by reducing your expectations you are less likely to be disappointed. Any nice surprises are a bonus but not to be relied upon.

By reducing your expectations of him, he will be able to relax a little, not be so anxious when he knows he is meant to do something to please you, but hasn't worked out what it is or how to do it.

The Husband Says:

I sort of agree with Karen's thinking here, but I would be being unfair, and I would be taking advantage if I expected Karen to lower her expectations forever. I want to please. I want to fulfil expectations. But I need to understand the expectations first.

So would you settle for: "Lower your expectations, at least for a little while"?

Lying

It is a myth that those on the autistic spectrum do not lie; it very much depends on the person, their level of anxiety and the situation.

There is a certain art to lying, both for NTs and for those with an ASC. For us NTs it certainly comes more naturally and it is skill we learn from a young age. Indeed, child psychologists say it is a milestone that every NT child needs to pass at the age of four, though it is not one that gets checked with the health visitor. It is possibly one that should be, as our son passed all of the traditional milestones but I think alarms bells would have been raised much sooner and we could have had an earlier intervention.

L

Different Types of Lying

Deliberately

This is the kind of lying that takes planning to get it right. Aspies are not good at this as they either miss out something really obvious or get caught in the nitty gritty and use too much detail.

Omission

This is something our AS partners are accused of on a regular basis. However, I think they are getting a bad press. The lying by omission is more to do with thinking that have already told you something or it is connected to their theory of mind where they assume you already know, as they know. They are generally more open and honest than we would like to be so they do not bother with being tactful so have no need to do this. It takes up too much brain power.

Defensive

This is the most common form of lying for our Aspies. This happens when you ask your Aspie a question and he or she immediately denies they know the answer. They often assume you are accusing them of something when you are not so they immediately leap to their own defence and deny any knowledge of anything, just in case they get into trouble.

Outright Denial

This is something that NT children do when they are very young. When they are caught in the act of having eaten a bar of chocolate but deny it even though the evidence is literally all over their face. It takes your Aspie much longer to achieve the mental maturity to realise that they have been caught out and the best thing to do is admit it.

The Husband Says:

Sometimes it is necessary to tell a lie to protect someone else from harm. See White Lies.

But Aspies are often spectacularly poor liars; perhaps in being slow to spot facial expressions (the big give-away for liars) we are poor at spotting other people's lies and therefore think that lies are easy. You would think that with all this putting on an act that Aspies could remember the lies that they have told and maintain a cover story, but this is surprisingly tricky - it is the weaving together of truth and fiction where you will come undone.

If you must lie, then the "sin of omission" - not telling something that someone else might consider important - is the simplest, dare I say fool-proof lie?

L

M

- ✧ Making Assumptions
- ✧ Man Cave
- ✧ Marrying into a Different Culture
- ✧ Marrying your Dad
- ✧ Massage
- ✧ Medication
- ✧ Meh
- ✧ Meltdowns
- ✧ Memory
- ✧ Mental Exhaustion
- ✧ Mental Health
- ✧ Mental Processing
- ✧ Metaphor
- ✧ Mild Autism
- ✧ Mind Blindness
- ✧ Mirroring
- ✧ Misplaced Guilt
- ✧ Missing Language
- ✧ Misunderstanding of Intention
- ✧ Moderation
- ✧ Motivation
- ✧ Moving Furniture
- ✧ Moving House
- ✧ Multi-layered Meltdown
- ✧ Multi-tasking
- ✧ Music

M

Making Assumptions

We neurotypicals are guilty of making assumptions about most people, their actions and most situations. We use the knowledge that we already have and use that to predict what will happen in a given and typical scenario. This is an ability we have which can often stop us from worrying about the unknown.

This is an ability that those on the autistic spectrum can only dream of. It is very much part of their 'taking life literally' outlook. They find it difficult and some people just cannot transfer previous knowledge of a situation from one occasion to another. Just because the quiz night went well last time and was enjoyable does not mean the same will happen again the next. They may of course tell us that they are pragmatic but we NT wives' will see this as a rather negative outlook. I for one usually expect things to go well unless I have prior knowledge. I am not always right.

This lack of previous knowledge transference shows up in many everyday tasks. When, as a NT mother, I asked my AS son to help lay the table, I got cross with him for only getting his own knife and fork out. It dawned on me that I had not been specific enough with my language. I should have asked him to lay out the cutlery for the whole family. If you wonder why your AS husband is reluctant to do certain things for you, it may relate back to when they did something you had asked but then you criticised them for doing it wrong. In fact, who is at fault in this situation? The person who gave incomplete instructions or the person who carried them out to the letter?

We NT's have to be so careful with our language but we are not used to doing this. We pepper our language with metaphors and similes and leave out what we believe is unnecessary obvious information.

NT   Never assume that Aspie's know what they are doing, particularly if it is a new situation, no matter how trivial. Be aware, if they make a mistake, not to be too hard on them (regardless of whether they are an AS child or adult). They are not mind readers.

It is safe to assume that you can never assume.

Man Cave

I think this alone could save most marriages be they typical or otherwise.

Be it a garden shed, home office with a closing door, a loft with a Hornby train track or time spent tinkering on the car, every man deserves to have a place in his home he can call his own.

David is not really a car tinkerer. Indeed, he probably shudders at the thought as he will be mentally dragged back to his teenage years when he was forced to fix cars and change bicycle tyres at the family run petrol station. It did teach him a lot about being practical and he did amass a lot of tools but he tries not to get them out too often these days.

A man cave, especially one combined with a tool shed has multiple uses. The male of the species feels great pride, and bristles with testosterone, when he lines up his tools. Asking him to do a task which will allow him to display his fine and shiny tools means that you might get something fixed and he feels useful (while having quality time to himself and the radio). He even gets thanked.

Marrying into a Different Culture

At first I didn't think this applied to me but actually when I stared to think about it, it does.

I was born and bred in Wales to an English mother and a Welsh father. We moved to the north east of England when I was 17. Looking back now, I realise I had quite a sheltered and mostly happy upbringing in a nice, leafy, middle class part of Cardiff. We went to church twice every Sunday and I sang in the choir until we moved. My father was an only child and, though my mother wasn't, we didn't often get to see our cousins who lived in the big smoke in England. I had good friends in and outside of school and I used to spend a lot of time outside playing in the park, climbing trees, paddling in the stream and walking my dog.

David on the other hand, was brought up in a council house in Gateshead for the first 13 years of his life and attended, what sounds like, quite a rough school (particularly for such a delicate little boy). His father worked in the local Ordnance factory and it sounds like there wasn't a lot of money to go around. David's mother is one of eight siblings who are all still very close. David has barely mentioned any friends that he had at school and he certainly hasn't kept in touch with them.

So twenty years ago, a Welsh girl and a Geordie lad met and fell in love over common grounds of sense of humour and taste in music. I'm not sure I could quite use the term exotic about myself, but I suspect he found me interesting and different from anything he had experienced before - and he wanted to know more.

So what is the relevance of this article? Marrying into a different culture means that some of the quirks and idiosyncrasies you spot in your partner are put down to having a different upbringing and background, and not at first down to personality. Misunderstandings may be seen as due to lack of common ground or language. Because there appears to be a reason, you are more patient and tolerant at first. You even find it endearing. After years of this behaviour, you realise that you know each other well enough, and have enough common history together, for these

M

continuing difficulties in the marriage to be caused by differing backgrounds any more. They are caused by thinking differently.

The Husband Says:

This article seems to me to be a thinly disguised piece on class, so I'll go with that...

Karen exemplifies the middle classes; upper middle most likely. I'm an example of class mobility - starting with working class roots and trying to be accepted as upper-middle. Now the upper-middles are the hardest bunch to crack - they have the strongest and most developed social norms that the Aspie has to learn by rote. If you need a text-book, try: Watching the English: The International Bestseller Revised and Updated

Now the upper classes: they are easy to get along with. English-eccentric is almost the full specification for Aspie-in-hiding. The upper classes are so relaxed about their social position that the social norms bubbling up from the middles just melt away.

The Wife Replies

The fact he didn't understand this article is rather poignant isn't it?

Marrying Your Dad

Sometime after I had married David, my mother commented that I had married my father. I did not take this as a compliment and I'm still not sure how it was meant. I did at the time disagree with my mother, but deep down I knew she was right.

What is it about daughters marrying a man like their father? I did look up to my dad when I was little. I was more of a daddy's girl than my mum's. As well as lots of cuddles, we would fight terribly. We still argue now and I find him most annoying, but I love him dearly.

I suppose David had a lot of the traits I admire in a man; hard working, intelligent, lots of dark hair but he also had traits where he was, and is, completely different to my own father.

So I was brought up, unbeknownst to everyone within it, in an Aspie household. The love was there but maybe not as effusive as in my friends' houses. For example, even though my parents constantly bickered, I always knew they loved each other. That's not a bad thing to want to emulate. Perhaps my parents long lasting marriage (until my mum died in their 38th year) was something I subconsciously want to emulate and has given me the resolution and determination to try and keep my own marriage together. I know my mum had a to put up with a lot and, in hindsight, I have a lot of sympathy for her.

Massage

This may seem strange in relation to someone who is sensitive to touch. However, it is all about the right kind of touch.

Our Apies like to know what is going on and be in control. If you give them notice and let them be in control, they can find massage very enjoyable and very relaxing.

It may be a learning curve at first, as you will have to work out how much pressure they like in certain areas. Some will like only a very light touch whereas other will prefer "the firmer the better".

It is a way of being intimate with your partner, whilst being quiet and relaxed and, if their libido is low or they are wary of sexual intercourse, it is a way of being with each other without the threat of Sex.

The Husband Says:

As Karen says it might seem odd. But for the hyper-sensitive, having a firm massage that can be controlled is completely different from for example, tickling, and can help to calm down hyper-sensitivity. Likewise, hypo-sensitivity can to some extent be "reactivated" by the touch of massage.

Try it. Go to an expensive spa and see how professionals do it. Don't be worried about THAT either; professionals have seen it all before and you will be (to begin with) so anxious about THAT happening that THAT can't happen at all. There's a lot of myth and bravado around this subject.

Medication

Asperger's Syndrome by itself does not need any medication. It is neither illness or disease. It is a difference in the way the brain is wired and there is no cure for that. For many 'sufferers' they do not require a cure either.

For those who have a Co-morbid condition, such as ADHD, there can be a requirement for medication.

Antibiotics and Asperger's

We are increasingly told by the authorities that we are becoming resistant to antibiotics and that we should not be taking as much as we are, especially for common ailments such as a virus, as antibiotics do not fight viruses.

There is another reason not to take antibiotics when not entirely necessary; this being that antibiotics not only destroy the bad bacteria that have caused any infection or illness, but also they destroy the good bacteria in your gut. There are

M

billions of good bacteria in our gut and we need them for good health and to reduce inflammation in our bodies. Inflammation is the cause for many serious illnesses such as Crohn's disease and cancer, but it can also affect our brains and the way we think.

I am not in any way suggesting that inflammation and antibiotics are the cause of autism. I am however suggesting that, when you already have a different perspective on the world to the majority of people, you need to keep your thinking skills at optimum capacity. Having your thinking affected makes you moody and irrational and even confused at times.

Of course, we all need antibiotics from time to time if our body's immune system cannot naturally protect itself. In which case, we need to take precautions after we have finished a course of antibiotics, and replenish our stock of healthy bacteria in the gut. This can be easily done by taking a probiotic supplement or drink.

The Husband Says:

Two points from an Aspie, and additions to what Karen has said:

I don't like the idea of taking medication (drugs) that might affect mood or personality (psychoactive). I see that as some aspect of losing control, and I like to think that I am in control.

For years I used to suffer from recurrent tonsillitis and I'm also allergic to the usual anti-biotic to treat this - penicillin. Having reduced stress levels and with Karen giving me a selection of vitamins, I don't seem so prone to tonsillitis anymore. Of course your mileage may vary...

Meh

What is this?

This is what my Aspie family describe with perhaps a shrug of their shoulders when they just don't care.

You will have noticed your partner often works on the extremes of everything. He either obsesses about things or completely ignores them. He is highly excited or desperately miserable - or at least these are the things you notice.

This is because a lot of the time they don't react to the dull, mediocre and every day. They don't react because they are not sure what they are feeling. There is a wide chasm between misery and ecstasy. Those two they can relate to so they often dwell in those areas because they know what they feel like. The rest of the time life can just be a bit Meh.

If pushed to, I can identify all kinds of feelings while I sit here typing right now. I know I have other things to do. I know I have to keep quiet while David is on a conference call and though I am not anxious about it I am being careful not to draw attention to myself. I'm keeping an eye on the clock waiting for my daughter to come home through a storm and though I'm not worried exactly, it will be nice to know she is home safe. I am aware of lots of little thoughts and feelings bubbling away in my mind. I'm not sure your AS partner is.

The Husband Says:

I completely "get" and agree with the concept of 'meh'. But what is a mystery is the connection between 'Meh' and penguins, and taking this one step further the fondness with which Aspies hold penguins. Is it a Linux thing?

Meltdowns

I can only describe what an autistic meltdown is like from my end. It often comes completely out of the blue, or so I think at the time, and it varies very much in strength and what triggers it. It can be as little as yelling at me for being in the way when he is driving to a full blown meltdown where he is in tears and gibbering with distress.

I know it is terrible as an autistic person to have a meltdown but I will let David describe what that is like. I can only describe how I feel being on the receiving end of it. Certainly in the early days of our marriage when he would shout at me for reasons I felt were unjustified, I would shout back at him. I am a quiet person but I will not be treated badly and will stand up for myself.

NT

I eventually realised that this would escalate a situation and I had to learn to be more mature, less reactionary and try to calm and defuse the situation. It is very hard to do when you have someone screaming at you, especially in public. It is also very bewildering to be on the receiving end of one of his tirades when you know, or thought you knew you had done nothing wrong. In the many years before I knew he had Asperger's, I thought that I was going mad because situations just didn't make sense.

The Husband Says:

I've procrastinated by about a week so far on starting to write this article. Karen says I don't need to write about everything, but this topic is so important, and I think so misunderstood by NTs that I feel I have to commit electrons to screen. So here goes...

First off for Adult Aspies, the term 'meltdown' doesn't at all describe what is going through your head (or not) at the time of the unwanted behaviour episode. Infants have tantrums when they don't get their own way. NTs might mistake adult Aspie 'meltdowns' as the same thing. They are not. There is no logic behind an infant tantrum, only unmet desires, where manipulation of the parents through guilt, noise and bluster, might get the child their own way.

M

Adult Aspie 'meltdowns' are different (at least from my perspective).

My so-called 'meltdowns' usually stem from two areas of thought and behaviour. First, and perhaps the easiest to explain, is when anxiety levels in a given situation reach such a height that I am barely able to function anymore. This is a disablement of cognitive function caused by that flight or fight adrenaline response - the Aspie act of trying to appear normal slips, logic fails, and I simply don't know what to do. It's unfortunate at this stage that the thing that has triggered this maximum state of anxiety is a debate or argument with someone else. I feel like I'm no longer able to keep up my side of the discussion so even a simple debate becomes an argument. The Aspie desire to 'win' is not diminished; I tend to continue arguing. I'm likely to shout to try to make any last remaining (possibly desperate) points to somehow 'win'.

NT
To help me resolve this type of meltdown, try to think of something that will reduce the pressure that is leading to the anxiety. Don't force an immediate decision. Time and space generally works.

The second type of so called 'meltdown' are worse. Here I'm not particularly anxious, but instead some carefully planned activity starts going wrong. In particular, the situation is going wrong in a way that I can't control and can't plan for and my logical approach to the unknown is clearly failing. To break the cycle I need to make a neurotypical style 'jump' - a leap of faith, that by doing something seemingly illogical, the situation will get better instead of worse. The outcome appears to be much the same - I go argumentative, but now (when carefully analysed) my arguments make no sense whatsoever. I'm flailing around looking for a solution that will get me out of this problem and I'm unwilling to listen to others - I'm responsible, I have to fix this, but I've got no idea what to do. You NT's just 'wing-it'; I need to form a plan but my cognitive functions are just not co-operating with me to allow me to do this.

Can you help me resolve the situation somehow? Well I'll be acting to your eyes really irrationally, but I won't have the forward momentum to actually carry out such an irrational plan. Perhaps you can give me alternatives or an 'escape plan' - let's change the plan we had embarked on so radically that the old planning clearly no longer applies; help me analyse a new route out of trouble. This is going to take time; possibly a change of environment.

Worst of all is if you are on the receiving end of a 'double whammy' meltdown, where not only am I extremely anxious, but I also run out of 'plan'. Only time and space and a reduction in the pressure to perform is going to fix this one.

Can I repeat that these behaviours are not childish tantrums. You probably shouldn't 'give in' to a child in a tantrum and you probably shouldn't back down from a proper NT stand-point on a child's manipulative behaviour. I strongly believe that the vast majority of adult Aspie meltdowns are not at all a child-like tantrum ploy to gain control, but a genuine 'brain-lockup' where, in desperation, there is just no logical course of action to follow.

You can help with strong leadership and by giving time to resolve a new course of action by allowing me to see through the fog of anxiety. There is no magic, instant control-alt-delete for

M

an Aspie meltdown - time, space, an emergent new coping strategy and a post-mortem long, long after the event are the only way to go.

Let's return to the series of meltdowns that Karen described under the anxiety article. Let's see how these were 'double whammy' types...

The whole sequence started on a family holiday in London. We had meticulously planned to do lots of things and not quite achieved a few of them due to massive crowds in the school holidays and over-ambition! The hotel we had stayed in should have been OK (it was budget), but had dropped the ball on quite a lot of things - our kids were on a different floor to us, I found I was unable to visit them to make sure they were OK, and they didn't answer their phones to open the door to me. The hotel was also slap-dash on their fire safety and I became anxious that this was an accident waiting to happen. So I was really on edge. The hotel was adjacent to a big municipal offices and leisure centre; the hotel offered free car parking but the council offices didn't - so the broken barrier at the hotel was an open invitation for the council workers to avoid paying to park. I was unsatisfied by the hotel at checkout, I was driving a new car that I wasn't really 'getting on with' and finally, a local woman criticised my parking quite vocally and abusively in the car park. My planning for the drive to our next stop just disintegrated under the strain. I really didn't want to be there at all. But I had no choice other than to transport Karen and the kids to our next destination; in a car I hated; in an environment full of hostile people; with a family who were resentful that I wasn't performing at 100%.

My social cup was already full arriving in Liverpool at my sister's. I tried to act neurotypical and normal, but it must have been clear that I was troubled. I just wanted to get home and probably never drive that car again. I was disappointed - I had picked that car out as comfortable and somewhat a status symbol that I deserved. The reality was that people on the road seem to have a hatred for BMW and Audi drivers. I'd become an Audi driver and, in my mind, now I was a target for some really terrible driving. You can read the 'body-language' of car drivers and they were all hostile to me. So on the way home, those Audi-haters had even more 'evidence' of my short-comings. In the end, I used Aspie-logic, in the middle of a meltdown-whilst-driving to drive slowly in the inside lane of the motorway with all the trucks who were at least giving me space. As I got closer and closer to home I began to relax a bit (but not much), but Karen just did not understand what was going through my head through all that period. In the end I was able to explain, but it's still one of the most anxious and embarrassing periods of my life.

To round out the story, what has allowed me to drive and enjoy the car? Well, Karen reminds me that most of the people I meet in the car, I will never see again, so what should I care about what they might think? The other thing - we have a second car, a very anonymous Toyota that does not attract any of the unwanted Audi-hating attention, and I enjoy driving that to work when I'm not putting on the social-status-by-car-type act. A lesson to learn? Don't try to project your desired personality onto a car - quite the reverse is going to happen - the public is going to take your choice of car to directly reflect what they think your personality is.

(M)

Memory

Retentive Memory

From a very young age, we realised our son had a very good memory. He learned his colours in moments when I taught them to him as a tiny tot and he remembered them the next day when he showed his grandma. Even now, at the age of 16, he will turn to me and say, "Remember when we went to France in July 2008 and I was terrified of the wasps hiding in the wall?" Not only does he have a good memory he has a very specific memory that remembers details for a very long time.

My long term retentive memory is not great. I am most envious of the rest of my household for being able to recall facts so easily. I was never any good at exams at school, even with my favourite subjects, as the pressure would get to me and I could not recall anything. I came into my own when I was able to play to my strengths with coursework. My first degree was all coursework and no exams so I did well. My family on the other hand actually find revision really quite tedious and unhelpful. We soon learned with our eldest, who has recently taken his GCSE's, that getting to look over information he already knew was completely pointless and demotivating for him. Our strategy was to give him a test paper and find the gaps in his knowledge and work on that. The gaps in his knowledge were usually in areas that hadn't been explained well by the teacher or that he had not understood the first time.

We played to his strengths by drawing diagrams and taking him out to places and explaining in situ the history and geography of the place. Our Aspies need enthusiasm and visual and intellectual stimulation to succeed.

Short Term Memory

There is nothing wrong with their short term memory. However, if they were not listening to you or have absolutely no interest in the topic they will not remember it.

NT If you want them to remember to do tedious chores, you need to make them a visual reminder. Telling them in the morning to come to the parents evening that night is no good. Ideally you will have had it on a prominent calendar for them to see somewhere. One of the best ways to remind David is that he puts it in his works calendar as he always checks that - work is a priority to him.

Text reminders on the day are generally no good as he steadfastly ignores all texts and phone calls from me during a work day. He did look a little bemused when I pointed out recently that, if I wanted to contact him in an emergency, I wouldn't be able to get hold of him. In days gone by I would have known his office phone number off by heart. As he moves around a lot with his consultancy business, one would naturally assume that, since he has his mobile with him at all times, that he would use it occasionally as a communication device and not just a time piece and music player.

The Husband Says:

A few points on how my memory works and how people perceive me as a result:

As Karen says, us Aspies often have excellent short and long term memory, but with some limitations. I'm a very visual thinker; I can manipulate a lot of numbers simultaneously in my head, but I do that by 'writing' them on a mental blackboard so that I can 'see' them to work with them. I'm also a spatial thinker so the positions of these images relative to each other is important. My mental spatial awareness is rather good, if let down by the usual co-morbidity of physical.

Rather embarrassingly, as a visual thinker, I can spot people in a crowd who I have met before (albeit fleetingly) but I can't recall their name. I have no easy means to link the picture of their face to the arbitrary construct that is the name they have been christened with.

It is very easy to mistake a good memory for genuine intelligence. A big chunk of standard intelligence testing relies on short term memory in its various forms. I don't think I'm spectacularly clever, but I remember lots of stuff. If I can manage to make linkages between these pieces of trivia, then I appear clever.

If something doesn't make sense or doesn't fit into a pattern, then I struggle to remember it. My memory is not for arbitrary factoids, it is for stuff that links together and is likely to be useful.

Mental Exhaustion

As neurotypicals we have no idea what it is like to be Asperger's. Even now, with all my knowledge, insight and experience, I still do not know. I will never know. I get little snippets here and there and I am recognising the signs more and more and I am sympathetic to them.

Within my family the signs are there threefold, though they often appear in different ways. On the outside, when we leave the house, we often appear as a normal happy family. On the whole we are, but there is a lot that goes on behind the scenes to help the good times happen.

David is a master at faking it and preparing himself mentally for a difficult time ahead. He will cope with this by planning well in advance and thinking things through very carefully. I have noticed our daughter does the same. Like her father she plans what she is going to do and when she is going to stick to it. I have learned to back off when I try to make impromptu plans with her and I discover she has already mentally prepared plans for the day.

M

Avoiding Mental Exhaustion

All this planning and preparation is very wearing for them. Not only are they doing normal physical and mental tasks that we NT's do every day, but on top of this they have to work extra hard to 'appear normal' socially, keep up their high standards of perfection and, due to their lack of intuition, try to figure out the status and desires of everyone they meet.

By the time they get home from a typical day, my Aspie family just want to disappear to their respective zones. These days they will tolerate a little questioning from me about their days, even occasionally volunteering information if it has been an especially good or bad day, but pretty soon they escape to their rooms to 'switch off' and not have to worry about other people for at least an hour or two.

For our daughter, it is a case of shutting her bedroom door and either going on YouTube or devising role play scenarios with her myriad of tiny characters. I have never been invited to join in. It is very much her world, with her rules where she feels safe and in control.

Our son has his PC set up to the highest quality that he and his father can devise for gaming. The day fibre optic broadband arrived in our rural village was a day of great celebration! Our son is not particularly into 'shooty' games but prefers strategy and world domination. Probably in a similar vein to his sister but his is virtual.

Their father will come home and often tell me about his day and then he will check his emails and Facebook. We share a study so his office is not a complete sanctuary. Since we have moved to a larger house, he disappears into the smaller living room where he has set up a Smart TV and arranged the furniture and lighting exactly to his choice. I rarely venture into this room. It is a man cave where the Grand Prix is shown loudly and on an enormous screen, or he watches mind-numbing American series like Storage Wars.

It isn't that I am not welcome in this room, but I can tell he doesn't really feel comfortable if I just join him when 'his' programmes are on. He wonders why I am there. Occasionally I will ask him if we can watch a particular programme together, usually some Friday night comedy which we both enjoy, but otherwise I feel I encroach on his down time. It has taken me a long time to learn not to step on any of their toes. Ours is a very quiet household at times. Indeed, I like my own space, but I do also crave adult company and chit chat. I generally get that from my many friends and when I need a soft cuddle the dog usually obliges.

I have learned to accept this and even encourage the situation so they get to recharge their batteries. Once they are recharged they are bright, articulate and interesting individuals and a joy to be with.

M

The Husband Says:

Just a quick note on the difference between mental exhaustion and taking a quick break to recharge batteries. A good night's sleep or a substantial time to reflect can sort out true mental exhaustion. Don't mistake this exhaustion from the 'context switch time' needed at the end of every major piece of work - like a working day. It takes time to swap from work-persona to family-persona; perhaps half an hour. After that though your Aspie might come back bright as a button. We sometimes call this decompression time - like a deep-sea diver getting the nitrogen out of their blood, a little quiet time between tasks or events works wonders.

Mental Health

 Looking after the Wife's Mental Health

It is vital for you to look after your mental health. Living with an Aspie man is a daily struggle. I mention elsewhere that I wondered for a while if I was depressed but, on discussion with my GP, we decided I wasn't but that I was under a lot of pressure. I was at such a low point that I seriously considered whether antidepressants would work for me.

However, I knew realistically that popping a pill would not change the difficulties in my life and I knew deep down that, if I could change these, that my life and health would improve. I do however, have plenty of friends who rely on antidepressants and feel that they have made a positive impact on their life and coping abilities.

Recent research suggests that depression could be caused by inflammation in the brain as inflammation is caused by intolerances to certain foods and leaky gut syndrome. It is worth looking at your diet as this could naturally lift your mood. I can testify that cutting out gluten and dairy makes me happier and healthier and a much more tolerant person. Within an hour of eating a chocolate chip cookie, especially those lovely chewy ones, I become an irritable monster and it can take hours for these feelings to disperse. I can't allow myself to feel like that, so there are certain foods or combinations of food which I avoid - unless I am prepared to face the consequences.

Looking after your Aspie Partner's Mental Health

I need to point out to those of you who are new to the condition of Asperger's Syndrome that this is not a mental health condition. It is not a disability but a difference. However, due to the way this difference is treated by peers and other adults over the years, Aspies can be bullied and get depressed and have other comorbid conditions just like NTs can.

M

If your Aspie has been treated well and positively and helped with their anxiety they may never have a mental health problem.

Quite often Aspies are diagnosed with depression but my husband has a theory about this:

The Husband Says:

...I don't think I've ever been clinically depressed. I think that the black cloud of anxiety that Aspies often drag around can look like (or be co-morbid with) depression, but it's nowhere near as deep as a genuine depression could be. Now, doctors tend to define conditions like Asperger's or depression according to the bunch of symptoms that are presented - they currently can't diagnose on root cause because mental health cannot be readily measured with an instrument like a ruler or an x-ray machine - so to them a comorbidity is a long way to a diagnosis.

Back to this core message from me: Yes, I'm wired up mentally a little differently to you NTs, but No, that doesn't mean I'm 'broken' and need drugs as a chemical crutch to support me and make me 'normal'. I don't think any Aspies would like the level of loss of mental control that psychoactive drugs bring along. We are proud of our mental faculties - they are just different, not wrong. I don't want my faculties dulled - just pointed in the conventional direction if they are troubling the NTs.

Someone to listen; someone to talk to who understands. That helps calm the symptoms of Asperger's, in a way that I suspect a true depression isn't dispelled by just talking.

Mental Processing

Your neurotypical brain processes about eighty percent of its information subconsciously, with minimal cognitive effort.

Not so for your AS brain which, because of delayed processing, deals with eighty percent of information on a conscious level.

A typical day requires so much more effort for your Asperger partner than it does for you and this leads to his nervous system becoming taxed and overwhelmed.

The Husband Says:

I've theorised elsewhere that my automatic and innate processing of mood, behaviour and emotion is present, but weak and delayed to the point where it is virtually useless. My principle coping strategy these days is to work to try to understand what an NT might 'see' in a given situation - to take extra time (and effort) to 'process the scene' and almost forensically piece together what the clues are trying to tell me. That's hard work.

M

Metaphor

Quite often we Asperger Wives are married to grammar Nazis and pedants. They love order and grammar and punctuation come under this banner. Their love of words and the addition of literal thinking means they take great delight in metaphors and similes and the play on words.

As they tend to see things from the literal interpretation and not the common metaphorical meaning it brings a whole new light to phrases such as "Toasting the Bride". This presents much mirth in our household.

Mild Autism

Asperger Syndrome is often described as a as mild autism spectrum disorder. There is nothing mild about this disorder. The reason it is described as 'mild' is that people compare it to Leo Kanner's version of autism which is extreme, non-verbal behaviour.

Having AS means that you can appear normal to society and therefore society has high expectations of your social and communication skills and expects you to act like the majority of the neurotypical (NT) population, i.e. 'normal' as it is regularly referred to.

Most people with Asperger's work out from an early age that they are not 'normal' and that they have difficulty carrying out or coping with everyday situations. They know long before they receive a diagnosis. Their awareness of being different creates a huge amount of anxiety in everyday situations. This is very hard for them to cope with as they feel judged and inferior to everyone else.

Couple this anxiety and with additional sensory difficulties, which make experiencing everyday situations like shopping or going to school very difficult, then you can start to see that this is not a mild condition at all.

The Husband Says:

You neurotypicals do like to hierarchically name stuff. To do that, you feel like you have to enumerate thresholds of how big or how far or how orange a thing is. So whilst I'm accepting that all conditions can be measured on a spectrum, you struggle with how to name different apparent severities along that spectrum. So everyone is autistic - depending on how you measure 'autism'. Now here's the rub. We don't know what the chemical and physiological condition of the brain 'is' that corresponds with 'autism'. You see a bunch of symptoms and you try to say that with this, this and this symptom you must be autistic, not because you have identified some physiological process that is broken or different compared with NTs. So now that we acknowledge that we are only talking about symptoms, then 'mild autism' is just

M

the symptoms recognised as being of autism, but less 'far away' from the state of being considered neurotypical.

Thus we enter the debate between the differences between autism and Asperger's, starting with: are there any? I'll leave that for the commentary on another article...

I'll pre-empt. I think autism and Asperger's are different. Sometimes they appear to be similar.

Mind Blindness

Term developed by Simon Baron-Cohen. It means in short an inability to empathise or put yourself in another's shoes; a shortage or deficiency in "Theory of Mind".

Mirroring

NT

Mirroring is an unconscious copying of someone that you respect. You will notice NT's copying the body language of people they like. For example, if someone crosses their legs or takes a sip of wine, if you like them you will also do this. It gives out signals of admiration, respect and comfort.

Your Aspie partner is less likely to mirror your body language unless he consciously takes notes of what you are doing and thinks that he too should be doing this. This is because he is not comfortable in his own skin or confident in his social abilities. He knows that you are comfortable and well versed in non-verbal communication and therefore he takes his cues from you. This is why many of the things he does comes across as awkward or delayed.

Motivation

In an Aspie marriage you can use this mirroring to your advantage. You will have noticed that nagging your partner rarely gets good results, or you get the desired results but with a big dose of bad grace. They do not enjoy being constantly reminded that they have responsibilities, especially when they are not confident in doing them. Generally if they enjoy something or are confident in their abilities, you will not have to nag them, in fact they will often jump to and solve the problem or complete the task straight away. This actually gives them great satisfaction.

Where the mirroring, or perhaps I should call it 'Delayed mirroring', comes in is when you lead by example. By carrying out an activity, such as going for a bike ride, you will actually inspire your partner to do so. However, if you 'spring' the fact that you would like to go on a bike ride with him, he is likely to be reluctant to join in. Unless he is an avid cyclist, he may be daunted by the task ahead. Seeing you going off for a ride and coming back flushed and happy will inspire him to consider doing this task, unless he is completely averse to the outdoors and exercise. He will see that you have got something positive out of the experience and feel that he wants to take part too. The tactic here is not to nag him at all but let him come to his own conclusions. Let him look up routes and if he wants to, take the lead. Once he becomes interested in something, regardless of whether it was his original idea or not, it may become all consuming. However, if you are keen to do activities together, this may be the price you have to pay.

The Husband Says:

Here's a handy tip founded in basic studies of body language. In an uncertain social situation, if you are with someone you trust and know, then consciously mirror them. Neurotypicals who are supportive of each other and agree with each other, subconsciously mirror even very fine details. So if you want to look like you fit in and agree with the current consensus, then mirror your NT partner. Don't be too self-conscious - it is actually pretty difficult to over-do this.

Karen talks about a form of macro-mirroring of whole behaviour patterns. I guess this is more properly setting an example.

Misplaced Guilt

The Husband Says:

I think Aspies suffer from this a lot. We have unrealistic expectations that perhaps someday we can 'cure' ourselves and become neurotypical with the absolutely perfect act of being normal (whatever that is). We set ourselves that goal of average-person behaviour and we fail - we are just not wired up that way. There is a guilt of not being normal, of not delivering what our partners seem to want - neurotypical normality.

But in a mature Asperger marriage, I think partners like Karen are able to come to terms with Aspie behaviours; probably far faster than an Aspie could ever perfect a normality act. So the misplaced guilt of not being neurotypical has already been superseded by your NT partner making account for and accommodating your foibles.

That guilt you are feeling? It is probably misplaced. Just what is this 'normal' people speak of?

Missing Language

This comes under the Theory of Mind umbrella. You wouldn't think that getting ready to leave the house was so complicated. Even when we all plan to leave at the same time, I have to wait for everyone to be ready. When I find David at his desk,

M

I tell him that I am ready to leave and he will then tell me that he is also ready to leave - but he doesn't tell me unless I ask. At times, we have both been waiting for each other to say that the other is ready, and since I have been burned many times in the past, I am patiently waiting for him to make signs that he is ready to leave the house while it turns out that he is waiting for some type of cue. Unfortunately, he missed my cues of being dressed with shoes on and bag in hand.

I have informed him that we need to communicate with each other over vital information that the other cannot read from their mind or body language. If he wants me to know that he is ready, then he has to tell me.

The Husband Says:

Karen speaks a lot of sense here. NT to Aspie communications need to be clear, complete and precise because the non-verbal cues that NTs use all of the time are lost on the Aspie.

But this whole area is a bit of a minefield. What does 'clear language' look like that isn't condescending or degrading? Let's take Karen's example of going out. Now my smart casual dress for going out looks rather like my work garb. Karen will need several attempts to choose the right outfit. She's come downstairs - I haven't changed, so in the land of non-verbal communication: (i) Am I ready to go out?; (ii) Is this the final choice of outfit?; (iii) Should I comment that Karen's outfit looks great and make a move for the car?; (iv) Was Karen coming downstairs to ask my opinion of an outfit she wasn't sure of rather than to signal time to go?

Looking logically at this puzzle suggests that, instead of looking at the news on the computer whilst I wait for Karen, I should change my behaviour - perhaps go to the bedroom and talk with Karen on choice of outfit? This all boils down to modifying behaviour - what would an NT do?

Things that do work - Ask 'Will this do?' with respect to my clothing, in good time to change if the answer is negative (and this line could be inviting a negative response, which might be for the best anyway). This also gives Karen a chance to explain her current status on the process of getting ready to go out.

As Karen points out, this all falls under 'Theory of Mind' - just because you can't see the progress towards being ready to go out (because it is happening in a different room and you can't see it) doesn't mean it isn't happening - don't just assume nothing has happened - if in doubt, ask!

Misunderstanding of Intention

Scenario:

The Asperger husband and NT wife are tidying up their house to put it on the market and they have an estate agent visiting the following day. The husband would rather be in his office working. His wife is busy cleaning and occasionally asking for help with technical or heavy items. It had been agreed in advance that the husband was to set up the power washer which the wife would use to clean the paths. Unfortunately, a small but significant piece of the washer had broken whilst in the shed. The husband becomes extremely stressed as he knew his wife wanted the garden to be perfect and it, being a Sunday afternoon, would not be possible to fix.

The wife though disappointed, decides to use an ordinary garden hose and a brush, and proceeds with the job whilst her husband has spent over an hour searching for a replacement piece of equipment. The wife, pleased with her work, especially once the sun has dried out the paths, cheerfully suggests to her husband that he should take a look at the garden. The husband makes no comment but instead begins vigorously brushing the same area, intermittently shouting demands to his wife despite the fact she is now up a ladder cleaning windows. The wife compliments her husband upon his work but still he is in a bad mood. The wife, by this time, is finding it very hard to maintain calm as she has taken the brunt of her husband's mood for everything which was beyond their control.

In this typical scenario, the wife tries to establish equilibrium when something minor goes wrong. Aware of her husband's catastrophizing she tried alternative solutions.

Much later when he was calmer, the wife asked him why he had redone her work. He said she had told him to go and see how awful the garden was. He felt he was entirely to blame and had tried to rectify the situation. The wife replied 'remember you told me it would look better when the sun came out? I only suggested you look at the garden because I thought that you were right'.

She had wanted to raise his mood by pointing out that he was right, but he was so immersed in his self-imposed failure and guilt, that he misinterpreted what his wife had said. The wife realised that in order to have avoided the situation escalating, she should have been more specific. She had assumed that, when she had suggested that he look at the sunny garden, he would remember his earlier comment and be pleased with the result. However all he heard was criticism.

NT How to avoid this happening in the Future: Be aware that your husband is constantly analysing situations. He will be constantly looking for the good and bad in everything, regardless of how trivial you may think it is.

Before tackling a task together, try and think it through first. He will appreciate your planning and, once he knows what you intend to do, he will most likely be happy to help or, if preferable, let you get on with the task.

Consider your language with him and be patient. Be concise and clear in your instructions to him if you have not tackled the task before. Pay attention to what he says and, when you have finished, tell him he has done a good job. He will appreciate it. As a NT you may think it patronising to point out the obvious to him but, unless you tell him he has done a good job, he will not know and he will worry that he has let you down.

The Husband Says:

I don't have anything insightful or clever to add to this - it will be common sense to you now that Karen has pointed it out. Treat this as Karen's final exam - if you can navigate your way through this minefield scenario then you really know your Aspie well.

Moderation

Everything in moderation except moderation. This is a NT mantra which I understand and, though it may not rule my life, it makes a lot of sense and I try to implement it where I can.

Not so for your Aspie. Indeed, I am not sure (though they may nod wisely at this philosophical quote) that they really understand it, and they certainly cannot carry it out.

The Husband Says:

Karen is correct. Aspies are not moderate, centre-dwelling, people. We are polar - to one extreme or the other, and we polarise other people's opinion either to join us at one extreme or to be repelled to the other.

There are only a very limited set of circumstances where extreme opinions are valid. The world is not some large debating chamber with a line of argument to be 'won'.

Motivation

David likes to say that I am a 'starter' and that he is a 'finisher'. When he says this it is not meant as an insult. He doesn't realise that it hurts me. He thinks it funny, but I know he also gets annoyed with my half-finished projects.

It's true, I do start projects and run out of steam on them. Often with children I just get distracted by the daily grind. The school runs, feeding them, breaking up fights, and so on. I can see how it looks but I don't like the way he judges me for not getting things finished quickly.

Also, people work better in a team, and we are not a team. If I want to start a project in the house, he will tell me to do it or hire someone to do it. He never suggests doing it together. When people work together they motivate each other. I know for example; it is completely pointless to tell my daughter to tidy her room. Even though I know she prefers to have her room tidy and not strewn with painful tiny

M

little toys and dirty clothes, she is not motivated to do it. When I offer to help she jumps at the chance of us doing it together.

The Husband Says:

Well I wasn't expecting that. Clearly something we have to work on as a couple.

I'm not being disrespectful when I say that that there are 'starters' and 'finishers'. Some people that I put on a pedestal leave a trail of unfinished business in their wake - but without them starting off loads of threads; motivating; cajoling to start; then so many of these projects would never come to fruition because us finishers would never dare get going on something so large and daunting.

So we could turn out to be an ideal pairing - a visionary starter and a diligent finisher. I think our problem is different - we cannot agree what to start. I prefer the comfort of the status quo and Karen seems to like change. I do need Karen to tell me when to stop. Like lots of Aspies with an eye for detail, my own standards of workmanship don't live up to my own expectations. So I really need my NT starter to tell me when I've done enough and finished a task otherwise it will just keep going on and on with me progressively gilding the lily.

The Wife Says:

Writing this book and App has taken a fair amount of team work. However, our roles have been clearly defined. I am the main author and creative director with the educational know how. David has been the technical support and provider of inside Asperger knowledge. I could not have done this without his unique skills.

Moving Furniture

When we were going through the diagnostic process for our son at the age of nine, the consultant psychologist spent a few hours asking us a lot of questions about his behaviour. The one that sticks in my mind is when the psychologist asked me about when our son comes home from school and the furniture has been moved around, does he get upset? I laughed and said, "no he doesn't even notice but he", and I pointed at David, "freaks out if I do it".

This happened shortly after we moved in together. David had a lovely little first home on a new housing estate. I loved it as it was tidy and calm compared to the busy, untidy house my family lived in. I would get home from work earlier than David and, as this was in the pre-internet days, sometimes I would get a bit bored. I decided one day to move the sofas in the front room around. David came back shortly afterwards and did an almost comic 'double take'. He could not process what had happened. Unbeknownst to me, I had violated his carefully thought out space. He was quite cross with me and, even though I didn't understand I did put the furniture back again. It didn't stop me from doing it again, but the next time I involved him so he had prior notice.

M

We have moved house several times over the years and, when we have found a house we like, I have always been able to imagine where our furniture would go. David on the other hand cannot imagine it at all. It always amused me that he would use his CAD packages from work to draw up a plan of the house and then he would even create little sofas and beds to see where they would fit on his scaled plan.

I have noticed there is an estate agent who offers this service for free - which is a great idea. I wonder if they have an Aspie on their team?

The Husband Says:

I wonder if there is a Theory of Mind thing going on here. I crave the status quo: a comfortable stability without change. I'm uncomfortable with leaving 'my' space or territory and then coming back, expecting it to be how I left it, only to have it all having changed. I have to learn the properties of my new environment.

Does this have links to my co-morbidity of mild dyspraxia? I need to 'learn' the relationship between a space and my body within that space, to avoid being so clumsy and stubbing toes on the furniture.

And then there is the link to motivation; experience has led me to believe that every time a furniture juggle starts that it will be left part completed and I'll have to finish it off.

Karen tells me that I don't have a very good sense of visualisation as to how a room will look when it is finished. This is odd because one of my Aspie traits is excellent spatial awareness, but also the use of measuring tape and CAD package to ensure that the rearranged or newly bought furniture will fit. I wonder if this is just Karen's way of saying that we don't communicate between us the plan and the desired finished effect that Karen is looking for. We shouldn't assign blame, but who's communication failure is that?

I didn't have any of these problems when I was a bachelor. Furniture stayed where it was put.

Moving House

We have moved house several times in our married lives. Each time has been more stressful than the last. Partly it has been because we have had more responsibilities and more stress e.g. children, but also the way the housing market has been in the last 15 years has added a lot of difficulties regarding selling one property and financing the next.

I have always been the instigator of the move and David has always been the resistor. He doesn't like change but sometimes he can see the benefits of change. He does not like setting things in motion and he really doesn't like it if it involves large amounts of money. It makes him nervous.

Hard Work

Be prepared to do most of the work yourself. A lot of what is involved in moving house is keeping it clean and tidy and dealing with people, be they estate agents or house viewers. David likes none of this. He has never been motivated enough to really make the effort to help me. Even when we were given just a few hours' notice of a viewing, in the ensuing panic, David would still only put in the minimum amount of effort to look like he had "helped" but would then stop and leave me to carry on alone. This is not conducive to a harmonious relationship but I have learned to grit my teeth and get on with it. I knew that it would be worth it in the long run.

I have proved myself right as the house we have moved to is an almost perfect autism-friendly house. Though we have neighbours, we are detached and neither are particularly close. We have our own private drive that is not easy to find so we rarely get cold callers. No one parks in our parking space and it is very private. In the last few months since moving here everyone is much more relaxed.

Different Perspectives

It took a long time to sell our last house due to the stagnant housing market, and at times I felt despondent, but I did not give up. It took some time to convince David that we would have to drop the price of the house we were selling if we were ever going to move. This was very difficult for him but now he has no regrets about doing so.

He was only able to see the fine detail and not the bigger picture. I believe that it is my job to be the provider of inspiration and hope within the family when they cannot see it.

The Husband Says:

I never really want to move house. I get comfortable where I am and moving house is incredibly stressful - not just for the neurotypical reasons, but for the Aspie ones - like setting off a whole new cycle of unresolved and uncompleted change. Given my own way we would be a family of 4 people in a tiny little 2 bedroomed house.

Having said that, the most recent move was the least worst that Karen has organised. This time we used the professional removal men and we left plenty of time to achieve the move. The technicalities of the paperwork were awful, but as Karen says, the house we have moved into is very close to a dream home for Aspies. This latest move has also resolved a lot of overhanging tensions - the last house was a project house and the ethos of the project was finally vindicated by the new owner being exactly what we had re-modelled the house to suit. This last move represents a large dose of closure for me.

But moving house triggers off the whole moving furniture thing again. There is a curious variant of this in the current house, in that the electricians have left us with a logic puzzle of which switches operate which lights. This one is worthy of the Krypton Factor.

M

Multi-layered Meltdown

What is this?

You've had an accident and you've broken your arm. It's going to take up to six weeks to mend and you can't drive the car. He suddenly has to nurse you and take over everyday tasks. At first he is helpful and sympathetic but it doesn't last.

He gets frustrated with you because he's helping you get dressed but you are just crying out in pain. He has to cook the meals and make sure the kids get to school while you just issue instructions.

He becomes very short tempered and starts being mean and unsympathetic. He notices that you managed to make a cup of coffee with just one hand so he stops doing this for you. You proved you can at least do that task yourself.

You ask him to go shopping for food and give him a list but he is gone for hours and comes back with the wrong things. He is rude to your family and friends who come to see how you are and he gets short tempered with the children. Everything becomes your fault as if you had deliberately hurt yourself. You end up with an injury, in pain, obstructive, bad tempered help and having keep him and the children calm in this maelstrom of chaos and emotion.

He is not coping. The person he loves most in the world is Hurt and he feels inadequate. When he tried to help you dress you cried out in pain so he must of been doing something wrong so he isn't going to help you get dressed again. He doesn't want to hurt you.

He's suddenly overwhelmed by the amounts of tasks he has to take on board. He thinks he is no good at these tasks which is why he doesn't usually do them. Everyone is relying on him and he is expected to function when his normal calming routine has become non-existent.

It gets to the point he is so emotionally stretched he can't even follow simple instructions on a shopping list. It is one extra task too many. He knows he will get it wrong and it is a self-fulfilling prophecy.

This is where you get the blame as your injury is the catalyst for all this.

What to do

1. No matter what, try and stay calm. He will mirror your actions so if you freak out so will he.

2. Try and get some help in from someone he trusts and respects to ease the burden of responsibility on him but you might not want them staying over as he won't feel like he is getting any space from having a 'stranger' in the house.

3. Thank him for the things he does do for you.

4. Make visual plans and timetables so he can see what time your daughter needs to be taken to gymnastics or the bins have to be put out.

5. Remind him this is just a temporary blip and you will get better.

6. Get a gum shield for the amount of times you are going to have to bite your tongue and grit your teeth.

7. Remind yourself he is only this stressed because he loves you dearly.

Multi-Tasking

As mentioned previously in Motivation, David says I am a Starter, not a Finisher, as it drives him mad when he comes home and there are lots of tasks started and, in his eyes, not finished. I have to hold my hands up here: I get lots of ideas and enthusiasm for things and sometimes, once I've started them I realise they are beyond my capability or my patience, but mostly I always have the intention of finishing off a task, just maybe not as quickly as he would like.

It is hard for someone who is so focussed and singular-minded to understand how it is possible to have many jobs and interests on the go all at once. As a creative person for example, I do get bored really easily. I usually have more than one book on the go at once. I flit from task to task as I get bored of one. Sweeping the kitchen floor is so tedious. Why not have a cup of coffee and a ten minute read of a book to reward myself for doing such a tedious task? It recharges me with enthusiasm to complete the task.

As a mother of two children and also a dog owner, there is always something to distract me other than my own whims (oh hang on a minute I've just been interrupted by my teenage son who was desperate to tell me essential information about killing a robot in his new game). Right where was I?

Oh yes I get easily distracted. Tasks are not always finished within an acceptable time frame. I do try harder to get things finished or even not to start certain tasks - if I know they will annoy David sufficiently. This App isn't all about changing his behaviour but also looking at my own, to see what I can tweak to improve life.

The Husband Says:

I talked a lot about how I think Aspies are poor at multi-tasking under 'interruptions'. Perhaps I should go into more detail as to why, here...

Aspies are very task orientated with detailed plans leading all the way to completion of any given task. Closure on a task is also very satisfying. Thus anything that diverts away from completion or closure is unsatisfying - like getting another task that has to be done, especially

(M)

if all the tasks are expected to be worked on in parallel and completed together. That's a planning and logistics nightmare.

The way my Aspie mind works is that if all the materials for the task are at hand, then the fastest and most efficient way of getting it done is to perform the activity from start to finish according to my plan and without interruption. Working efficiently is very satisfying and soothing. Every interruption comes at the cost of a context change - a process where I have to stop working on the plan for this task and 're-load' the plan for the other task and pick up the thread where I had left off. Each context switch thus has a cost which, in my Aspie opinion, is high. So I minimise the number of context changes and that leads to single-task-to-completion behaviour.

Some would call it obsession.

Music

As Escape

Music is a big part of our lives. My daughter and I are particularly musical, i.e., we sing and can play instruments, whilst the men in our lives have no interest in this area at all. To me, the two choirs I am in are my escape into another world where no one talks about autism, and I can think about and enjoy my time being creative and mixing with other like-minded people.

Perfect Pitch

We suspect our daughter, who is a lovely singer, may have perfect pitch. This is supposedly, but not exclusively, an Aspie thing. I actually wonder whether she gets this trait from her dad as he has an extremely good ear but, because it is so precise, he will not sing, ever - this is for fear of making mistakes. He doesn't mind pointing out other people's mistakes though.

How Much we Have in Common

David and I bonded over our mutual love of certain bands and albums back in the mid 1990's. Garbage, Oasis, Sleeper, Ocean Colour Scene, and many others. We had very similar CD collections. It would always give us something to talk about or listen to in the car. It seems such a small thing now but at the time it meant a lot. He does not really share my love of classical music but he was not brought up with it, and I am happy to keep it as something of mine.

Putting it in Order

Used to be a problem with CDs. Now it's just a frustration that Media Player puts my music in the wrong order! Don't get me started on the Amazon MP3 Downloader or iTunes!

The Husband Says:

That last little bit about getting the music collection in the right order? Coming from an NT? That just shows we are all on the spectrum somewhere!

- ❖ Naivety
- ❖ Narcissism
- ❖ Need to Know Basis
- ❖ Neurodiversity
- ❖ Neurotypical
- ❖ Never Assume
- ❖ Noise
- ❖ Not Invented Here
- ❖ Not Letting Things Go
- ❖ Not Trusting my own Mind

Naivety

Trust between spouses is of course vital but the AS husband can put himself into social situations unwittingly causing his wife to have doubts about his fidelity.

The man may know that he is just walking a young work colleague home after a night out, but perhaps not even the young female colleague is sure of his intentions. To the AS man, he is being chivalrous. To his wife, when he comes home late and drunk having been to a young lady's house on the way back from work, this can appear suspicious.

He on the other hand, knows that he did nothing wrong and in fact, as far as he was concerned, he did the only right thing in seeing that someone was safe. Surely his wife knows this? No, she does not know this. Even now maybe after ten years of marriage a wife cannot know entirely what is going on inside her husband's head. He knows he is being faithful and it does not even cross his mind that his actions would be misconstrued in this way. So he cannot understand the coldness in his wife when he eventually arrives home. Neither is he aware that his colleagues may be talking about him behind his back when he gets to work on a Monday morning.

The Aspie's lack of Theory of Mind (i.e. he is assuming that other people all think and behave like he does) can cause many problems in a marriage. The wife gets cross because she cannot understand his actions and he does not think it worth explaining because "surely it is obvious"?

The Husband Says:

Neurotypical partner take note: your Aspie, whilst naive, is loyal and faithful. Why can I say this with such confidence? Well, us Aspies have to learn all of these social conventions, including those around fidelity. We come across as naive because we are trying to distil a complex set of interactions down into the simplest possible rule set that we can follow, and that rule set is often not sufficiently detailed to deal with complex emotional subjects like relationships involving more than two parties. That's the reason we come across as naive - we are employing KISS (keep it simple and stupid) in our models of how emotional topics should work. We borrow some of your neurotypical language in mirroring and we deploy your sophisticated language as if we were using a dictionary: with a poor understanding of finesse - we are clumsy where you would be sophisticated.

An example: A few nights ago we watched 'True Lies': you, me and our 16 year old son. In the scene where Jamie Lee Curtis undresses to her underwear, our son could only look away and you were amused by a pair of Aspies with no language available to us to describe a very humorous but very sexy part of that film.

Some adults, even with school long behind them, bully Aspies over our naivety. A few years ago I was working alongside a female lawyer. I was teased by male colleagues that I was having a relationship other than a professional one with her. I still lack the sophistication of language to describe the relationship as otherwise and I know that I came over as flustered

N

and embarrassed whenever the subject was brought up, which to the NTs would indicate guilt. Even NTs can mistake anxiety and embarrassment for guilt.

Having a strong and trusting relationship with an understanding NT is the antidote to all this anxiety.

Narcissism

Narcissism is an extreme interest and admiration of oneself. Asperger's can often be mistaken for Narcissism as it is an autism spectrum disorder. The word autism comes from the Latin auto or self. These men and women can come across as very selfish or egocentric. Their first thoughts are for themselves. They often do not spare a thought at all for people on the periphery of their lives.

It may be possible for someone to be autistic and narcissistic but I suspect that is rare. Many AS men may come across as uncaring on the surface but underneath they care very much. It is easier to pretend that you do not care.

The Husband Says:

It's quite logical that there are probably a vanishingly small number of narcissistic Aspies. I have a lack of self-identity when it comes to inter-personal behaviour. I've had to construct a rough and ready surrogate model to plug that gap. I couldn't be proud of such a shoddy job and exercise such self-praise and self-love with such an obvious limitation as to be a narcissist. Now perhaps a less self-aware Aspie might manage to be a narcissist, but I believe the boundaries between Asperger's and classic autism depend on levels of self-awareness of one's own condition. I know I'm a bit broken; narcissists don't.

Need to Know Basis

This is a common problem in our marriage, not that David has noticed.

He gets wound up about something such as not getting paid - which is a fairly regular occurrence being self-employed. He tells me in great detail about not getting paid and what he has had to do to get his invoices paid. Understandably he is worried as we have a roof to keep over our heads and children to feed, but David will convince himself we will be out on the streets if he doesn't get paid soon. He can't see reason and catastrophizes. Once he has calmed down a little, he realises he just has to wait until the money lands in the bank. I try not to mention the subject as it will just bring it to the fore and upset him again, or he will think I am 'having a go at him' for being a failure. I never think this.

So I wait days/weeks for him to tell me we have been paid, during which time I am being particularly careful with money. Eventually I may say something that triggers a response from him and he will happily tell me that the money landed in the business account a few days ago. He has been feeling relieved and has been happily settling bills all this time without telling me.

He does not see this as a problem. I have asked him time and again to keep me informed, but it does not occur to him in his relief that I need to know.

Perhaps it is partly my fault as I stay outwardly so calm about it causing David to think I am not worried. If I was storming up and down and pulling my hair out, perhaps he would remember to tell me.

NT This is where I am meant to give you sound advice on how to improve this. I could go on about lists and better communication but none of it lasts. If you have found a better way that lasts for more than a week or two or you constantly giving him the Spanish Inquisition, then please email me karen@asperger-marriage.com

The Husband Says:

This failure to communicate appropriately is not deliberate. It has roots in failures of Theory of Mind. I get so fatigued at having to track who knows what (the state of all the objects in everybody's minds, whether they should know about change, should assume change or whether they have to be explicitly informed about it) that I give up explicitly passing on information. Neurotypical theory of mind means that you NTs figure out stuff where us Aspies haven't caught on and we look silly telling you what you already know, so we stop communicating to you what you probably already know. You then think we are keeping secrets.

The solution - something that Aspies hate - the idle chit-chat of NT conversation. Neurotypicals maintain a burble of conversation on the seemingly trivial because being social means making noises to each other regardless of the information content - which is often low.

AS *So Apies should drop into conversation stuff that we already know that we suspect that the NTs in our lives already known. In the guise of conversation this information passing is no longer redundant.*

But easier said than done. It requires effort to maintain social chatter.

Neurodiversity

Neurodiversity is an approach to disability which suggests that diverse neurological conditions appear as a result of normal variations within the human species.

We recently discovered a great advocate of this thinking called Steve Silberman, an American author and science journalist, who has taken the time to write a fabulous book called "Neurotribes". This book celebrates the different ways of thinking, especially in autism.

N

However, Steve Silberman is Neurotypical and the Neurodiversity movement has been led by people on the autistic spectrum who believe that their difference in thinking is not a disease and does not need to be cured. There are tensions even between groups whose desires are the same.

Neurotypical

NT You are probably neurotypical.

Neurotypicals are those persons without an autism spectrum disorder (or other neurologically atypical patterns of thought and behaviour) perhaps 96% of the population if prevalence statistics are to be believed. Of course everyone is placed somewhere on any given spectrum, so neurotypicals are at the far left of the autism spectrum. There is considerable debate about at what threshold a diagnosis of Asperger Syndrome, high functioning autism and classic autism might be positioned. To a great extent, the actual position does not matter unless having a particular label is important to that person.

In slang, the opposite of neurotypical might be "Aspie" or neurodiverse.

Never Assume

NT You can never assume anything about your Aspie partner unless it is part of his daily routine.

Be direct with him. That is all he needs.

The Husband Says:

Perhaps the subtitle to this book should be: 'Never assume, it makes an ass of u and me.'

But that cuts to the very heart of an Aspie in a relationship. There's so much of the innate NT sensing of mood and behaviour missing to the Aspie, that we have to make assumptions to keep moving and keep processing and continuing to function. It's a fine line between making guesses to fill in the social gaps and 'assuming' that all things should be that way. You can't ask me to never assume, but you can help to fill in the gaps for me.

N

Noise

Sound can be a major sensory issue for everyone on the spectrum. Loud music, crying babies and munching, can all drive an Aspie to distraction or even anger. I remember being on a plane with my son and there was a baby crying. Morgan got more and more agitated and angry that someone would bring a crying baby on to a plane. I had mixed emotions about it as I felt empathy towards the parent who would be having an awful time with their child, fully aware that all the passengers would be affected by the sound, whilst at the same time agreeing with my son that it was indeed annoying - but sometimes these things are unavoidable. We managed to resolve it by turning his headphones up particularly loud so he could hear a sound of his choice.

Remarkably though, I do not feel that it is the volume of noise that is the problem. I think it is more likely that it is the lack of control over their environment that is the problem. They don't like the other person's music and they certainly don't have the ability to block out the noise of a crying baby. They don't have the natural ability to "switch off" from being completely immersed by external noise - the response that we NT's can use in stressful situations to protect ourselves.

Controlled Volume

I'm sure David and other Aspies do not have an aversion to high volume of music when it is music they either like or are in control of. David worked as a sound and lighting engineer when he was at university. It was a clever way of being in control of a situation and making sure all the sound and lighting worked, without having to be amongst the dancing masses in a sweaty student union. What they do not like is sudden, unexplained noises. For an already anxious person, this can tip them over the edge. If you know a loud noise is coming you can prepare for it.

A few years ago we started attending 'autism friendly' cinema screenings. These intentionally had the lights up and the sound turned down but, as a consequence, all you could hear was whispering, munching, and crisp packets being rustled. I did not enjoy the experience though I'm sure it was helpful to many. When it was the 25th anniversary of the film "Back to the Future" and they were showing it in the local multiplex, we decided to go to a regular screening instead. We thought Morgan would enjoy this and, because I had seen the film so many times, I was able to give him advance warning about loud noises or nasty situations about to happen. He thoroughly enjoyed it and just put his hands over his ears when I told him to. That way we all felt in control.

The Husband Says:

Karen has it right. I like 'noisy' when I can control the level of noise.

N

I wonder if us hyper Aspies worry if there isn't any noise at all. A steady background thrum of conversation or traffic is soothing. I think I might worry if I couldn't hear anything at all - would I think my hearing to be broken?

I don't believe that my miss-spent youth has significantly damaged my hearing, but I wonder if the very quiet high pitched noise I can hear all the time is tinnitus and an Asperger's co-morbidity?

Not Invented Here

NT "Not Invented Here" implies that the idea or suggestion has been rejected on the grounds that the person rejecting it did not think of it themselves first.

Give it time for the planted seed to germinate.

If you want the suggestion to be adopted, then perhaps you might have to sacrifice your role as 'inventor' of the idea to the person you want to adopt it. Then it will be 'invented here' and miraculously become acceptable.

Not Letting Things Go

NT If you don't let go of all previous arguments you will end up full of bitterness and resentment. Be kind to yourself and Let It Go.

The Husband Says:

I'm particularly guilty of this and it prolongs the arguments we have. It is easy to preach the common sense to "not flog a dead horse", but it is much harder to put into practice. The passage of time and patience (not an Aspie strong point) seems to fix this.

Not Trusting my own Mind

When we first met, I had just left university and was a lowly temp at the successful engineering company where David was working. I was easily impressed by someone with a car, a mortgage and a proper job. He was definitely a step up from previous boyfriends.

I enjoyed his intelligence, worldliness and generosity. I put him on a pedestal. I naively believed everything he said. I excused the niggly, quirky parts of his character.

N

After marriage, this carried on for a while but, as I got to know him better, I started to see the darker side of him more often. Yet he was so forceful in his beliefs, and so confident sounding, that I still felt he was superior to me in intellect and, therefore, he knew best. I saw this as love and admiration for him.

So when slowly, he started picking on me, lashing out, and putting me down, it was hard not to still believe that he was right. He was right most of the time. When he misconstrued things that I had said or done, and blamed me for things he had or hadn't done, or twisted things that I said, or was paranoid about the neighbours, I started to doubt myself. Maybe I had said that. Maybe I was wrong. Maybe people really did think like that about us.

It was a miserable and bewildering time. It led to a loss of my confidence but it also led to a lot of arguments between me and David. I hadn't entirely lost my spirit and sense of self. Some things were just so weird for me to comprehend that I buried them deep in my mind. I was very much in denial about the state of our marriage.

The Husband Says:

You are quite right about this Karen.

I wonder if I can explain why it feels important for an Aspie to be right, to be vindicated, to 'win' every argument? This is probably going to sound like a string of excuses...

I get the interpretation of social nuance so wrong, so often, that on my specialist subjects, I want to make up for this and always be right. Even when I'm wrong. The worst thing for me is when someone points out in a public way that I am wrong and comprehensively so. Is there middle ground you NTs can lead your Aspies to? I am far from totally comfortable in my social skin; can you give me space in private to make mistakes so that my public ones are less obvious?

N

- ✧ Obeying the Rules
- ✧ Obsessions
- ✧ Occupational Health
- ✧ OCD
- ✧ Offering to Leave
- ✧ One-Track Mind
- ✧ One-upmanship
- ✧ Opinion
- ✧ Organic Food
- ✧ Organisation
- ✧ Organisational Skills
- ✧ Overfunction
- ✧ Over Delivering
- ✧ Over Sharing

Obeying the Rules

Rules are there for a reason. They bring order to the world. Without them it is chaos. People just do what on Earth they like and are unpredictable. This is why Aspies love rules. They know what to expect and to keep the status quo they obey them almost without question.

There are no exceptions.

One of David's biggest bugbears is when other road users do not adhere to the Highway Code. Often in the UK, and it seems particularly in the North where we live, people are fond of flashing their headlights at you when they think you should manoeuvre. In busy traffic a thoughtful resident of our local town may flash David to say they are letting him through. This kindly person has no idea of the thought processes going on in the car they are trying to help.

Even if the way is clear, David will not take advantage of it. It is not in the rules. He will sit there and ignore the increasingly insistent flashing of the other car, intent on moving when he is ready and not before.

I used to find this exceedingly annoying and because I am empathetic I would then feel guilty that my husband was basically being rude to other drivers whilst David saw it as sticking to the rules.

As he says, "If everyone obeyed the rules, we would all know where we are."

The Husband Says:

As Karen points out, rules are important, but there must be a hierarchy of rules stretching from commandments to guidance. So-called 'common sense' is how NTs arrange rules into a hierarchy. Us Aspies have a nasty habit of trying to follow all of the rules all of the time.

AS *Perhaps the following quotation from Harry Day, adopted by Douglas Bader should be adopted by all Aspies: 'Rules are for the guidance of the wise and the observance of fools'. That's not an encouragement to break a commandment, but a suggestion to get the hierarchy right.*

Obsessions

This is one of the main criteria that a clinician will look for when diagnosing someone with an Autism Spectrum Disorder.

The Obsession or Special Interest is often misunderstood and people think that those on the spectrum are just obsessive, but NT's fail to see the reason behind the obsession.

The Husband Says:

It's fine to have special interests, even a positive benefit to the household if, as is common, special interests can be harnessed to something productive like DIY. There is a danger of crossing the line from special interest into obsession. Listen to your NT if she is worried about you. Take a break.

Occupational Health

 Who are Occupational Health and what can they do for employees on the autistic Spectrum?

Occupational health is there to keep employees physically and mentally well at work. This means if they know that your partner has an autism spectrum disorder they can help them in areas of work which make them feel ill or uncomfortable. For example; if your partner's place of work is keen on 'hot desking' and this makes your partner stressed when he is going to work as he doesn't know where he is going to sit or what he is going to find, he can speak to Occupational Health about it. After a short assessment they would most likely grant him his own permanent space.

Obsessive Compulsive Disorder (OCD)

'Perfectionism is fear in shiny shoes'

Some AS people have an Obsessive Compulsive Disorder and some people with AS like their routines - people may believe they have an OCD when they do not. An Obsessive Compulsive Disorder is something that can severely affect someone's life to the point of disablement. The disorder can make people very miserable and wish they did not have it. Those with particularly bad OCD should seek counselling or other alternative therapies such as hypnotherapy from an expert.

The difference between an Aspie who likes his routine and order and someone with OCD (with or without a comorbidity of Asperger's) is the compulsion part. Someone with Asperger's can take great pleasure from seeing all their tins lined up neatly and alphabetically in the cupboard. It becomes an OCD problem when they can't leave the house or believe that something bad may happen if the tins are not all neatly lined up. For those Aspie's who have an obsession with tidiness and order, this is not harmful. It can be annoying for them if other people around them are untidy, and it can possibly be difficult to live with, or it may actually be a plus side to your relationship! If the obsessiveness brings calmness to their lives, then there is no problem to be cured.

The Husband Says:

I'm glad I'm not an obsessive compulsive. I'm driven to finish stuff and my eye for detail has me wanting to finish things properly 100% and not just 95% - nearly there. I'm sure Karen would help me get professional help if I became compulsive.

I suppose that's the diagnostic dividing line. I'm happy to see a job completed well. I'm not compelled to do it all over again as a routine.

Offering to Leave

Sometimes he may feel overwhelmed by your presence and the stress of normal life that having a wife and children brings in to it. Sometimes, temporarily, the thought that he could just leave it all behind may become attractive to him.

Most likely though, when he suggests that perhaps he should leave, or that it is okay for you to leave the relationship, he is doing this because he cares for you. He feels that this is the only answer. He cannot see another way to improve things.

He forgets that you married him because you love him so, for him to suggest that one of you should leave, cuts like a knife to the heart. It is not a solution it is a rejection.

How will the Wife Understand he is Doing this Because he Cares?

Women can be fickle and, though I have not done this, I know of instances where the husband has behaved so badly (but naively) that the wife has asked him to leave. Once the cause of the outrage had been explained to him, he admitted that he was in the wrong and then packed his things and left. The wife was devastated. She didn't really want him to leave. Surely if he loved her he would have fought for her? Why did he just do as he was told and go out the door?

In his eyes he was doing the best thing for her. He was doing what she asked of him, which was to leave. What she was really saying was, 'You've hurt me badly and I want to show you how much you've hurt me by asking you to leave.' Instead he has compounded the situation by taking her words literally and doing as she's asked. He does this out of his own love for her and his guilt and shame about the hurt he's caused her. Instead of building on her shattered self-esteem and proving to her that she is worth something to him and worthy of fighting for, he has walked away.

She chose him as her protector and, when he doesn't do that, it is devastating for her. He on the other hand, because he is not a fighter, and believes he has her best interests at heart, does what he is told and leaves.

What he then can't understand is why she starts crying and getting even more angry with him. He has done what she asked? He did all the right things. Yet, she is still not happy.

At this point he may turn from sad and defeated to angry and blaming her. He does not understand her. He is sad, lonely and frightened. What do animals do when they are scared and backed in to a corner with nowhere to turn? They attack.

The Husband Says:

About thirty minutes. That's how long it takes.

In the midst of a meltdown, with the adrenaline flowing freely and my mental faculties compromised, I'll do the calculation of: if Karen and the kids would be better off with or without me. That calculation hasn't got the 'social and emotional' properly factored in.

So Karen goes out with the dog to relieve her frustration with me. I mistake that for her doing the same calculation and finally deciding to do the 'right thing' and leave me.

It takes about thirty minutes for me to realise the social and behavioural benefits of being in a stable relationship with Karen as leader and guide through the social maze.

After sixty minutes I'm worried that I've gone and blown it this time. But to date, every time, Karen has forgiven me.

Thanks, x x x.

One-Track Mind

This is so infuriating for us NT's to witness. No deviation from the path no matter how circumstances change.

This causes all kinds of trouble in the natural course of daily life when unplanned things happen and, especially, when you are parenting.

However, you need to have sympathy with your AS partner. He is terrible at making decisions where the subject isn't logical. He will have spent precious thinking time considering, analysing, calculating, weighing up and, reluctantly discarding, every option presented to him.

Careful thought and consideration was given to his final decision and then some "unthinking NT" wants to suddenly disregard that effort and change it on a whim.

Perhaps you can now see one of the reasons why he was irritated with your change of plan and why he is determined to forge ahead with the original. Any sudden diversions need to include equal consideration as the original plan.

The Husband Says:

Case in point with a hint of irony: we are now rushing to finish the first release of the app and there is lots still in my plan to do. You are doing a great job of buffering and pushing away distractions so that I can get on with what I do best. But I was quite brutal and said that for the time being I'm finished contributing to the creative parts of the project - that was my plan - I need to concentrate on other things - but you can't help but sneak in a quick review of a new article here, or a bit of mission creep on icons there. All those things contribute to getting the app finished, but they divert me from completing my responsibilities and promises of delivery on the app. As a result, my stress levels rise and that whole adrenaline flight or fight thing kicks in.

Us Aspies make careful plans. We want to be punctual with our deliveries. We are completer-finishers and want to end the plan with all the detail stuff done. That gives us remarkable focus that looks like a one-track mind. We can change focus to other tasks but that comes at a cost - a broken plan and the time burden of re-planning.

One Up-manship

This is a classic example of lack of reciprocation that AS men just do not understand;

Telling your partner you are tired will most likely invoke a reply you do not expect (at first) or want. Expecting your partner to give you some sympathy in this area will not happen unless you explain to him first that you need some sympathy.

Having spoken to David about this I asked him why his response was always to reply that he was also tired. He told me that if I was tired then basically he felt it was his fault and he was failing in his duties. He would always respond with the answer that he was also tried to prove to me that he was a good husband and that he too was working hard to provide for me.

AS The irony is he just has to give a couple of platitudes or a hug to make me feel better. Instead his reaction to my little sigh, provokes frustration and anger in me making me feel worse. Knowing the psychology behind his response is both interesting and a relief. If you delve further into his psyche you can actually find just a loving man who wants to do his best for you.

The Husband Says:

I need to know I'm putting in enough effort and not slacking. Perhaps we need another little flag to wave, this one with the legend 'enough'. Perhaps I also needed to figure out that there are some difficult things in our relationship that only Karen can do and that no matter how much I'd like to do them for Karen, she has to do them herself. That would be so much easier

to understand if 'ownership' of the task were made clearer. Otherwise I'm going to see a challenge to do it badly and with poor grace.

There's another facet to One-Upmanship that Karen doesn't explore above. I don't know if it is a feature of my personality or the Aspie parts of my personality, but I am tempted to the dark-side of competitive one-upmanship. My gadgets are better if they are more expensive, shinier and perform better than other people's. Aspies seem to be the first to instigate or join an advocacy war. "My Samsung Android phone is better than your Apple device because..." Is that the same part of personality that can lead to need to "always be right" and potentially aggressive behaviours like road-rage?

Opinion

We NT's like to use other people as soundboards for our thoughts. It is a normal thing to want to know someone else's opinion, whether you agree with them or not it can be a learning experience and can focus your mind.

Unless however, you want to know the ins and outs of a chemical reaction or the torque of a Bugatti Veyron, don't ask his opinion. He will see it as a trap! Even if he knows the right answer he will want to give you the answer that he thinks you want to hear. Therefore, you will just see fear in his eyes or an overreaction to a simple question. Particularly if you are asking him whether you look nice or not.

The Husband Says:

You want opinions? I've got plenty.

I think us Aspies are proud to expound our knowledge and once you get us out of the field of cold hard data, it is easy for us to mistake our own opinions for unassailable data. The condition makes you judgemental; trying to sort out the difference between someone looking a bit unhappy and genuine disgust - that creeps back into the world of questionable fact. You NTs are by comparison fence-sitters.

As for questions with social consequences, yes, they are all traps. They all fall into the category 'Does my bum look big in this?'.

It's also ironic that with a study of people and body language to make up for our lack of innate sense, that we can easily see people weather-vaning around to other people's opinions. Is it irony that we are some of the worst people for weather-vaning for acceptance ourselves?

Organic Food

No one really knows what the exact cause of autism is. Most experts now believe that it is a genetic condition. Certainly when looking at both my own family and my husband's family we can see genetic links going back generations.

However, modern life does seem to be exacerbating the worst excesses of autistic behaviour. The mass use of pesticides cannot be a good thing for our health. I used to think that being Organic was just a way for people with too much money to show their superiority over those that cannot afford it.

However, the more I have read and the more I have observed, I have started to wonder whether the population as a whole, and not just those on the autistic spectrum, are being slowly poisoned by these pervasive pesticides.

Organisation

I am not a naturally tidy person. I admit it here and now. I was not brought up in a tidy household. This probably had something to do with the fact that my mother was married to an Aspie who had no intention of helping her around the house, and that she had four children to contend with. Yet my life is not chaotic, no matter what it looks like to David. I have never lost my phone, keys or purse for long. They always turn up. I have a saying that 'They are not lost; I just don't know where they are.' Therefore, I don't panic about something I have mislaid.

Most Aspies are naturally disorganised however, some realise as they grow up that the only way to succeed is to be particularly organised and they force themselves into routines which they stick to rigidly.

In our hallway, amidst the chaos of shoes and bags strewn across the floor you will always find David's chest of drawers where he has neatly hidden his wallet, keys and watch which he offloads the moment he comes through the door. On his way out of the door he goes through the ritual of putting these items about his person and generally checks again as he is about to shut the front door. He does on occasion, when particularly anxious, rush out of the door with none of these items in his pockets but he doesn't get far as he can't get into the car.

The Husband Says:

The comfort blanket of routine.

Not only are my keys and wallet in the top right drawer of the cabinet, I have developed almost a tic, in that I pat each of my pockets containing keys, wallet, phone like a certain supermarket advert. It's comforting. Us Aspies really are creatures of habit.

Is this a Theory of Mind thing? I know exactly where I left it, nothing can interfere with it, so it will be there when I go back to it. All will be well in the universe.

Organisational Skills

Your husband may need help with organising his life. He is probably either extremely organised and gets thrown when routine changes, or he has no routine at all and is completely disorganised, losing things, forgetting appointments or where he has put important items all the time. This is due to his lack of executive function (see Executive Functioning). If he is highly organised, you may be surprised to find out that when he was younger he was extremely disorganised. He will have developed and learned strategies to help him appear normal and get on in life. However, you are the loose cannon in this relationship and you probably, unknowingly, regularly ruin his routines and therefore his feelings of safety.

NT
If your partner gets easily upset at changes in routine and spontaneity you must learn to be sympathetic and understanding. There is a strong reason why he has developed this way of living. Unlike you and I he can't just turn up somewhere unprepared. He can't just 'wing' it. He won't be able to read the situation in a room like you and I and he has no natural social skills to deal with the unexpected.

If, on the other hand, he is extremely forgetful and disorganised there are ways that you can help him to remember. See Lists

The Husband Says:

David's Top five technological crutches for appearing organised:

- *Google Calendar. Everybody's calendars on every electronic device, synchronised and updated by magic. Including my son's college lecture timetable, my daughter's singing lessons and my hotel bookings.*

- *Little pictures of people that appear on my phone when they ring me. Three rings are enough to remember from their picture who they are and what we last talked about. On the fourth ring they get to talk to my voice-mail.*

- *TripAdvisor. Find me a decent steak within walking distance of here; now show me the map of how to get there.*

- *Sub-folders of my e-mail Inbox. Move stuff to subfolders by subject once it's done. Leave it in the Inbox when it isn't.*

- *Google search. Typing a few words into Google search when you don't know the answer to see if there still is wisdom in crowds.*

Over Delivering

Most employers love this trait in their Aspie employees, though most don't know they have employed an Aspie.

David is a regular over deliverer. He finds it hard to gauge when to stop. Work generally takes him longer than he planned. He is a fairly good judge at how much work he needs to do but as he is a perfectionist he finds it hard to hand in anything that isn't perfect.

There are a number of reasons for this.

1. His eye for detail. Unlike us slap dash neurotypicals, he is aware of every tiny mistake and inaccuracy. He is also very hard on himself if he finds a mistake in his work. David would generally get cross with himself and grumpy with me because of this, so as an Aspie wife I try not to interfere. I would rather he took longer and was satisfied with the work he handed in than have to put up with his mood.

2. Self-esteem is crucial to his wellbeing. He worries that his employers will think he is not good enough. As a self-employed contractor, work life is always a little precarious. He is generally on a high when a project has gone well but can be in the depths of despair, or even very angry, when a project has gone wrong or people have not listened to his advice or ideas.

Over Sharing

This is when you share too much personal information with an acquaintance or friend.

Your NT will usually know when and where this is appropriate and where the personal and social boundaries are. The only time they will be less inhibited is when inebriated or angry. Sharing personal information is fine with the right people, in the right forum. For example, talking about sexual dysfunction with a relationship counsellor is fine, particularly as you know this will go no further, but over coffee with someone you haven't known very long could be embarrassing for you both in the long and short term. I once was in a friendship with a woman whose marriage eventually ended in divorce. Several times over coffee, (not even wine!) she regaled me in detail about her disastrous sex life. Way too much information at any time really.

Your Aspie may find it hard to judge when to share personal information, who with and how much personal information to give. The hierarchy of social relationships is extremely complex and ever-changing. It would be impossible to keep track of without a complex computer programme that was constantly updated. Our NT minds keep track of all our relationships. We treat our friends differently depending on who we are sitting with and whether they are going through a good time or not. We change our language so it is less offensive or more humorous depending on the situation. We NT's find this relaxing and fun but the more I write about how complex it is, I can see that to someone with no social understanding it is way beyond comprehension.

Scenario: our Aspie doesn't want to be left out of a conversation and, he can overhear other people sharing rather 'rude' information with great hilarity, so he shares the story of an intimate moment between himself and his wife that he finds funny... and assumes other people will too. He doesn't even notice his wife go red in the face and then pale, though he may eventually notice her silence and her sudden 'unexplained' bad temper.

Socialising and trying to fit it is a complete minefield for our Aspies. We must be patient with them and not get too mad with them when they make a social gaffe.

The Husband Says:

Been there, done that. Perhaps after all these years we can begin to laugh about it!

In general I think that Aspies tend to compress the scale of social interaction. So it's a much shorter distance between what we think is a humorous episode and an explicit revelation.

Aspies - let's be careful out there...

Over-function

Over-functioning in a relationship (and under functioning) are terms defined by Murray Bowen as part of his analysis of the family unit. In what he considered to be a properly functioning family relationship the load or work of the relationship is equally borne by all of the parties to the relationship. Where one partner is working harder they are over functioning; where another partner is doing less than their 'fair share' of the relationship work then they are under functioning.

In an article in The Guardian on 13th November 2015, Oliver Burkemna extends this theory:

"Faced with a challenge, you either switch into fixing mode, taking control, attacking the to-do list, and offering supposedly helpful advice; or you pull back, pleading for assistance, hoping others will take responsibility, and zone out. Put that way, it sounds like OFs are the productive (if slightly irritating) ones, while UFs are freeloading losers. But the true situation's much murkier, and more interesting, than that."

"OFs and UFs get stuck in a mutually reinforcing trap. The OF takes on more than his or her fair share of responsibility for (say) housework, parenting, or finances, because otherwise they don't get done. But that just reinforces the UF's

dependency, so now those tasks really don't get done, and the OF must do even more. The relationship curdles, each accusing the other of either laziness or nagging."

Burkemna offers some advice:

"Breaking the pattern is tough, because the OF needs to step back and do less, which means potentially letting bad things happen and tolerating the resulting anxiety. (Harriet Lerner, who popularised the OF/UF idea in her book The Dance Of Anger, calls this "hanging in": neither taking on the other's responsibilities, nor checking out emotionally.) And don't expect the UF to approve at first, either, since being pushed toward more responsibility is anxiety-inducing, too."

The Husband Says:

I don't think that Bowen and Burkemna have extended their work to cover the often atypical relationships in an Asperger Marriage. I think they are right to consider both the OF and UF position as being borne out of anxiety but I don't think that they consider that the OF and UF state can exist in one person at the same time.

I think Karen would agree, that on tasks and responsibilities where I am comfortable that I tend to over-deliver (OF) to reduce my anxiety by making sure that stuff "remains done". Simultaneously, on other tasks where I am by no means confident, I try to pass the responsibility to others. But am I genuinely underperforming (UF) in this case, or am I just in garden-variety Aspie avoidance?

As for Bukemna's "solution", anything that is going to increase my anxiety is going to be near impossible to implement. I might be able to change, slowly and painfully, with a tremendous deal of support from my partner. I'm also interested to see what Karen's opinion is of Harriet Lerner's book which seems to focus on the ability of the female partner in the relationship to effect beneficial change; will there be any specialist advice for Asperger Marriages?

- ✦ Paradox
- ✦ Paranoia
- ✦ Passing the Phone
- ✦ Pathological Demand Avoidance
- ✦ Patience
- ✦ Patronising
- ✦ Pedantry
- ✦ Perception
- ✦ Perfectionism
- ✦ Personal space
- ✦ Perspective
- ✦ Persuasion
- ✦ Pervasive
- ✦ Pets
- ✦ Phobias
- ✦ Physical Differences
- ✦ Pick your Battles
- ✦ Planned Spontaneity

- ✦ Planning
- ✦ Portrayal of Aspies
- ✦ Positive Qualities
- ✦ Praise Him
- ✦ Pregnancy and Childbirth
- ✦ Presents
- ✦ Pretending
- ✦ Priorities
- ✦ Procrastination
- ✦ Progress
- ✦ Prosopagnosia
- ✦ Proxy
- ✦ Psoriasis
- ✦ Psychology not Personality
- ✦ Public Displays of Affection
- ✦ Putting on a Pedestal
- ✦ Putting out the bins
- ✦ Putting things in Order

Paradox

My husband is a complete paradox. However, I didn't really know this when I married him. I thought I was marrying a man with just one side to his personality. I must have been blind, or rather I think he credits himself with being a rather good actor!

The man he let me see was the one who was jet setting and brave. This was the man who was sent at a moment's notice to the Far East or the Deep South of America, to climb up the side of enormous ships on a skinny rope ladder in the middle of a stormy sea, or finding a nest of termites on a piece of electrical equipment he had to fix, or being held at gun point in a Korean airport because a ship mate had an unusual item in his luggage. These were the stories that caught my imagination and made me think he was an interesting and exciting man.

However, stories are always much more exciting when told in hindsight. I'm sure if I asked him to be honest and told me exactly how he felt when climbing up that ship, now that I now he suffers from vertigo, it would be very different. At the time he was trying to impress me - and it worked!

These exciting things that happened were all related to because he is dedicated to his job. He is not the sort of man who seeks out adventure whereas I, though not exactly a thrill seeker, would love to be more spontaneous and have our own exciting stories to tell.

He is a very good narrator; he is good at telling the truth whilst embellishing it in such a way as to make himself look good.

The reality is that he likes to plan everything to the smallest detail. He is risk averse and worries too much about consequences. He can talk the talk but, realistically, he will avoid doing anything where he does not know what the outcome will be.

The Husband Says:

Climbing up the side of a ship whilst suffering from vertigo might sound far-fetched, but consider this: I really, really liked my job. I was surrounded by derring-do extreme sports enthusiasts. I wasn't going to come home with my tail between my legs having failed to climb a ladder (albeit a rather extreme ladder).

Now that I can avoid such stupidity, I do. Can you imagine the stress and anxiety level of having to go to a ship in a small boat where when halfway you can't see the shore and you can't see the boat for the waves, and all that you have in the way of safety gear is your laptop computer wrapped in a bin-bag?

This is a demonstration of how far Aspies are willing to go to appear whatever flavour of 'normal' is prevalent within the group they find themselves. We want to fit in, we will follow the crowd even if it seems daft on analysis to have done so. And no, it doesn't make much sense.

P

Bringing back the relevance of our relationship, perhaps you need to challenge me to do the things you want - it will raise my stress and anxiety levels, but you are able to shape me to your model.

Paranoia

Paranoia is characterised by delusions of persecution or a tendency for irrational suspiciousness or distrust of others.

The combination of low self-esteem and cynicism in an Asperger personality can lead to apparent symptoms of paranoia at times. Like most things it depends on the current mood of the individual and the circumstances. With his naturally negative thought processes, David will always assume the worst and think that people are 'having a go at him' or that they think the worst of him when they do not.

His 'paranoia' is fed by the extent of the stress and anxiety he is under and how much he understands the social situation or difficulty he is in. The more panicked and anxious he gets, the less he is able to rationalise and understand what is happening.

This can lead to extremes of emotion such anger, in David's case never directed at himself, or deep sadness and confusion.

What to do?

NT Keep calm. Your actions, especially when he is under extreme stress, will give him a light to follow in the dark. Try not to take personally anything he says in anger. If necessary, walk away, but you must resist from shouting back at him. He won't be able to begin to rationalise until he has calmed down.

Once he is calm, do not make a fuss about his behaviour. Explain as best you can without using negative words like 'paranoia' what actually happened. If you don't know, it is probably best to leave the subject and let them ruminate on it themselves.

The Husband Says:

Is being a bit of a pessimist a full blown clinical paranoia? Probably not. I haven't progressed to taking action against those who are supposedly threatening me. But a mistrust of other people's motives (because I struggle to 'read' their behaviour into motive) is a co-morbidity of Asperger's and paranoia.

I don't have issues with paranoia, only issues of trust with people who I haven't got to know fully enough. It takes me longer to trust people than most neurotypicals. There's a lot more measuring and assessment needed.

P

Passing the Phone

Or passing the buck.

The phone rings and it is not a business call so, once he has established what it is about, he will generally tell the person on the other end of the phone 'You need to speak to my wife.' There are many telephone calls that he could quite easily deal with himself but he prefers not to. It isn't like he doesn't have any interest in the conversation so he then he sits and eavesdrops on the conversation he has refused to have. Very frustrating.

The Husband Says:

Yes, passing the buck.

For what I think is good reason; not avoidance.

I don't have the movements of the whole household at my fingertips. I'm a poor social secretary. Most phone calls seem to be to setup meetings and, since I'm the anti-social one, that call is probably not for me.

I don't think it's just an Aspie thing, I think it is a bloke thing - that the 'phone is used to communicate the here and now and urgent, probably because with our Scrooge-McDuck personalities, we begrudge the money for the phone call being spent on idle chit-chat (despite the call plan giving us free calls on an evening). Just look at the Japanese attitude to answering the 'phone - 'Mushi-mushi. Hai! Hai! [Phone crashes back onto receiver]' - that's the pinnacle of efficiency - 'Caller: Get on with it; Yes. Yes. [ends].'

If I held onto the 'phone and had an in depth conversation with one of your friends, you would be suspicious.

The Wife Says:

This is where we fall down in our relationship and understanding as I am not a jealous person and have never given him any reason to think I am.

Pathological Demand Avoidance

The National Autistic Society website states that PDA is "now considered to be part of the autism spectrum. Individuals with PDA share difficulties with others on the autism spectrum in social aspects of interactions, communication and imagination. However, the central difficulty for people with PDA is the way they are driven to avoid demands and expectations. This is because they have an anxiety based need to be in control."

The Husband Says:

If I can't be in charge of the game, I'm not playing. Sounds familiar?

Once again another spectrum aspect of conditions. When does pathological demand avoidance and its relationship to anxiety turn into plain old laziness avoidance?

Patience

Patience is a finite emotion without the gift of understanding. Early on in our relationships we tend to be tolerant of our loved one's little quirks and foibles.

The quality of being patient is: the bearing of provocation, annoyance, misfortune, or pain; without complaint, loss of temper, irritation, or the like.

I have a fair amount of patience and I often give the impression of having more than I do, though inside I may well be getting irritated by a situation.

I am lucky that my NT personality is strong enough to know when I have to be patient and when to let my frustrations out. It is not worth my shouting at David or the children as none of them can handle it. The poor dog occasionally gets the brunt of my frustrations as do my very patient friends.

How to find Patience

 We'd all like more wouldn't we?

First of all, you need space and time to yourself, be it giving the dog an extra walk, a yoga class or going to a local coffee shop and using their Wi-Fi. You always need a quiet time to be yourself if at all possible.

Educate yourself. Read up as much as you can about the condition. If you can get inside his mind and understand how he thinks you will become more tolerant, but it will take time.

The Husband Says:

I can be patient when I have set the time aside to be patient. I usually feel driven and under time pressure and that leads to severe impatience. But when an 'appointment' has been made, Karen tells me I'm not a bad tutor - something which requires a lot of patience.

I suppose it's all in the planning. Is there such a thing as spontaneous patience in the NT world?

P

Patronising

What may be patronising to me may not be patronising to David. We had a discussion about this after I had written a Social Story describing how to make your wife a cup of coffee in order to make her smile. I was worried it may be viewed by him as condescending but he thought it was very good. The only thing he wasn't so keen on was the hips on my stick figure didn't align in one picture.

The difference is that I was worried it would be patronising as it actually felt patronising doing it. But I was looking at it from my point of view, not his. He said it was actually very useful Hints and Tips into a mysterious Neurotypical world. There currently are no written rules and any insight into this is gratefully received.

However, he did point out, woe betide any NT who tries to tell him how to install Windows 10.

The Husband Says:

Karen hasn't mentioned this and I think I should bring the subject up. People say that sarcasm is the lowest form of wit. They are wrong. There's a level far beyond sarcasm and that is being patronising. It is so low a tactic that it can't even be considered on the spectrum of humour.

And sometimes, when I'm trying to win an argument, I choose the thermonuclear option - to be patronising. When I do this, I deserve all the fallout that I get.

There's a fine line between passing on useful information and being patronising. I don't think I could be a teacher, for many reasons, but one of them is that their material is so patronising to someone half-way intelligent.

And then there is being accidentally patronising. Us Aspies can easily fail to judge the level of an audience, mainly because we haven't empathised with them, and what sounds in our head to be a clear and appropriate explanation is just more teaching Granny to suck eggs.

Pedantry

Ok I hold my hands up here. I am a bit of a pedant. This is related to my love of words, books and reading. I have always loved writing and I have always loved proof reading. I seriously considered becoming an English teacher for a while due to my love of correcting other people's work.

We are all on the autistic spectrum somewhere and this is possibly one of my traits. However, this could set off the nature/nurture debate as I was brought up in an Aspie household where pedantry was rife. My children are just as bad.

Recently I referred to learning something by 'osmosis' and I was corrected by my son who informed me that I couldn't possibly have learned it by osmosis unless water was involved. Since no water was involved I learned by diffusion. Thank you Morgan. I stand corrected.

Most people however do not take quite so kindly to being corrected. An Aspie should learn to hold back on correcting someone, particularly someone in authority when they perceive them to be wrong.

The problem is that most Aspies have a phenomenal memory (See Velcro brain), an eye for detail and an overwhelming urge to be right. This is a killer combination at Quiz Nights, especially as there is a prize, but does not otherwise endear them to people.

The Husband Says:

Ah, sweet irony of being able to correct Karen's formatting error in the title of this article.

Pedantry is wonderful when harnessed for proof reading of technical documentation and sign-off for projects. Ambiguities resolved; the world is a better place. But pedantry is a dreadful weapon when wielded to suppress a lesser intellect (see patronising). It is OK if harnessed together with permission and good humour, but ripping into another's work just for the sake of it wins no friends. Your social problems just multiplied. Beware.

Perception

Due to the differences between you and your husband's theory of mind you will often see or remember situations and occasions differently. He may remember a family event that was fun for you quite negatively, because someone in the room disagreed with his opinion.

Most NT people would be able to move on or forget about something like that but your husband will most likely ruminate about it, even if he never mentions it to you. There will be many reasons that will affect his mood which unless you are an emotional detective you will never be able to fathom.

The Husband Says:

Perception depends on viewpoint. Karen cites theory of mind as a reason for differences in perception; can I add another factor - the thinking and memory style of the person making the perception and recollection. I'm a visual thinker - I will remember more vividly what I believe I saw; the arrangement of people and things in the room where the event occurred. Many of the words will be forgotten and the mood and behaviour would be lost on me to begin with.

There is a growing body of medical thought that what I perceive as timing problems in my thought processes are seen by other Aspies quite literally as distorted vision. I get the full picture but don't always know what to do with it; others get a distorted picture like a television set with a fault. That this is a timing fault is confirmed when Aspies with visual disturbances are given coloured glasses and the disturbance settles down - the coloured glasses make the visual processing system of the brain work harder which would even out the timing errors.

One of the latest papers is: Ludlow, A., Taylor-Whiffen, E., & Wilkins, A. (2012). Coloured Filters Enhance the Visual Perception of Social Cues in Children with Autism Spectrum Disorders.

I wonder if this is why I think my vision is improved when I wear a pair of sunglasses, even when it is not sunny?

Perfectionism

I recently saw a headline that described Perfectionism as 'fear in shiny shoes'.

I thought that was a perfect explanation. My observation of my little family (David and our two Aspie teenagers) who all have AS to varying degrees; is that they are all perfectionists but in very different ways.

David likes to prove to everyone that he is right and better than everyone else. This stems from a fear of feeling inadequate in other areas of his life. Not only does he always want to do a job well but he wants to be the best at that job and we are not talking just within his engineering community here, but in the world. It seems to be his way of measuring his self-worth.

He has achieved this and is well known and well thought of in his varied areas of expertise. However, he has confessed to me that he ends up making a rod for his own back because, once he has proved how good he is at something, he has to continually keep up that quality of work - which is exhausting. Worse, at first he received admiration from people for his capabilities but after a short amount of time people start taking his expertise for granted. One of the main reasons David likes to do well is so that he can continually be praised. Being continually exceptional at your job is even harder when the praise is less forthcoming.

It seems a little sad to me that he doesn't get such a feeling of self-worth from being a husband and father. This is actually the most important job in the world and is not measured by bank balance, and perhaps therein lies the problem.

Note to David: in conversation you mentioned that you naturally an over deliverer.

In our son's case, and to lesser extent with David the old 'head in the sand' option is very tempting. If concerned that he is going to fail at something it is better to ignore it, not bother and therefore you won't have failed. This technique may work well in some areas of life but not when it comes to passing exams.

The Husband Says:

I think we need to tease out two types of perfectionism here: the perfectionism of a complex activity fully completed to the best of one's ability (even though it might not be fully perfect in every area) and the perfectionism that is quality; that an object being worked on is so refined that it can no longer be improved - it is perfect.

The two conflict with each other. Perfectionism is a curse because it leads to failure to complete perfectly. I think I'm like many Apies - we pattern match so anything that doesn't fit into a visual pattern stands out like a sore thumb. We see these patterns where others don't so we become fixated on the one bulb that is flickering or the displaced ceiling tile or the slight differences in width of the grout line in the tiling.

There's no magic cure for this; by all means harness it in DIY projects but please NT's, don't let it change from over-delivery to becoming an obsession for your Aspies; call them off when it is Neurotypical-good-enough.

Personal Space

This isn't a problem for every adult Aspie. I think that many people with ASC become aware that they are encroaching on people's space as they grow up. I suspect they will have been told once or twice, possibly unkindly. We all know what teenage girls are like!

However, you do occasionally come across someone who will stand too close, making it uncomfortable for the person they are talking too. We all unconsciously have our own zones which we don't like certain people to come into. It is actually a cultural thing and we British are particularly stand offish compared to many European countries.

Like many issues with autism this can be traced back to sensory problems.

The Husband Says:

Edward T Hall made the first studies on how much personal space people need and the consequences of personal space being invaded uninvited.

This diagram is rather interesting since it shows that when I'm driving the car, if another car enters my 'public space' of about one car length, then perhaps that is too close for my comfort too, since I temporarily 'own' this piece of road as my public space.

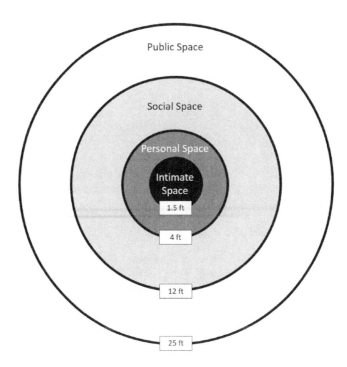

That I, as an Aspie, am anxious when my personal space is invaded (and I am not an unusual Aspie in this respect) rather leads to the undoing of Baron-Cohens theories on autism and the amygdala area of the brain. The amygdala is clearly implicated in reaction to personal space infractions, but Baron-Cohen suggested that autism was related to an abnormal amygdala. My amygdala seems to be working fine, so autism must be more complex than Baron-Cohen was suggesting...

Perspective

It is safe to say that David and I view the world from vastly different perspectives. I'm sure we would anyway, as most normal couples do from their male and female positions, but we cannot empathise truly with each other. We will always be second guessing what the other thinks and why.

Persuasion

I have to spend a lot of time having to persuade my family to do anything. They are not keen on change and the unknown. I am the family motivator. This is my role and I accept that.

Consequently, however, as I am the one who always gets things started, no one within the family tries to persuade me to do something unless it is for their personal gain.

e.g. "Mum can my friends have a sleepover."

"Karen will you make me another cup of coffee?"

I would love for my kids to ask me to take them to see an exhibition or for David to try really hard to persuade me to do Go Ape. I never have much to resist against. It's a strange thing, but I miss it. I think it must be the human need for attention. It is actually quite pleasurable when people try and persuade you to do a thing even if you are scared or not interested in taking part. It is not the taking part that counts but the being persuaded to take part.

The Husband Says:

I don't 'get' the whole thing about roller coasters or horror films or anything where you need to be persuaded to participate to enjoy it. I wonder if thrill seeking is a neurotypical thing? Me? I can take it or leave it. I'll do theme park to keep the peace, but my heart isn't really in it. How is scaring yourself witless any kind of fun?

So I don't understand why or how I should be persuading Karen to do the dangling in the trees inches from death that is Go Ape or the zip wire across the top of a Welsh slate quarry that can only end in tears.

But if that's what you really want darling...

As for other stuff, I need to work harder on the planned spontaneity.

Pervasive

There are some psychologists who, despite being educated that Asperger's is a pervasive condition, believe quite wrongly that the condition does not affect an Aspie's every thought and every action.

Recently a friend went to an AS counselling expert (who charges a lot of money per hour) to be told that her husband was quite capable of paying her romantic attention if he wanted to, that he just didn't want to. Personally I believe that this is totally wrong and, certainly, it was devastating for the female partner in particular to hear.

I do not, for one moment, believe that this psychologist is right. The AS brain is wired differently from NT brains and it is also wired differently from the classically autistic brain too.

One of the reasons I wanted David to be given his right to reply on here, instead of me just putting my singular theories out, was so that you could see right into his brain and exactly how he thinks. He thinks very differently from us NT's. He does a good job of pretending that he doesn't, but his EVERY action is driven by the fact he thinks and feels differently to us. To the point that some of his writing has still been a shock or revelation to me now - and in fact I don't understand all of his answers. I considered editing them, but I want people to see exactly what it is like, warts and all.

The Husband Says:

Pervasive is an accurate description. As us Aspies get older, we develop more and more coping strategies, but if you relax and let the strategies slip, then the anxieties return and our social problems return.

In the example above, the real problem is that whilst not being as romantic as his NT partner wants, there is no 'school' you can go to that is itself socially acceptable to learn how to put on this act.

This leads to an interesting philosophical argument: is an 'act' of romance equivalent to 'real' romance? Would that same misguided therapist then go on to say, if the Aspie partner did do something romantic 'it's all just an act' and undo all the hard work? Probably so.

I hope as Karen points a spotlight at adult Aspie-NT relationships, that some of her successes with me can also be shared for other Aspies and their NT partners. Let's not dwell on the negatives from the nay-sayers.

Pets

It is often recommended for children with ASD, or for the family, to get a pet. The child can lavish all their love on a 'constant' in their life. It calms them down and stops them from ever feeling lonely, unloved or different when at home.

Added Responsibility

A pet, however, can be an added responsibility and, as an adult, there may not be the time or space to have one.

When I first met David, I was dismayed to find he was not an animal lover at all. Despite living in the country, his family had never had a pet whilst growing up. The only animals in their house were the rodents that they trapped and killed!

So he was a little reluctant when I first mentioned getting a dog. Rather selfishly, I presented him with an ultimatum. I would give up my job in London and come back to the north east to marry him if he allowed me to get a dog. I had owned and trained dogs from a young age but hadn't had one for a few years and I desperately missed that side of life. It never felt right going for a walk by myself.

P

David was sufficiently in love with me that he would have agreed to almost anything, and he was very keen to have me living back at home again. Neither of us really enjoyed the long distance relationship we had had for over a year. He readily agreed, so I gave up my job in London and the first thing I did was start looking for a Welsh Springer puppy.

It was a good job I was prepared to take on all the responsibility of being a dog owner by myself. I had told David I would do it, and I did. He did enjoy the benefits of having a puppy and, though he wasn't able to admit it, he became fond of Dylan very quickly. Having a dog added another dimension to our relationship and we started to become more of a family than a partnership. David's mother, who was so keen to have grandchildren at first, was a bit wary of the dog but, by the time we came back from our honeymoon, she didn't want to give him back.

The Husband Says:

A pet sounds like a great idea, but I'll warn you of a few Aspie down-sides.

Karen had an expectation, that I have never met, that I would walk her various dogs. I have a couple of fundamental problems with this. First of all, Karen's Welsh Springers have a definite character and bond to their owner and they are quite stubborn. I worry that the dog will run off and ignore my commands to come back. Some of Karen's dogs do that with her already, and it is maddening. The other problem I have extends to babies too: I have a hyper sensitivity to some smells and textures. There is no way at all that I could clean up the poop from a pet given that it would be warm, smelly and squishy with just a thin plastic bag for protection.

A cat might be considered better at first thought - but if you look at the psychology of pets, cats are far too selfish and self-serving to be good companions for humans.

We do have a rule in this household for pets - nothing in cages or tanks.

Phobias

A phobia is an unusual, maybe irrational, fear that causes a large amount of anxiety in a person and, often, they will go out of their way to avoid their phobia. A phobia might be an experience that is tolerable to most people but is completely intolerant to the few. Due to their extreme sensory processing, it is fairly common for people on the autism spectrum to have a phobia or two.

Common phobias for those with ASD are fear of thunderstorms, vomiting, bees and wasps and crowded places.

Recent research with autistic children, using exposure therapy and virtual reality, has shown to make a positive impact on these fears.

P

The Husband Says:

I'd never really thought before if there was a link between my hyper-sensitivities and phobias. On reflection, it seems logical, and a couple of scientific studies in 2014 confirm the link to autism.

Let's pick up a medical dictionary definition of 'phobia' and check if my supposition is true: 'A phobia is an intense but unrealistic fear that can interfere with the ability to socialise, work, or go about everyday life, brought on by an object, event or situation.' Now something like my poor balance leading to a fear of heights through falling is entirely realistic so the unrealistic bit doesn't fit, and there are few to zero situations where I would be unable to socialise, work or go about ordinary business. I'm not confined to the house by a fear of heights, so it does not qualify as a phobia. Perhaps I am lucky in this respect.

So it turns out I don't have any genuine phobias, but I do have raised anxiety as a result of some of my hyper-sensitivities.

The Wife Replies

David suffers from vertigo but he does not have a real phobia. A real phobia would have stopped him climbing the Eiffel Tower, the Leaning Tower of Pisa and going up the side of ships on rope ladders. He doesn't like it but the end result is worth it. A phobia will stop you in your tracks.

Physical Differences

During my first assignment at university we had to do a reflective piece. I chose to look at my son's early years to see whether, in hindsight, there were indicators that he was on the autistic spectrum. I dredged up some video footage from when he was at Preschool. He was taking part in a performance of the Enormous Turnip. It was quite unusual for him to take part in something like this, even at the tender age of three. I had expected him to sit it out, but I think the staff must have practiced with the children a lot and he actually enjoyed playing a part. His part was Boy. I guess he thought he knew the part quite well. All the other kids were dressed up as farm animals apart from the oldest and largest child who was the Farmer. The part demanded that he go and fetch a 'fox' to help pull up the enormous turnip. In his excitement, Morgan ran across the stage to grab the 'fox' who happened to be his best friend. He ran on his little tiptoes, flapping his arms wildly.

As his parent, all I saw was my little boy excitedly taking part for the first time and enjoying it. What I did not see was that the toe walking and arm flapping were prime indicators of ASD.

As he got older the arm am flapping got less pronounced but the toe walking continued. He still does it today, particularly in bare feet. What I also now note, is that his sister has always 'floated' across the floor like a little fairy. She too walks on her toes. When she was a trainee ballet dancer, I assumed this came with the territory. It was pronounced enough that it was often remarked upon, but in a positive way as she was a pretty little girl. It is different, of course, when their six foot, two tall father also does it though. I wouldn't say he floats but there is a definite bounce in his step.

The Husband Says:

It is only recently that literature reviews have been carried out to try to establish if there is actually a real link between autism and gait disorders. The best summary paper I have found is: Kindregan D, Gallagher L and Gormley J 'Gait Deviations in Children with Autism Spectrum Disorders: A Review' Autism Research and Treatment Volume 2015

Picking the bones out of that, it seems that three mechanisms are in action: us Aspies are making up for balance and proprioception issues by shortening stride length and increasing the spread of our feet apart, the former meaning that toe contact with the ground in stride is accentuated.

The second effect described is one of timing, which again I can understand - if my mental processing of social issues is delayed and disturbed then it could be the case that my self-timing of measurements of my own gait might be disturbed and delayed leading to unusual patterns when walking and running - simply my timing is 'off' leading to my toes being on the ground longer than usual.

The third effect is one that I can't see a logical reason for, but seems to be present in the data - Aspies seem to have weakened ankle joints which mean that it is harder to lift toes off the ground by flexing the ankle. I know I have weak ankles by the number of sprains I get, but how this is causally linked to autism remains a mystery.

Pick your Battles

Every day, if not every hour, something will arise in my household that could be deemed autistic behaviour. Some of these things are endearing, some slightly irritating, most I don't even register any more. What I do notice is rudeness, bad moods and unreasonable behaviour.

When this happens I need to assess whether this is something that my Aspie family are justified in doing. If for example, as has happened recently, we have been left hanging by our telephone provider who keeps insisting that our son's new Android phone is on its way. It was ordered over a week ago, so I think David is justified in getting a little cross over the phone to the call centre. Whether he should be insulting the poor call handler, I'm not so sure about. I suspect if he didn't insult them he would get a better service. However, when he is het up, I choose not to step in and point this out. It won't help.

However, I recently decided that I had spent too much time worrying about my family and not about myself, so researched and started on a Low Carbohydrate, Healthy Fat (LCHF) way of eating. David for the time being has decided not to join in with me. I know he is focussing on other projects at the moment and he is not ready to take on one of mine, even though he knows he really should.

Part of my new way of eating is high protein and low carbs, so for breakfast I have been having scrambled eggs in the morning and thoroughly enjoying them. This morning I asked him if he would like some eggs and he suddenly looked really guilty, "Ah, I threw them out yesterday, they smelled off," he confessed.

I sigh and point out that this was before we went shopping yesterday and he saw me buying high protein food, so he knew I was sticking to this way of eating and he could have mentioned that we needed more eggs. I gritted my teeth and decided not to lose my temper. I have no proof one way or another that the eggs were off so I can't legitimately protest that. I did feel that I was within my rights to point out what he HAD done wrong.

"Do you think that this was one of those 'Need to Know' moments we were talking about just yesterday?" I asked. He paused for thought, and then admitted that it probably was. "I've been bad," he confessed. Hopefully he will now remember to tell me when we are out of eggs. I am not confident of this. Because of his situation non-transference, he may not be able to apply his new found awareness to a slightly different scenario, e.g. if we have a 'bacon out' situation. Possibly, once he joins me in this way of eating and it applies more to him, he might be able to do this.

In the meantime, I will try and continue to be patient and not too disappointed as he racks up one by one his Need to Know situations.

The Husband Says:

I'm going to tackle the topic of 'pick your battles' in a slightly different way. Writing this book and app can lead to a sort of revolutionary zeal where you want to change everything for the better and NOW! So bearing in mind that my Aspie condition has its roots in anxiety, stubbornness and resistance to change, you probably don't want to try to change too many things all at once: pick your battles or you will not win the war.

NT *Choose battles that are going to show that this programme works. Choose one big thing that you would like to change and work at that; measure the improvement, point out the improvement. Then and only then tackle another topic. Make clear what, where, when and how you are changing things. Explain and communicate clearly.*

A last thought. Calling them 'battles' is probably missing the point too. Opportunities for change?

P

Planned Spontaneity

This does not compute to the Neurotypical brain. This is David's phraseology.

The Husband Says:

This is a clever strategy from Karen. The Aspie (me), plans in great detail a surprise activity for the NTs in the house. To avoid upsetting the other Aspies, they are included in the planning for the secret surprise. To the average NT, it is the gesture, the surprise, the spontaneity that they will recognise and cherish. They will not recognise the planning that has gone into the spontaneity - don't be down-hearted for not receiving praise from the NTs - they think that spontaneity comes naturally and requires no effort.

You will need to sneak a look at a diary (if there is one) to avoid clashes with other events. You might need lots of flexibility in your spontaneity to cope with diary changes.

Don't try too hard to be "spontaneous". It's the little things.

So what planned spontaneity can you do to impress your partner? Make a bucket list. Here are some to get you started...

- Breakfast in bed. Full on Cooked-English if you are brave, but it's the thought that counts so toast, coffee and orange juice will be just as effective.

- Do a domestic chore without being asked and don't seek praise afterwards; let the completed task speak for itself

- Give a present when it isn't a birthday, Valentine's Day, Mother's Day or Christmas. Wrap it up or it isn't a present.

- Arrange a family day out; broad timetable - not too prescriptive - things can go wrong.

- Book a table at a favourite restaurant

- Book a spa day or beauty treatment - perhaps even try a massage for yourself too.

- Make the bed and put chocolates on the pillow. Can be risky if you have a dog with bedroom access or food intolerances to chocolate. Choose wisely - flowers might be better with a vase on stand-by.

- Child minder and over-night hotel stay, but not when the kids are too young since everybody else's screaming children will make you immediately need to come home to yours.

- Suggest a date and a broad destination for a holiday - but don't make the plans because you will need everyone's buy-in. Just the idea that you *want a family holiday is enough.*

- *Cook a meal from scratch. The recipe steak and stilton parcels never fails (provided your partner is an omnivore).*

- *Hide some ice-cream or ice-lollies at the back of the freezer for just the right moment - perhaps after a shared chore is done on a hot summer day?*

There's lots more. Apply logic to what will be enjoyable and what can be planned in advance but kept a surprise. If in doubt, ask another NT to keep a secret and test-fire your plans with them to iron out the bugs.

Planning

Helps to avoid stressful triggers, eradicates uncertainty and therefore reduces anxiety all round.

This should preferably be done together. This is definitely a Need to Know situation.

The Husband Says:

Forward planning is the number one best coping strategy for an anxious Aspie. We get to rehearse what our 'play' or 'move' would be given particular circumstances, and we get to try to figure out all of the possibilities that could occur.

As with all things, there are down-sides:

Aspie pessimists will always concentrate on the worst that can happen, rather than the enjoyable that can happen

There is the disappointment when real life takes you 'off plan' to something you hadn't thought of

You can spend too much of your life planning for things that will never happen - that is a waste.

Most Aspie plans are far too full of 'stuff' that has to be done leading to further disappointment.

Portrayal of Aspies

Aspies have always been written about in book and portrayed in the media, they were just never identified as such.

I used to identify with George from the Famous Five for two reasons; one, I wanted to be a boy and two, her father (Uncle Quentin as the others called him) was like mine, always working in his study and grumpy. I felt a connection.

The Husband Says:

- *I'm very fond of Jim Parson's portrayal of Sheldon in "The Big Bang Theory". Recommended for a box-set binge.*

- *Avoid "Scorpion". Trite and thin.*

- *Hugh Laurie as Dr. Gregory House in the eponymous "House MD" gives good value. Just don't expect to be able to behave like that and be forgiven.*

Positive Qualities

There will be times these days when you wondered what you ever saw in him and why you married him. It is actually good to think this and remember why you did. He must have had good qualities for you to be attracted to him in the first place, let alone marry him. It is hard to see at times but the man you married is still there. You just have to find him.

Reasons Why I Married David

As a young girl I had three requirements for a husband:

1. He had to be tall. Tick.

2. He had to be intelligent. Tick; and

3. He had to have dark hair. Tick. (Okay, its more white these days but at least it's still there.)

Those qualities are fairly superficial but I managed to get them anyway, so not a bad start. At thirteen I obviously wasn't too bothered about whether my ideal man was reliable or faithful or would be a good father. Perhaps I assumed those qualities would come naturally.

The Husband Says:

It's important as the Aspie in the relationship to consider this article carefully. When the air seems thick with perceived criticism, remember that she chose to marry you. She saw things in you that she wanted then and probably still wants now.

Did you do stuff when courting and wooing that you don't do now? Is that because you think you are more mature and older people with kids just don't do that? Or perhaps you think that you achieved that goal and once done it stays completed? It won't do any harm to dwell on these things and talk about them.

In my experience, us Aspies have qualities that any partner might want - we are generally loyal, solid, reliable, task finishers with an eye for detail. These qualities might get disguised by a mountain of less desirable qualities. Make the best of what you have got.

Praise Him!

NT
   I cannot emphasise this enough. Like a flower that needs watering regularly to keep it alive, so his ego needs watering with praise every day. I look back at when things started to go wrong for us. It was probably when I realised the pedestal I had put him on was crumbling. When I started to see that he wasn't superhuman, and in fact was quite defective (I don't believe he is defective now, but that is what it felt like at the time).

Was it after he stopped trying, or when my attention was turned elsewhere once our son was born? I can't answer that exactly but it was around that time.

Our son was a difficult baby and I had very little help from David, I don't suppose I had cause to give him any praise and, perhaps, gave little thought as to how he was feeling at that stage. It wasn't that I ignored him but obviously my attentions were concentrated on our beautiful (but very difficult) child.

If I had my time again, I would do things very differently. Looking back the signs were there but I missed them. If he put up a shelf, I was to immediately praise the quality of it. He didn't just 'want' to be appreciated but 'needed' it too. He worked harder and harder and all I did was complain that we never saw him.

Bolster his ego. When he has done something well, make sure you tell him. That is what you would do with your child when he achieves, or how you would praise your dog for good behaviour, hence, though it may seem patronising, why not do the same for your husband? Tell him how much you appreciate him coming home from work early to help out with childcare or revision. Thank him for doing a good job. We make these two vital mistakes in life: assuming that he knows we appreciate his hard effort and that he doesn't need to be told. He doesn't know that we appreciate him unless we verbalise it and he does need to be told. He will be much happier if you show him in words and actions how much you still love him.

David occasionally tells me he loves me. Usually after I have done something for him that he really appreciates. He is giving me just the signs without the words, I don't necessarily return them. His way of really showing me he loves me is by doing things for me. If I don't show appreciation for the fact that he has just cut the grass (because he didn't want to; he only did it for me and because social convention says you shouldn't have a jungle in your front garden), then by me not saying a simple "Thank You", I am basically rejecting his love.

From there you can see why he may start to become cold and distant with you. Perhaps you are just with him because you wanted someone to cut the grass and have babies with. You have to prove otherwise.

The Husband Says:

I'll give you an example from my working life as to the power of praise with Aspies:

I worked in a company with four directors. One dealt with performance, pay and results. He would reward my hard work with pay-rises and bonuses. At the end of a job successfully delivered, another director would say a heart-felt thank-you. His appreciation was worth far more to me than the money.

Now it is also difficult for an Aspie to receive praise. We are often shy, self-effacing and modest when praised. Don't mistake a coldly received praise as one that has not been fully received and appreciated. The payoff will last for days and days afterwards.

Pregnancy and Childbirth

Neither of us had ever been through this before so, in some ways, we were in the same boat. Pregnancy happened early on in our relationship and marriage, so we hardly ever fell out and he was, mostly, supportive of everything that I did. David came along to ante natal classes. There was no discussion about that, I just expected him to come. It was a good thing that he did, and he was able to learn without feeling silly as there were plenty of other scared looking fathers-to-be there. He didn't ask any questions but he did take everything in.

He took great care of me during my pregnancy with Morgan. He never complained when he came home from work to find me asleep on the sofa and I hadn't cooked tea. He put up with my funny moods and gripes. Luckily for me I went completely off alcohol, but I also couldn't stand the smell of it and wouldn't sit near David if he had a drink in his hand.

He was wonderful through my whole labour. I'm sure it was very difficult and tiring for him but he was very supportive throughout. I couldn't have asked for a better husband. In some ways I'm glad I didn't know about his diagnosis back then as I may have given him the option of not being there - which he may have taken. I assumed that, as my husband and the father of our baby, he would want to support me. He knew his role and he performed it perfectly. That was the easy bit before the child arrived.

P

The Husband Says:

It shouldn't come as much of a surprise that the Aspie husband could be quite useful and well behaved during pregnancy. There are clear goals and a plan and a timetable.

From my direct experience, we know that child-birth is a very important time for our partners so we brace ourselves and put up with the blood and sounds that would normally have us running for the hills. We try to be organised but, if your coming out of hospital outfit isn't in the battle bag, expect us to select a fashion disaster of an outfit for you when it's all over.

What's more difficult is the relationship with the baby as it fledges into a child and adult. We don't intuitively know how to bond socially, so we need a good tutor. We recently acquired another niece and it was good that Karen went to visit her sister just to be there and be supportive and pass on some hints and tips in the first few days. It might be good to seek this support out when the time comes for you. Perhaps one time when you want your mum or mother-in-law to be around.

Presents

I think I've mentioned elsewhere that, shortly after we first got together, David went to Japan for work for about six weeks. I missed him terribly and looked forward to him coming home - though I had no idea when that would be. I gave no thought to presents as, being brought up in an Aspie household, this really wasn't the norm to expect such a thing. My grandmother did bring us back an orange from Jaffa in Israel once!

So David arrived home unannounced and it was wonderful to see him. Once we had celebrated his return, he turned to his large travel bag and brought out a few items. He had bought a popular Japanese toy for my little sister and some genuine Sake (and Sake cups) for himself. He handed me a vacuum packed package that, at first, I didn't know what it was. It was dried fish! Needless to say, I threw it out of the cupboard three years later when we moved house.

Perhaps, if I'd made more fuss then, things may have improved a little but I was too polite and, to be honest, rather amused by the whole thing.

David is an incredibly generous person and has always enjoyed treating me to nice things. At first I was very uncomfortable about this and wouldn't let him. On the other hand, when I think back, these 'spontaneous' purchases were things I had admired which he then offered to buy for me. If it came to forethought and planning a surprise present, he failed significantly. I think birthdays were generally a meal out, which of course he got to enjoy too.

It didn't occur to me for quite some time that he didn't know what to get me.

This ruined the run up to Christmas one year as he had a meltdown or, as I saw it at the time, an abusive argument about the fact that he hadn't bought me a present.

I hadn't raised the subject but he shouted at me that he was too busy working to have the chance to go out and buy me something. He was genuinely upset and wouldn't accept the fact that I wasn't bothered. It's nice to get a present but not necessary at our age. Particularly when the kids are small - Christmas is about them. It's hard to describe now, so many years on, the barrage of verbal abuse I endured over this one thing that he wouldn't let go. He couldn't understand, and I suppose I found it hard to explain, that all I wanted for Christmas was harmony not expensive perfumes.

I learned after that to be more direct about what I wanted. I would give him specifics and deliberately not buy certain things for myself. Of course this often back fired as he was still working ridiculous hours and still didn't have the time to go shopping for me. Thanks goodness technology has moved on and we have the wonders of internet shopping now.

Presents from the Children

Until recently, I never received presents from the children as that would have meant David organising them. It would have meant making the decision and planning to take both children shopping to look for something for me. He would have been in sole charge of the expedition. I expect the idea still makes him shiver with horror. So I have never received a birthday present or a mother's day card from my children except the ones they were forced to make at school.

Okay, cut the violins!

Until recently that is! My lovely daughter has realised that mummy would like a present every now and then, and for the last couple of years she has insisted on dragging her poor dad out around the local town to every shop that sells anything a mum would like. What do they do to help filter gifts out during this process? They know I like purple.... So far, I have received two purple necklaces and a purple vase. I love them dearly but I do wonder if I will ever get anything in another colour ever again?

Still nothing from my son yet and he is now sixteen.

Pretending

As an Aspie wife you spend a lot of your time pretending everything is fine. You stamp down on your emotions in order to get on with your day. There is no time for emotions. The children have to be fed and got to school, appointments with doctors have to be kept and everyday life has to be dealt with. With a smile on your face. If someone suspects what is wrong it is hard to tell them as it is very likely they will not understand.

You also wonder what will happen if you open the flood gates just a crack.

The Husband Says:

There is an irony that whilst you are pretending everything IS normal, I'm pretending to BE normal.

What is 'normal'? Does the world collapse if my pretence fails and people figure out that I'm not wholly 'normal'? Can I get away with being quietly eccentric?

Pretending all the time is really tiring and stressful.

Priorities

NT Your priorities will rarely match with his priorities. Remember he does not instinctively realise that, just because it is bin day and he is the only one home, he needs to put the bin out.

He can and will (temporarily) make your priorities his priority if you ask him and explain to him their importance and how to them. Don't expect him to repeat this action without reminding him first.

He cannot read your mind but that does not mean he doesn't want to help you. Remember he struggles with empathy and theory of mind.

However, if he is ruminating on something very important to him, that will be his main priority. Don't get angry with him. Appreciate that this is the way he thinks and motivates himself. Once his priories have been acknowledged, you can help him analyse what are perhaps more realistic and more immediate priorities of married and family life.

Procrastination

There is a certain amount of reluctance for an AS male to get on and do a job requested of him, particularly one he doesn't like. Of course, this could probably be said of any man and indeed of any woman. However, your AS individual can take procrastinations to Olympic levels. This comes across as very irritating to the wife and looks like he is both lazy and doesn't care. But is it really that simple? After all, the way he demonstrates that he loves you is usually not by telling you but by showing you.

There is no doubt that in the general population if you don't want to do something you put it off, however I believe there is more to it in the Aspie population.

Their thought processes tend to take a lot longer. They have to mull over every eventuality. What, to you and I, might be a simple question with an obvious answer

P

does not seem that way to an Aspie. The neurotypical instinct will mentally reach for the answer that feels right but when you have AS you are constantly bombarded by many answers that could be right. Which is the right one? They do not have the instincts that we have, the ones that automatically filter out what feels wrong. The process of filtering is called Top Down Modulation. They have to sit and think it through logically.

Putting off doing a task, even a simple task, is a way for the AS husband to think the process through and so, when he does do it, he does it once and he does it right. To him there is nothing worse than having to carry a job out twice, after all it is boring and repetitive but possibly, even worse, it means he did it wrong in the first place and that means (in his mind) he is a failure.

Many Aspies have poor Executive Function, which is basically the ability to plan and carry out tasks. Personally, I have to distinguish between procrastination from human laziness and innate ability to procrastinate, and what I call mental paralysis, not understanding where to start and feeling overwhelmed, which leads to the excuse finding of typical procrastination. Breaking a task down, making to do lists and building routines around tasks can help with the mental paralysis.

NT Left to their own devices, they find it very difficult to structure their time. They get absorbed in topics and what, to you, are mindless unnecessary tasks. Helping them to forward plan and schedule in events and activities, where they can spend quality time with you and your children, will help them and you. They will know, when they have entered the event onto the wall calendar or their phone diary, that this is something important to you. They will be reminded by phone and they will be prepared for it. They will most likely enjoy the day with you.

The Husband Says:

Procrastination can be linked to avoidance. Procrastination IS avoidance when it happens in the middle of a task. Delay to the start of a task is less likely to be procrastination and, as Karen describes above, the problem of lack of top down modulation or the need to plan endlessly rather than just "know" how to start and get on with a task.

I see this all the time in myself and my son particularly. When faced with an English literature essay, that first sentence is nearly impossible to write. Creating the essay plan is like getting blood from a stone. But once the writing starts in earnest, it comes tumbling out in a massive torrent. But don't try to stop it or dam the flow part way through - that leads to a stopping point; a break where the doubts might surface and procrastination on the re-start might occur.

When writing these observations and comments from my perspective, I did quite well working alphabetically for a few weeks. Then life got in the way and I paused at 'P', somewhat appropriately perhaps? That pause stretched into weeks and clear procrastination. But I'm back on it now and it's a sprint to the finish...

P

Progress

I want to give you hope and encouragement by sharing with you our progress.

We have come a long way in the last few years. Before our son had his diagnosis I was very unhappy. Not with our son but with the state of our marriage. The only thing keeping us together was that the kids were young and I wasn't well enough to deal with both the kids and a full time job. I often considered it.

I felt like I was in an abusive relationship but I couldn't voice it. Something wasn't right but I didn't know what.

Since that lightbulb moment when I was reading Tony Attwood's "Complete Guide to Asperger Syndrome", where he described our relationship down to a T, David and I have come on leaps and bounds. The first and probably most important step, was David himself believing that he had the condition. That way we could keep moving forward - and suddenly I didn't feel quite so alone in all this.

I spent three years learning, living and investigating Autism and its spectrum whilst doing my Masters. David was mostly encouraging and a great help. He would listen to me when I came home with a great piece of information and, during the third year, where our marriage and the way he thought was my main focus, he tried really hard to be as open with me as possible.

It was a hard slog where every day had a different challenge for us both. We realised we loved each other enough to want to put the work in.

We still have our off days and creating this App is particularly stressful for us both, but we both have an end goal and want to make it a success.

What has most impressed me about David is that he is now getting more understanding about how he ticks. Even better, is that he has started to realise how his violent mood swings affect me and the kids. There have been a few occasions when he has recently had the forethought to warn me that he has something really stressful coming up that he needs to concentrate on, and that he will be like a bear with a sore head.

This is such progress from a few years ago when he would just bite my head off for no apparent reason and I would often never even find out why. He can't change his personality completely but it is so helpful just knowing in advance that I have to be extra careful around him (because he can't afford the brain power to "fake being nice" - as he tactlessly put it once).

I appreciate his warnings on two levels. First, that he cares enough now to tell me he is going to be hard work so that I can prepare myself; and secondly, many of the times he isn't being grumpy and short tempered with me, means he is trying hard not to be like that because he cares for me very deeply.

Prosopagnosia

This is the inability to recognise familiar faces.

No wonder it is hard to socialise if this is one of your problems. It happened to me the other day that I was in the supermarket minding my own business when the woman in the queue started talking to me. She obviously knew me and I didn't recognise her at all. She saw my blank expression and laughingly played an air violin and said, "Do you remember me now?" It was my daughter's old violin teacher. It had only been year since I'd seen her and I probably didn't recognise her because she had had her hair cut and we were out of context. Very embarrassing though.

The Husband Says:

I don't have any difficulty recognising faces I have seen before (true prosopagnosia). I think this is the case for many Aspies. Just because I struggle to recognise the emotion from a facial expression doesn't mean that I can't remember the actual face. I see a change to the arrangement of their facial features, but fail to understand what that arrangement (expression) means - even though I know I've seen it before.

I'm very 'blind' to associating names with faces - but this is not prosopagnosia.

Proxy

Having a partner and family they love means they can be part of that family and reflect in their glory.

As a wife with a social life, David likes to hear about my escapades and gets the lowdown at the end of the night. He gets the juiciest bits of gossip from me and enjoys my night out without having to leave the house himself.

He will reflect mine or our children's experiences to extended family or colleagues as if he had been there himself, making him seem like the life and soul of the party.

NT Don't get resentful about this as I have done. Let him have his moments of being 'normal' even if they are stolen from you. It is a small price to pay if it bolsters his fragile ego.

The Husband Says:

Another accurate observation from Karen. I'm cheating with my normality act and using information from Karen to embellish stories so I appear neurotypical. I just omit any indication that I was not personally present; there is no lie per-se, I just don't shatter the NT illusion that I'm telling an anecdote about a time where I was actually present.

It's a coping a strategy - an Aspie 'passing off' a good story as their own.

Psoriasis

This is a nasty stress related skin condition that gets worse over time. David suffered from it for years. At first we didn't know what it was other than little red patches on his arms or on his chest. He was constantly picking at it. Then I realised it was in his scalp as well.

I bought treatments for him to use on his skin, but either he didn't use them or they didn't work. He discussed my "quackery" with our GP who had little interest in the sore, red and bleeding skin on David's back, chest, arms and scalp. At least that is what David reported to me.

On further research, borne out of desperation, I discovered that psoriasis could be a symptom of Vitamin D deficiency. I persuaded David to start taking 2000 iu of Vitamin D3 a day. After a month or two we noticed a little difference in the condition of his skin. On further research, I read that if you are deficient in Vitamin D3 you need to take quite a high dose to catch up and not just the Recommended Daily Amount (RDA). I doubled his dose and noticed that his skin was improving further. The sore patches that had started creeping down his face were clearing up, his dandruff was a little improved, and the worst bleeding patches on his back were at last clearing up.

Further research on Vitamin D3 pointed out that D3 should not be taken alone for long. To enable D3 to work better you need to also supplement your diet with about 400 mg or Magnesium and Vitamin K2. David takes a glass of orange juice with these vitamins every morning now and his psoriasis has completely cleared up.

I would like to add, though I am qualified in Autism I am not qualified in nutrition or epidemiology or endocrinology, but I have read a lot of papers from people who are. I would suggest doing your own balanced research before deciding to supplement either yourself or your partner.

The Husband Says:

I have no idea if there is any scientific reason why Karen's 'treatment' works. I am, however, a living example that it does, at least for me.

I don't think psoriasis is a co-morbidity of ASDs. Psoriasis IS made much worse by stress. Is it the vitamins amongst the food supplements that Karen gives me each morning that have almost eliminated my psoriasis? Or is it the reduction in stress in the coming to terms with my Asperger's that talking with Karen and writing these words has yielded? I have no idea. But even if I'm seeing placebo effect from the food supplements, these are very much cheaper and do no harm compared with the expensive antibiotic and steroid creams that could be prescribed and would probably have done no good. I was lucky to have Karen.

P

Psychology not Personality

Your partner does not choose to be difficult. It is his psychology which makes him less understandable to you.

Don't expect your partner to always act his age. When he is confident and knowledgeable he will be the most adult in the room, but when he finds himself in a new situation, he can be badly behaved and childlike. If you can recognise this as a sign of insecurity, you can help him out in such situations. Don't necessarily expect to be thanked or appreciated until sometime after the occasion. He needs time to work through his thought processes and decompress.

The Husband Says:

Now that's an interesting debate. Is personality something that is hard or even impossible to change? Does external personality depend always on internal psychology or mental processing? Of course this is the case. Personality is the 'average' of someone's responses to the world taken over a long period of time. My psychology, my brain wiring, tells me what to do in the here and now, this time around.

So that allows me to have the hope that, as I continue to do better and better at coping with 'normality', my personality can slowly change for the better without the major components of personality that make me 'David' changing too dramatically.

Public Displays of Affection

Don't expect any more than hand holding.

David believes it is wrong to show affection in public. He doesn't understand the nuances of social interaction and what is right and wrong so apart from a hand shake when meeting someone, he will not kiss or hug and I am lucky he holds my hand at all.

Putting on a Pedestal

Putting someone on a pedestal means that you think very highly of them or even that they are perfect. This usually happens with first impressions or in love. It can take some time before the cracks start showing and your hero crashes to the ground. Sometimes they are up there for ever.

Just occasionally, I pop him back up there. He still has many traits that I find attractive such as his extreme intelligence without which the framework of this App would not have been made and it would still be an unfinished document on Word.

The Husband Says:

Putting on a pedestal can work both ways around. An NT wife might find an Aspie Husband near perfect in the early days. From my experience as an Aspie, us Aspies can find any NT female partner to be near perfect and worth putting on a pedestal just because they pay us attention and don't ridicule what might seem at first sight to be eccentric traits.

Putting Out the Bins

AS Here is a Social Story on the subject of putting out the bins.

1. Your wife asks you to put out the bins

2. Check which day and at what time the bins go out. Is it waste bin or recycle bin this week?

3. If the bins are collected early morning, put the bins out the night before.

4. If the bins are collected later in the day, put the bins out on your way to work.

5. Don't forget to close the gate to stop the dog from escaping.

6. Bring the bins in when you come home from work.

Summary:

The Husband Says:

AS *Better to take turns putting out the bins than to consistently lose at 'Bin Jenga'. A family rota might be good?*

The Wife Replies

Still waiting ....

Putting Things in Order

For an Aspie the world seems a much better, more predictable place when things are in order. Because of their reduced Theory of Mind, they cannot understand anyone else who either: orders things in a different way (to them); or worse, does not order something at all!

See Control

The Husband Says:

Putting things in order is really very important for Aspies who have special interests or, as you know them, obsessions. I've written elsewhere about my efforts to order my music collection - of course this has to be in the one true way of: artist, band or conductor with the word "The" removed, then in release date order with re-issues due to re-mastering or remixing being placed when remixed or re-mastered. Any other order is just wrong; like genre - who decides if an album is rock or pop? So by now you can imagine my frustration with Windows Media Player - it doesn't "get" any of these things about my collection of MP3s. One day I will fix it.

Why is the need for order so strong? We want to complete, or get to the end of, our collection so that our special interest (or obsession) is complete. It's like stamp collecting - how do you know you have got them all? Well you place them in order so that you can see if there are any gaps that need filling. But which order?

I'm drawn to a popular saying: "Standards are like toothbrushes. Everybody agrees they are a great idea, but no-one wants to use one belonging to someone else."

- ✧ Questions
- ✧ Quirky Personality
- ✧ Quitters

Questions

NT Conversation at home can be strained at time due to your partner's inability and disinterest in chit chat. However, if you want to engage your partner in a lively conversation, just ask him about his work project or his latest hobby. He will enjoy telling you all about it.

There are good ways and bad ways at asking your Aspie partner questions. Try and be specific. For example, instead of me asking him a generic, "How was your day?", I make the effort to ask, "How did the meeting for your bid go this morning?"

The reason for this is, asking them how their day was, is seen as a trick question and also an impossible one to answer. Unless they start by telling you what happened from the moment they left the house to the moment they got home again. Their inability to filter out extraneous information (top down modulation) suddenly turns what you consider a simple question into hard work. Pinpoint the area you are most interested in and help them filter out the general 'noise' of the day.

The Husband Says:

Can that question be answered? Are you inviting debate or is there a yes or no answer that you want me to give? How complicated is that question meant to be? I learned a lot about my Asperger's when trying to help my son develop exam technique for his GCSE's. What was the examiner looking for? Could that oh-so-simple answer really be worth 3 marks or was he looking for three separate points in support?

Sometimes I wish Karen's questions displayed a number of marks to be awarded for the correct answer(s).

I should make another point for you neurotypicals. When what you want is to ask for something - give a command - don't phrase your request as a question. MAKE IT A COMMAND! If, by asking me a question, you have some doubt about the answer (we aren't in school any more so you are not testing my knowledge) then, instead, if you want me to do something - just tell me to do it. Leave no doubt. Leave no space for misunderstanding.

Quirky Personality

Now that we know that autism and autism spectrum disorders are genetic it is easy to look back in history and recognise the talented and quirky members of our family trees.

Certainly in my own family my paternal grandmother was known as 'eccentric'. As a child growing up I just thought that that was how grandmothers were. However, my brothers and I adopted a lovely old lady who lived next door to us who treated us like a proper grandmother would. We used to sit and play card for hours and she would let me play hairdressers with her perm and feed her cat. My father's mother barely visited us and if she did she would criticise my mother or anything else that didn't come up to scratch.

I actually think now from learning more about women on the spectrum that my grandmother was a highly intelligent and misunderstood woman.

The Husband Says:

In my opinion there are lots of Aspies hiding in plain sight in the upper classes of the English social class system. Why do I say this? Well, a key coping strategy for Aspies is to put on an act - to try to appear neurotypical. In the upper classes a level of eccentricity is not only tolerated, it is almost defining of class. So some Aspies in the upper classes whose act is not perfect will just be labelled eccentric rather than Aspie.

Why do I raise the subject? Don't get hung up if you think your coping-act is not perfect. "Neurotypical" is such a broad classification that you can wear a pink shirt and khaki chinos and still be consider NT as long as you keep up a plummy accent and pretend to be upper class. Professing an interest in golf and jazz music is a risky strategy - you might meet a true aficionado - but you can pull off such an obscure "cover story" as long as you don't go too extreme and claim something easily disproved and suspicious.

Quitters

I would rarely describe an Aspie as a Quitter. There are plenty of things they will not do. This is because they see quitting as failing and they don't like to fail. Therefore, in order not to fail, they will not start something.

On the other hand, if they are very involved in a project, it is very hard to get them to think of anything else. It will be a matter of pride to get the project finished and to a high standard. As above, quitting is a sign of failure.

Likewise, they often do not have time for people who are Quitters and may be rude and arrogant about something they are extremely good at and others are not. Quitting to an Aspie is a sign of weakness.

They do not have the neurotypical concept of it is worth trying something at least once. Projects and activities are not always successful but if you don't try you will never know. To an Aspie it can be better not to know that they are a failure. The risk of ending up in a Quitter category just isn't worth it.

The Husband Says:

Please be kind to your Aspie. By all means challenge your Aspie to do things for you, and rely on your Aspie to find a way to finish the task to your requirements, but please don't set us open ended challenges that we can never finish. Define what success by completion means.

I need to be a bit more clear here. Aspies are often perfectionists. The lily will be gilded endlessly until it is absolutely perfect. As a neurotypical, towards the end of the task, congratulate your Aspie and enquire, as a progress update, just exactly what is being done to complete it and what parts of the task remain outstanding. If the last 5% is just nit-picking stuff that your Aspie is hung up on, then praise and declare the task complete then and there. Otherwise you will wait ... all day ... and all night ... and into the following day for a completion that is never coming.

Thank you.

R

- ✧ Rage
- ✧ Rant
- ✧ Reciprocation
- ✧ Reducing Stress
- ✧ Religion
- ✧ Repetition
- ✧ Resentment
- ✧ Resilience
- ✧ Retaliation
- ✧ Rigid Thinking
- ✧ Romance
- ✧ Routines
- ✧ Rules
- ✧ Rumination

R

Rage

I have Rage. I have rage for injustices for my children. However, I am adult enough and have enough emotional intelligence to know as and when to let my rage out and appropriately so. Generally, I will do this in a rant to understanding friends or in a well worded, many times rewritten letter.

However, a recent and very large injustice from my son's school and a late night encounter with a teacher in a supermarket, meant that this poor unfortunate teacher did get quite a lashing from me. I wasn't rude and I did apologise to her but I bet she wished she had never stopped to ask me how he was doing.

NT I don't think you should ever feel guilty about having a rage. Sometimes, due to circumstances it is just beyond your control. There is a reason you feel like this. What you need to do is let it out before the red mist descends.

The Husband Says:

I'm much more volatile than Karen and can fly into a rage much more easily and from a wider range of negative stimuli.

Until writing this, I hadn't really stopped to think where this volatility might come from. Several things spring to mind:

I don't like repeating myself. It is a waste of my precious time. If the message isn't sinking in the first or second time, why should I persist a third, fourth, however many times? Now if someone is deliberately goading me by making no effort that almost "deserves" rage. But what if I can't read their facial expression to determine if this behaviour is malevolent or naive?

I'm already working hard to contain my emotions and my anxiety from not understanding a given social situation. Why should I take on your problems too? It's all too likely that if you impose on me that my frustration will emerge as a rage.

If rage is defined by neurotypicals as an over-reaction to a situation, then perhaps rage is what you get when an Aspie coping-act collapses and all the anxiety comes tumbling out all in one go.

I don't think many Aspie rages are genuinely violent. They might look that way - they are a boiling over of bottled emotion, but I don't believe that harm against a person is intended. It can be that the release of anxiety and emotion is accompanied by some stimming to help to establish the direction in which "normality" might lie. In order for this stimming to be sufficient in the midst of a rage it might itself have to be extreme. Self-harm might be a possibility - a literal banging my head a against a brick wall.

So the best thing to do for an Aspie in a rage? Grab and hug tightly - that will help it pass more quickly.

R

Rant

Statistically it is much healthier for a man to be in a marriage than for a woman. The man offloads his stresses onto the woman and she is left in the role of carer whether she likes it or not.

Everyone should be allowed a rant from time to time. I believe it is better out than in. The question is how best to deal with it.

Controlled Rant

NT Choose carefully who you disclose your anger or personal information to. If you are the wife of an AS husband you must be careful, if you choose to talk to him, not to set off down a negative path where he feels responsible for angst. To be honest, I would avoid ranting at your husband at all as it is pretty much built in to them to take personal responsibility for your upset, regardless of whether it has anything to do with him or not.

Phone a Friend

NT Choose a friend who will have the time to listen and also understand your predicament.

Support Groups

NT If you can, try and hold onto your rant until you get to your support group. Group members will be most likely to listen and agree with you, or give you advice on your situation. Once you have had your rant, take a deep calming breath and try to listen to other people and give them a chance to have their say.

The Husband Says:

I think most Aspies quietly enjoy a good rant to the point where we think it should be an Olympic sport. Except that for something to be a sport you need to change your shoes... that's a rant in itself; I digress.

So a good rant is a release, and you neurotypicals acknowledge that. You look for structured opportunities to release that rant-pressure in an appropriate environment and way. Us Aspies tend not to be so aware as to the social conventions on discourse, debate and rant. It's all too easy to take a subject at a dinner party and go far beyond debate into a polarised, one sided, opinionated diatribe, making it competitive and ultimately offensive.

The dark side of the rant can be diluted to acceptability with humour. Provide a safety valve and do some "polite listening" with your Aspie - the kind of listening where you don't listen at

R

all and let it wash over you. Perhaps trigger off humorous ranting by listening to the Radio 4 Friday Night Comedy and triggering your Aspie to comment and debate - almost guaranteed to get a rant started and get it out of our systems.

Reciprocation

There are many different and subtle forms of reciprocation. Because they are subtle, they will just pass your Aspie husband by. He may unconsciously know when he wants you to reach out to him, but he has no idea when you would like (or particularly need) him to reach out to you.

Hugging is one of the most obvious ones. What is the point of hugging he may ask? It is for reassurance sometimes when you have had a bad day, but it may be just to confirm, without speech, that you love and want to be with that person. Hugging is about giving comfort with your body even when you may have nothing to say.

More Subtle Forms of Reciprocation:

On a recent occasion, we were on our way out shopping when I could not find my bag with my purse and car keys in. David was waiting in the car for me with the engine running but I still could not find them. I asked our son, who was playing on the PlayStation, if he had seen my bag. He replied in the negative. I started panicking inside, even though I knew I had brought it into the house the evening before. Eventually, I asked my son if he was sitting on it - there was nowhere else in the house it could possibly be. He said he wasn't but I checked anyway. He was sitting on top of my bag! I grabbed my bag angrily and stomped out to the car, where David and our daughter were still waiting for me. I knew he would already be panicking that we had been burgled and that we would have to cancel all my cards again! I flung my bag into the car foot well and crossly told David that our son had been sitting on it all along. He turned to me and said 'Why are you cross with me? It's not my fault!'

I felt like I had hit a verbal brick wall. I wasn't cross with David. I was irritated with our teenage son for holding us up for ten minutes and making me worry that my purse had been stolen again. What I needed from David was for him to say something along the lines of 'Teenage boys who'd have them!' or get cross along with me or make a joke about it. I needed my feelings validated. At which point my frustration would have been acknowledged and I could have calmed down and we could have got on with our day.

Instead, he completely misunderstood my tone of voice and thought I was having a go at him. Of course I wasn't cross with David and I knew in my heart of hearts if I'd given it a moment's thought that I should try and be calm by the time I got in the car because he always reacts like this. He never lets me release my emotional valve. He always cuts me off, or makes the situation worse, and then I just have to deal with my emotions by myself. It is soul destroying and lonely and the solution seems so simple; yet it never is.

This is what people with NT husbands never understand. It is so hard to describe, but because the event is fresh in my mind I am able to put it into words.

I'm not blaming David. He is not capable of dealing with it any better. The only way we could have coped with it together is if I had got into the car and told him I needed to vent for a moment and that I needed him to console me. Of course by the time we had gone through the rigmarole of the script it would seem pretty pointless.

 Perhaps a set of flash cards would be more appropriate; I am mad but not at you. Reply: I am mad for you even though I don't know what about but I am glad you are not mad at me.

AS It is very important to have one's feelings validated.

The Husband Says:

Reciprocation is one of the things that suffers from deficient theory of mind in Aspies. Taking Karen's example above, I wasn't present when Karen was searching for her keys - with poor ability to empathise and understand what Karen was feeling regarding possible lost keys, in my mind the trauma of potential lost keys just hadn't happened. I was not directly affected by lost keys so it hadn't "happened" for me. Now at the same time I was feeling guilty: I had been the last person to get ready and go to the car and I'd had a misunderstanding with my daughter about if she was ready or not. So I thought I was in Karen's bad books and wanting to take the blame for what I had assumed had gone wrong. So instead of reciprocating and joining in the general discussion of "how bad it is to nearly lose your keys and how unhelpful Aspie sons can be", I was looking to be blamed and shouted at for late running. That didn't happen so I was confused.

It's easy to see how misunderstandings like this can occur. We all want to reciprocate, but reciprocation itself is complicated.

Reducing Stress

NT How often have you heard a professional say that you need to reduce the stress in your life? If we knew how to do it, then we would have!

Reasons for Reducing Stress

- Feeling healthier

R

- Harmony within the home
- Happiness
- More energy
- Time to have patience and understanding

Reasons we get Stressed

- Bad time management.
- A bad relationship
- Being taken for granted
- Unhealthy life style
- Taking on too much work
- Not being able to say "No".

Over functioning in a relationship to cover for others under functioning

A few years ago I became very ill to the point that it affected my eyesight. I had no choice but to resign from several committees and take a step back. I was not physically capable of carrying out my duties for a long time. Though the condition was very distressing at the time, there was a small, hidden part of me that felt relieved that I now had a reason to say "Enough is enough, I can't do it anymore." It gave me the chance to step back and concentrate more on my family and my health.

Recognising the Signs of Stress

- Tiredness
- Irritability
- Uncontrolled weeping
- Mood swings
- Skin conditions such as adult acne or psoriasis
- Drinking too much
- Headaches
- Migraines
- Comfort Eating

You should try and stop before your body hits a wall and tells you "No more". I understand that, as a wife of an Aspie or a parent of ASD children, this may at first seem impossible. However, it is worth considering how your life would be improved if you actually back out from some of your other responsibilities. For many caring NT's this is a hard thing to do. Being selfish. Letting people down. However, do not forget that your health is very important for without you your family would not thrive. You are the main support.

It doesn't mean you can't ask for help. Look into respite care or ask family members to step in occasionally.

Reducing Stress for those on the Spectrum

It might be hard to realise or admit to yourself that you might partly be the cause of their stress. Either directly or indirectly. Directly; your criticism or impatience with them will only anger them and lower their self-esteem. Indirectly; his high expectations of himself and what he would like to provide for you, such as a nice house or car will add to his stress as he has to work hard to provide this.

If you can bolster his self-esteem and help him realise that he doesn't have to work quite so hard and have such high expectations of himself this may help calm him down.

Be careful you are not putting your own unrealistic expectations on him.

Try and get him outside in the sunshine. The exercise and natural Vitamin D exposure will be good for him. You may have to disguise this as an expedition to somewhere interesting, maybe related to one of his obsessions. I admit I find it hard to get David to leave his desk. He refuse point blank to come on a dog walk with me. He will on the other hand walk miles and miles without protest if he knows that we will find an old water mill that may have hydro power potential, which is one of his obsessions. This has the multiple benefit of piquing their interest and taking their mind off other problems, and the exercise will raise his serotonin levels too.

The Husband Says:

AS
Karen has examined the subject of reducing stress from her perspective in an Aspie Marriage from a Neurotypical point of view. These are my recommendations.

Lots of people will tell you that they strive and succeed on stress. I do too, but that is a lie. Deep down we are over-delivering to control and reduce anxiety and that stress is leading to further anxiety. A self-defeating circle of behaviour.

So a first stab at an Aspie marriage stress-reduction plan: Both agree that both are going to do less - at least for one day; Don't stress about under-delivery; Don't shift even more burden onto the NT wife; Plan and declare a duvet-day or family-film-night.

Things that work for my stress reduction:

- *Pursuing a special interest. Unless that special interest feels like work. I'm not sure if writing these entries for the app is stress relieving or the*

R

deadlines are stress inducing.

- *A DVD-box-set-binge; this might overlap with a special interest.*

- *Mind-numbing repetitive TV.*

- *Good food (beware comfort-eating obesity).*

- *Driving somewhere quite quickly with loud music on (careful!).*

- *Reading.*

Back on the subject of your special interest being work and stress relief, Douglas Adams had wise words on this subject:

"I love deadlines. I love the whooshing noise they make as they go by."

- Douglas Adams, in "The Salmon of Doubt"

Religion

David was very keen to get married and he was happy to do this in a church. I have always attended church and felt that a registry office wedding would be soulless and wouldn't have the same meaning for me at all. David was happy either way. He just wanted me to be happy.

However, he does not have a faith and, though he believes in the right for other people to have a faith, I think he is rather bemused why people would believe in a deity where there is no actual proof of such a thing. His logical mind will not let him believe in something so intangible.

He is very much a hatches, matches and despatches church attendee, and that is fine with me as long as he never objects to my own belief and the time it takes up in my life.

The Husband Says:

Given that my religion is science, I'll nod to those more wise than I...

"Religion is like a pair of shoes ... Find one that fits for you, but don't make me wear your shoes." - George Carlin

"You can't pick and choose which types of freedom you want to defend. You must defend all of it or be against all of it." - Scott Howard Phillips

Repetition

Repetition covers two areas in an Aspie's life. It gives both pain and comfort. It has to do with whether they are in control of the situation.

The most obvious area in our household is the pain given by the tedium of repetition. Having to do a simple task over and over again. The Aspie brain likes to be challenged.

Homework is a big issue in our household, especially with our son. Why does his teacher insist on giving him 20 maths questions for homework? In our son's mind he only needs to do the easiest and the hardest questions to prove he can do them. Why should he waste his time, and his teacher's time in marking them, repeatedly proving he can do this relatively easy task? To our son it is physically painful, even though it is a mental task. I have often sent letters back to the school saying that we had managed to get him to do the first few questions and the last one. I did not add that it took several hours to get to that point and that they, as teachers, were lucky to get any homework out of him at all.

Comforting Repetition

This is a different kind of repetition. It is doing something that you enjoy, where you know what will happen. It is predictable, familiar, soothing. Autistic children demonstrate this by repeatedly opening and closing doors (to their parent's distraction) or spinning wheels on toy cars or lining identical items up in a row. This kind of repetition distracts from the hurly burly of life, makes them focus, and calms them down. This can be related to their special interest.

The Husband Says:

I really don't want to disappoint old fashioned teachers, but...

"Extensive research has determined that new learning in healthy individuals is significantly improved when trials are distributed over time (spaced presentation) compared to consecutive learning trials (massed presentation). This phenomenon known as the "spacing effect" (SE) has been shown to enhance verbal and nonverbal learning in healthy adults of different ages and in different memory paradigms (e.g., recognition, recall, etc.)."

- Journal of Clinical and Experimental Neuropsychology: Volume 25, Issue 1, 2003, "Spacing of Repetitions Improves Learning and Memory After Moderate and Severe TBI"

So if you want to make your point, show me one example of each variation, WAIT SOME TIME, then show me one more different set of examples. That way it might stick. Don't try to make me learn by punishing me by making me do two dozen, all nearly identical for

R

homework. And if you try this stunt in your class-room, expect to get a reaction; a negative one.

On Karen's point that certain types of repetition can be soothing, think of it like this - those things that are being repeated are often sensory so this is stimming to calm the hypo or hyper effects of the sensory issue.

Resentment

It is so easy for this to build up on both sides. Why doesn't he help me pack the shopping in the supermarket and why does he disappear off to the toilet when we get home, leaving me to put all the food away? Over the years, petty instances like this build up either in silent resentment or in arguments.

Resentment is an insidious thing. It is silent and creeps up on you unawares. It eats away at the love you have for each other.

But what really causes it? Is it his apparent thoughtlessness and selfishness or is it the fact that you never sit down and discuss how you feel?

If you do not tell him how much his taking you for granted hurts you, he will never realise and it will continue. Never assume that he knows the consequences of his actions. He can discuss the finer points of law or how to fix an engine, but he doesn't know the workings of your mind.

NT
Try not to let your resentment build up to the point where you just want to scream at him. Try to avoid telling him how you feel in a heated moment. He will remember all the bad things you say and ruminate on them for hours, if not days. He will take it to heart, be hurt, and will be cross with himself - and this rarely results in a positive reaction.

Take your time. Think about what you are going to say and how you are going to say it. Give him advance warning that you want to talk. Warn him it will involve feelings. Let him prepare himself mentally.

I have a warning here because women are the ones that like to talk their feelings through and men, most men in general, do not. Unless you have made a plan and are determined to stick to it this approach will not work. You cannot let your anger and resentment get in the way of this conversation.

My recommendation for getting through to him is via letter or email. David in the past has actually thanked me for doing this. It means he can attend to the email in his own time, when he is ready. It gives him the chance to read it several times and understand the meaning of the email. He can have time to think about it before he approaches you and it gives him back a little bit of control which he is terrified of losing.

Again, be careful how you word your email. Try not to use words in bold, capitalised words or exclamation marks. Humour is fine if you feel he will take it well. Be succinct, possibly even bullet point and list in order of importance. Make it clear that you still love him and you are doing this because you want to stay with him.

The Husband Says:

THIS!

If you read one article in this app, read THIS!

AS *Echoing Karen's first paragraph, the NT in the relationship often becomes resentful that the Aspie is treating her with so little respect, with such disdain. That's not it: your Aspie is oblivious to the social harm he is doing. SO COMMUNICATE - this is the key. Communication establishes what is wrong and can lead to an agreed plan to put it right. And be aware that clarity of communication is essential to avoid the communication looking like blame.*

Resilience

I'm not sure that this is something that you are necessarily born with but it can be built. In fact, that's probably the only way to get resilience. All of life's little failures and knocks help to build you up to be a stronger person. Resilience is about getting back up, dusting yourself down and having another go, being ready for another day, looking at how to improve, not give up without trying first.

To have resilience in a marriage however, I believe you need to have had a firm foundation in the first place. A loving and mutual start to your relationship. Why would I bother getting back up and having another go if I wasn't trying to get back what was lost or hidden on the way here? There has to be something worthwhile to get back up for.

The Husband Says:

Resilience is something Karen has lots of. I have some measure of determination to try to finish things or see them out. Don't mistake determination for resilience. If something unexpected comes along, I am easily distracted to failure, whereas Karen is resilient - she diverts around the trouble and still reaches the goal.

If it were not for Karen's resilience, our marriage would have ended long ago.

R

Retaliation

NT
In a former relationship with an NT boyfriend, we would argue and bicker all the time. He would wind me up to the point I would throw books at him. He loved it. We were young and it was tempestuous and exciting. It didn't last.

From the beginning it was a much calmer relationship with David. I didn't have to push for attention as he always wanted to know everything about me. He didn't wind me up. He was always respectful and caring. He used my name when talking to waiters in restaurants. He used my name a lot. He was proud to have me as his girlfriend.

Sometimes though, I would forget that he was just a gentle soul and I would get wound up about things. Sometimes I would start an argument. He would just look bewildered or even frightened. He didn't understand what I was doing or how to act. He was terrified of losing me. I soon learned that I didn't have to over react to certain situations. He was quite good at fixing things for me.

The problems began later on in our marriage. When he was stressed and cross with me I would get stressed and cross back. He didn't have the ability to calm the situation down and so it would escalate. The situation was almost untenable.

Once we understood his diagnosis I learned not to retaliate. I told myself, no matter how much it hurt, that he didn't mean it. He couldn't help it.

NT
Retaliation just escalates a bad situation. Don't do it. Is your pride more important than a successful marriage?

The Husband Says:

Be quite careful with your Aspie. I've written elsewhere that I think that the Aspie view of the scale of social interaction is quite compressed, so it is a short distance from argumentative to vengeful to retaliatory.

I can be quite competitive, so I have to be careful to stop a discussion turning into a retaliatory argument. Sometimes I fail and Karen is either on the receiving end or has to help clear up the resulting mess.

Rigid Thinking

The nemesis for the marriage. He can't and won't see your side of the story.

R

If you did something once then he assumes you will do it again. I have been accused of ALWAYS doing something that I only ever did once. See "It only has to happen once to become the norm".

Rigid Thinking Patterns

Rigid thinking patterns are one of the many causes of arguments in an AS marriage. Because of his reduced Theory of Mind, where he cannot see your point of view, he will stick rigidly to his argument. The rigid thinking often comes out when an Aspie witnesses something that they believe to be wrong or unfair. They cannot see the other person's point of view and they will argue endlessly on that point, irrespective of whatever else is going on. They do not realise that they may have upset the people they are talking to or that it is inappropriate to have that type of conversation at that time. They will also be unwilling to change the subject until they have won their point. They will neither realise that everyone is bored or fed up of the subject and would like to move on. Many people will often concede the point just to move on, giving the Aspie the 'evidence' that they were right to stick to their point and win. It is very important to their self-esteem to win.

The Husband Says:

You say theory of mind; I invoke the scientific method:

"Insanity: doing the same thing over and over again and expecting different results." - Albert Einstein

If science is to work (and science is my religion) then if I repeat the same assertions in a repeat of an argument that I previously win, then I should win it again. Isn't that kind of how the law works, and the law is the very basis of our social norms?

Now I'm demonstrating that social science is barely a science...

Romance

Romance in an Asperger Marriage is doing something for the person you love without being asked.

AS Romance Tips for the Aspie

Your wife will want a small amount of romance, even if she says she doesn't. I certainly say I don't want romancing but then I have very low expectations. I wonder what it would be like if David surprised me with something really romantic? I'm sure I wouldn't mind.

R

There is more to romance than buying your wife some chocolate from Thornton's, but if you can't imagine anything else, then that is still a nice little gesture to let your wife know you are thinking of her.

- Let your wife know you are thinking of her. She wants to feel part of your life, not an afterthought.

- A surprise doesn't have to be spontaneous. You can plan them.

- Does she have a favourite perfume or expensive face cream? Is it running out? Why don't you check and surprise her with a new one when she is least expecting it. Being thoughtful is considered romantic.

- Be spontaneous (she doesn't know you have been planning it for weeks). Come home from work and tell her you have booked her favourite restaurant, for no reason at all. If your wife is NT she will be delighted.

- Reciprocation. Responding to her thoughts and comments shows her you love her.

- Tell her you love her.

- Give her a hug. These things might not be important to you but if they are important to the person you love then you should make them be important to you. This is what she does for you with her little thoughtful gestures.

The Husband Says:

Romantic posters before Aspie Marriage:

Romantic posters after Aspie Marriage:

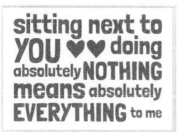

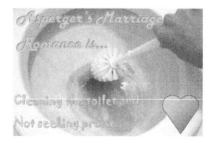

Routines

David likes to be able to plan ahead. He also likes to know what is going on in my head so very often the first question he will ask me in the morning is what my plan is. Sometimes I do have a plan. Sometimes I don't.

During the week we generally have set routines as the children go to school or college and they have their activities after. This is predictable for everyone so trouble only comes when these routines are disrupted. Holidays can be difficult if they are unstructured so we now prefer to make plans and stick to them.

The Husband Says:

You NTs love your spontaneity. Us Aspies like a plan. Somehow we need to meet in the middle and I'm finding the best way to do this is to keep a diary of appointments. But it wouldn't be an Aspie diary without a sprinkling of technology, so for the Aspie - try Google Calendar with all your events synchronised to every electronic device.

As part of her studies, Karen has been encouraged to keep a reflective journal - a diary of thoughts and feelings. I don't know if that might help a few Aspies, or if you are like me and need to see some direct payback from the activity of organising and scheduling into a routine.

I get really uncomfortable if my routine, or my carefully prepared plan, is broken by external events or people. Set this against Karen's desire for positive surprises, and we have come up with the concept of planned spontaneity; all the best bits of a surprise but compatible with an Aspie's routine.

'Routine' cuts all the way down to actions that have become so habitual as to be automatic. My patting of my pockets as I leave the house to check for keys and phone has become a habitual routine. Bad things happen if you break the routine - I hate trying to go a whole day without a watch or phone-clock to help judge the passage of time and to pace the routine. This is especially the case in winter when I do not see our house in daylight except at weekends.

Rules

Rules are there for a reason and need to be adhered to. They make sense of the world and, if everyone stuck to the rules, then Aspies might be able to reduce their need for control.

Unfortunately, the world is mostly full of neurotypicals who see rules as: there for their convenience but sometimes to be broken when they are inconvenient. This makes no sense to your Aspie and turns the world into chaos.

They need to be able to predict what is going to happen and when it will happen. David gets most infuriated when driving if people don't stick to the rules, even if it is someone flashing him to let him through and it is to his advantage. There are no grey areas. He will sit in traffic and ignore the kind neurotypical waving him on.

The Husband Says:

Yes, I'm a stickler for rules when they make sense. The Highway Code is a great example - it sets out the priorities for traffic so that everybody should know whose turn it is to pass through a constriction. Without the rules, you have what I can best describe as the traffic manners of Italy. That's scary. I haven't been quite so anxious as squeezing past scooters on a mountainous road on the Amalfi coast. I could foresee certain death and that wasn't going to be for MY family in the hire car.

But some rules are just arbitrary and I think deserve to be dismantled. Especially those nanny state rules on 'elf and safety. Like, what's the logic behind requiring reverse parking in the morning in car parks? That's the kind of rule I'll deliberately break in order to have the confrontation with the health and safety officer to prove his argument is without base.

Rumination

Rumination is caused by stress and anxiety and will often disrupt your Aspie's sleep. It is a negative thought process that dwells on past events and how the situation could have been changed. It is very difficult for your Aspie to get out of the downward cycle of rumination and constantly going over whether they were at fault. This can sometimes lead to depression.

NT It is worth keeping an eye out for your Aspies' ruminating behaviour. The best thing you can do for them is to jolt them out of their negative thought patterns by giving them something else to think about. Distract them, take them for a walk, watch a film or have a chat about something funny or positive.

Rumination can seem similar to worry, but worry tends to be about what is going to happen in the future rather than what has already happened that can't be changed.

The Husband Says:

I hadn't wrapped so many negative connotations around my ruminations. Karen presents all my extended periods of thought as somewhat negative.

But I spend a lot of time, thinking, ruminating, putting stuff mentally in order. It's good for my mental health to measure, order, organise and ultimately plan ahead so that what happened yesterday informs what I plan to do tomorrow. So if your Aspie is quiet, try to figure out if this is "good rumination" of forward planning to avoid unpleasant surprises, or "bad rumination" of dwelling on what coulda-shoulda-oula, but never happened. Break him out of latter cycle.

S

- Safety
- Sarcasm
- Saying Sorry
- Say What you Mean
- Secret Messages
- Seeing the World Differently
- Selective Hearing
- Self-Awareness
- Self-Examination
- Self-Harm
- Self-Medication
- Sensory Issues
- Sensory Processing Disorder
- Serotonin
- Sex
- Sharing
- Sharing of Household Chores
- Shooting the Messenger
- Shopping
- Shouting
- Showing your Love
- Showing your Weaknesses
- Shutdowns
- Sighing
- Simon Baron-Cohen
- Single Parent

- Situational Non-Transference
- Situation Avoidance
- Sleep
- Social Cues
- Social Norms
- Social Stories
- Spatial Awareness
- Special Interests
- Speech
- Spontaneity
- Stages of Grief
- Staring
- Start
- Staycation
- Stigma
- Stimming
- Strategies
- Stress
- Style
- Sunlight
- Support
- Surprise!
- Switching Tasks
- Sympathy
- Synaesthesia

Safety

This is a tricky one because though many Aspies are super aware of their own safety (overly cautious) they are less aware of the safety of others.

Another Asperger wife was very keen to point out her worries to me:

~ = ~

"For me there are two main issues/situations around safety with my partner of 10 years.

Firstly: Meltdowns. My husband has frequently 'lost it'. This started not long after we got married. These have come out of nowhere and often over very trivial issues, or so it seemed to me anyway.

Outbursts in the home tend to happen when he is overtired and/or hungry. There have been a number of outbursts in the car that have been very scary. He has screamed at me if I drive, pulling on the handbrake or slamming brakes on so hard I winded myself. He doesn't drive much these days.

These events are often quickly over but left me shaking and in a state of shock for sometimes days afterwards. Thankfully, these outbursts have dissipated with time, with me having counselling and going on anti-depressants.

I learned never to touch or shout back and eventually to remove myself from the room or even premises. But I always went back within a few hours. My husband is in denial about his moods. Deep down, I am sure he knows how out of order he can be. If I had my time over again I would leave the premises immediately after an outburst where my personal safety was threatened and stay away until we were able to talk, outlining very clearly what the issue was.

Secondly: the lack of empathy makes it difficult for them to assess when a person is ill and appropriate action to take. My husband has just offered me Lemsip for a stomach bug. A minor, even amusing, action but as I get older I get more concerned about this."

~ = ~

Safety wise in our marriage David has been a real mixture. On the whole he is overly cautious and worries about me. The day after I passed my driving test and ventured out on my own for the first time he was walking up and down the road looking for me, convinced I'd died in a multi-car pile-up.

It was before we had mobile phones and he must have felt completely helpless and out of control. Some people may say that those with ASD don't have an imagination but I present you with my terrified husband whose theory of mind and imagination were working overtime to create all kinds of horrific scenarios in his head.

S

Cars are often involved in areas of danger in our life and this winter we parked up in a city centre car park to go and see a show. It was dark, cold, wet and windy. I was huddled with my hood up and my head down, walking quickly towards the venue. A car drove into the entrance we were approaching. David grabbed my arm with great force in order to stop me. I had not failed to see the car, after all it had its headlights on but David assumed in his panic and concern for me that I hadn't seen it. I shouted in surprise and pain as he had really hurt me. It was accidental on his part I know but unfortunately the evening went downhill from there. I think he was upset I shouted at him when he was trying to save my life. In his panic he wasn't able to temper his strength appropriately and I was still quite bruised the next day.

NT All the above situations have a common denominator and that is they are all caused by anxiety, impairing judgement. If we can work on reducing their anxieties, these situations will happen less and less.

Sarcasm

They say that "Sarcasm is the lowest form of wit". This may be true but we NT's use it a lot.

It depends on your partner but some Aspies enjoying finding the sarcasm in your words and others will be offended by it. It also depends on their mood whether they find humour in it or not.

What is sarcasm?

It is normally used in a derogatory way about a subject, action or person. We tend to say the opposite of what we actually mean.

For if someone who knew I hated parsnip put some on my dinner plate disguised as potato and then after watching me gag asked me what I thought I may restrain myself to just say sarcastically, "Lovely".

However, the timing of my words, the screwing up of my face and my higher than normal inflection would indicate to my fellow NT prankster that I was not impressed.

If someone on the spectrum was following this exchange, would they understand what was going on? They may have seen and understood my unsubtle facial expression but they may not have grasped the nuances and intonation expressed in that one word which the other NT's in the room would innately get and find amusing.

S

Saying Sorry

If you have children, you will know how hard it is to get them to say sorry. I remember myself, as a child I found it very hard to admit when I was wrong. It wasn't until my early adult years when I realised that it was much easier to admit that I had made a mistake. I don't go out of my way to apologise to people, but I think it fair to hold up my hands and say that they were right and I was wrong. However, I do not give in when I know I am right!

AS **NT** The Aspie brain hates being wrong. I have only ever once known David say "Sorry" to me, unbidden, when he actually meant it.

What I don't think he realises is the effect his negative behaviour has on me. It is like he doesn't care that he has upset me or been rude to me. Not apologising for your behaviour implies you have no respect for the person you have wronged and it is hard to be in a relationship without respect and also it is hard to reciprocate that respect.

I know that he was distressed and that he doesn't mean to take it out on me but in the moment it still hurts. I have to go through a mantra of "He didn't mean it," and pick myself up mentally and carry on. It is hard work, lonely and soul destroying. Obviously, I wish he didn't insult me in the first place but I know he dwells on these things in retrospect as sometimes he emerges unexpectedly with an 'excuse' for his behaviour - but never an apology.

The Husband Says:

This was always going to be one of the more difficult articles to comment on. It's a big deficiency of mine and a significant problem for Karen and something for which there are no easy answers.

On the one hand as an Aspie, there is a temptation to go around apologising for everything - I'm not meant to understand social settings very well, so I must always be breaking the "rules" and should be apologising for them - right? That's a negative spiral itself and something that Karen really hates - a half-hearted apology when none was even needed.

But there comes the time and place when you inadvertently break some social convention, and perhaps an important one, where a proper apology is the only socially acceptable way out of the situation. There is a danger of misplaced logic here - I often believe that I did the right thing because it was the logical thing, but Karen reminds me that I made the situation worse by applying logic to a situation that does not respond well to a calculation of consequences and which set of consequences in the round is less painful.

Karen recognises a half-hearted apology from me for what it is - an attempt at damage limitation.

S

Perhaps the biggest problem in terms of 'apologies' for an Aspie, is that it is very easy for an NT to see insincerity in apologies. I know I am expected to apologise and I want it to be sincere, but it is the hardest part of acting NT to pull off. I usually miss and miss by a mile.

Apologies - very much a work in progress.

Say What you Mean

Communication is the main problem in your marriage.

NT Any easy fix, which is not actually obvious, is to always say what you mean. Be direct. Tell him what you want. Don't use metaphors or jokes until he is comfortable with your style of language and can tell what mood you are in.

NT Say what you mean and mean what you say. Tell him you will always do this for him so he can in fact take your words literally and not spend time trying to interpret and translate them from Neurotypical to Aspie.

It will reduce both your stresses and provide clarity in your relationship.

Secret Messages

We women are very good at expecting our men to know what we want without actually telling them. This is quite a hard job for a NT man to get right, but there is no hope for the autistic male who cannot even fathom a basic facial expression.

NT If you think you have dropped sufficient hints for what you want for your wedding anniversary, think again. Unless you have specifically said to him, 'Take me to [insert name] restaurant on our anniversary, I'll sort the babysitter out.' He will not realise that when you say in general conversation, 'Oh it's our anniversary next week wouldn't it be nice to go to [insert name]', he will most likely not register that he is now expected to get on the phone and book the restaurant. He might even reply 'Oh that's a good idea,' but he will probably immediately forget about it. In the meantime, you believe that he isn't getting on with organising your anniversary night out when in fact he's thinking about whether to display his Spotify music in order of genre or the day he made each one a favourite.

The Husband Says:

NT I'm afraid you have to be blunt to get your message across. I won't take offence; in fact I'll be quietly relieved.

Perhaps the best thing to do is to use the planned spontaneity strategy. At least that way you won't get Chinese whispers mixed with secret messages. With the broad parameters of your desire laid out, then your Aspie might surprise you with little details - he will be seeking perfection. But watch out for disappointment if things don't all work out for him and he thinks he has delivered in full your 'secret' desire.

If you do want a genuine surprise, then perhaps the best thing to do will be to share your secret with an NT confidant that you know understands your Aspie reasonably well and can coach him on the sorts of things you might want. Your husband might be quite surprised at an NT friend coming 'out of the blue' with suggestions, so coach the NT partner-in-crime as to what to expect!

All the better if you can arrange for a male friend to support your Aspie. Whilst male friends might not have the imagination to translate your secret desires in full, there could be very significant fall-out from a female-NT working closely with your Aspie to spring a surprise. Your Aspie might inadvertently do or say something quite inappropriate to your female-NT friend whilst concentrating hard on delivering the secret. Sort of "all blokes together" might work very well, allowing your Aspie to think that fulfilling secret desires is a general male failing rather than an Aspie failing.

Seeing the World Differently

Your partner's brain is wired differently to yours. He will never quite see the world from the same viewpoint as you.

Embrace your differences!

The Husband Says:

It's not that I want to see the world differently, it's just that I do.

First and foremost, my differing view on the world isn't wrong, it's just different. Is there a way that you can use my cross cutting viewpoint? Certainly in business this view from a different angle is valued; can it be such in a relationship?

At least consider your Aspie's "left-field" suggestions. Some of them have merit, even if a little unconventional!

S

Selective Hearing

Some wives think their husband rarely listens to them. I think this depends on the topic or possibly what is on their mind when you raise the subject.

For instance, the other day I was listening to the news and they reported a backlog in passport offices around the country. I wasn't too concerned as I was pretty sure our passports were up to date but, when David came home, I mentioned it to him and said we had better check as we wouldn't be able to get one in an emergency. He said he was pretty sure they were up to date, and we left it at that.

The following morning, he came rushing into the kitchen and announced that the passport offices had major backlogs and that we had better check the dates on our passports. I'm not sure I said anything. I was half amused and half annoyed. He later informed me that he had checked all the dates and they were fine for the next two years.

I don't know what he was thinking when I first gave him this information, he had just come in from work so maybe it wasn't the best time. It wasn't hugely important as we weren't due to go on holiday for a couple of months and we were both pretty sure our passports were up to date. What was it about hearing it on the news that made him panic, even though it was exactly the same information I had imparted the day before?

This is one of those occasions when, before I knew he had AS, I would have doubted either mine or his sanity.

The Husband Says:

I think that Aspies quite aggressively prioritise in order to cope with the barrage of decision making which is intuitive for the NT. I also think that people can mistake an Aspie memory (designed for facts, trivia and positions) for situational memory of what happened a few minutes, hours or days ago - I can remember lots of stuff but often forget what order it happened in (unless there is a logical order).

So if I'm concentrating on a task, I may be prioritising that task over listening to you, unless certain "trigger words" crop up that suggest your conversation has higher priority than what I'm doing. Bear in mind that staring blankly at a computer screen or out of the window might be me thinking deeply about something entirely unrelated to the computer screen or the scene outside the window.

In Karen's passport example, on the day that the passport office announced the massive delay that Karen seized on and reported, I was pre-occupied with other things that eventually I finished. The following day I was in holiday planning mode, and top priority became the consideration of dates on passports.

I think Aspies are slow to context-switch from one subject to another - seeking to complete one task before starting another, so this can lead to an appearance of selective hearing.

S

Self-Awareness

In some ways their self-awareness marks them out as having autism as they get easily embarrassed, especially over having made a mistake. Your Aspie will not always know when he has done something wrong but if the mistake is visual or aural they will know and be mortified. The problems come again with not knowing social conventions or not caring about social conventions. For example, is he a messy eater because he doesn't care that he has food on his face or is he unaware? Does he not realise that social convention requires you to wipe food from your face straight away or it is seen as something laughable by others?

The Husband Says:

Self-awareness. Now there's a catch-all topic.

Aspies are self-aware, but might prioritise awareness of surroundings since that might be where any threats and disruptions to the status quo are coming from.

With regard to the observation that Aspies can be messy eaters that don't care about dropped food, be careful to separate a possible co-morbidity of dyspraxia from the social stigma of having a stain on your shirt or a pile of food on the floor. Perhaps your Aspie hasn't "got a way out" of having made a mess rather than doesn't care about having made a mess. And you wiping my face looks like a public display of affection and we don't like those either.

On the subject of awareness of pattern, style and fashion, see my notes under Style.

Self-Examination

NT
It is very hard to be accurately self-critical as we are often our own harshest critic. However, we know ourselves best.

Now is the time to look inward and make some decisions about what you want out of life and your marriage; whether you are prepared to put the work in to try and make it a success; and, hardest of all, whether you may be partly at 'fault' in the relationship and there are improvements you could make about yourself.

We naturally go around in self-denial. It is easier not to look in the mirror and see our own flaws. It is easier to blame other people for things going wrong.

It takes two to make a relationship work and it takes two to make a relationship fail.

Be aware that this is not assigning blame. This is about self-examination and building self-awareness.

S

I recommend using a notebook and writing down your strengths and your weaknesses. Your strengths are very important here as well.

This is my list:

The Early Years	
Strengths	**Weaknesses**
Confidence	Impatience
Get up and go	Intolerance
Enthusiasm	Selfishness
Ambition	Ignorance
Independence	Lack of Empathy
Sociability	Quick to take offence
Caring	Defensiveness
Openness	Thoughtless
Relaxed	Temper
Giving	Tired
	Grumpy
	Untidy
	Inwardly Seething

After Twenty Years of Cohabitation	
Strengths	**Weaknesses**
Tolerance	Critical
Patience	Untidy
Resilience	Selfishness
Caring	Guilt
Thoughtful	Tired
Unselfish	Inwardly Seething
Self-Aware	
Understanding	
Educated	
Empathy	
Sympathy	
Giving	

I refer to The Early Years from when we met. I was 24 and had just come out of a long term relationship that ended badly. I had also just finished university and was keen to make my mark upon the world. I had not set out to find someone else to share my life with. I was selfish and not very tolerant of his issues, but in some way this seemed to appeal to David. He liked my enthusiasm and Joie de Vivre. He thought I was perfect and told me so. I knew it not to be true, but was happy to be told so.

By the age of 28 things had changed a lot. We were married and we had our first child. I had had my independence and was settling down. With motherhood, selfishness goes out of the window at least for a while. I started to grow up and not think of what I wanted so much, but what my family needed.

As David's behaviour got progressively worse, however, so did mine. Before children we had rarely disagreed, let alone argued. I was tired and ill and intolerant and he worked many hours and was hardly home. We had little understanding of each other. I aired my grievances not knowing how badly he would take this. In my previous relationship, my other half always bounced back very quickly from any criticism. I had no idea the damage I was doing to David's self-esteem.

I would argue back and stand my ground when I thought he wasn't being fair. In turn he would get more sullen and angry with me. It wasn't a good time.

Even worse, though there were times I was embarrassed or put in embarrassing positions by his stressed behaviour. How he insisted we left a pub half way through our meal because our two-year-old was being a little noisy. We were outside at a table, not inside disturbing serious drinkers. Or the time we were in a family restaurant when again one of the children was being typical for their age; he walked out and left me with the two kids after we had just ordered our food. I couldn't leave until after the food had arrived and I certainly couldn't take two expectant hungry children out of the restaurant. I couldn't see the car park and I didn't even know if he was still there. I felt abandoned and devastated and yet at the same time had to put a brave face on it for the children and the enquiring staff. I was not just upset but very angry. By this time though, I had started to learn not to retaliate verbally - but inwardly, I was seething. We never discussed it.

I should have been the one to communicate more but it was very difficult and I didn't know how. What a relief to finally realise what the cause of all our problems was.

Looking at the aforementioned, I realise that I have changed a lot in the last twenty years. A lot of it is positive but there are some negatives forced by our marriage and ill health.

I am definitely more patient. I believe tolerance has only come with education and understanding. I can cope with his outbursts now I know the basic, if not exact, cause. It is my reaction to them that can either calm him down or wind him up.

Recently the whole family suffered from a terrible bout of flu where we were all bed bound for days. Once we emerged from our sweaty beds, thinner, weaker and more emotional, David and I had an enormous row over nothing. He had said something very patronising that, ordinarily, I would no longer react to (as I have learnt that he doesn't mean it the way it sounds). However, even though I had told him I was feeling very emotional and my defences were down, he had not listened to me. For once I could not help but bite back. In my weakened state I did not have the mental capacity not to be offended and tell him what I thought. It was a big mistake, but it was unavoidable. It brought home to me now how crucial my behaviour is in the harmony of the household. My ability to stay calm against all odds is essential.

Years ago, I would have looked upon my shouting and standing up for myself as a strength, but now I understand it can be a weakness. It is much harder to let it go and not retort. It is harder to tell yourself it is his condition that makes him say and do the things that he does. It is harder to realise that this burden will always be upon you, that he is never really going to master it. He doesn't have the capability. I do, and I must make the most of it. I am the emotional sponge and if I do say it myself, I am the unsung hero.

Self-Harm

A Sign of Distress In Asperger's

This is a very private and desperate activity. It is often seen as the domain of teenage girls crying out for help but it is often well hidden and used to varying degrees by both sexes on the autism spectrum. The National Autistic Society website claim that about fifty percent of people with ASD will self-harm at some point.

The reasons for doing this vary from self-hatred to frustration and anger. Sometimes they feel it is the safest way to release their anger. I know some worry that, if they took their anger out on other people or property, that they would do serious harm. It is linked very much to low self-esteem and feeling inadequate and not knowing what to do about it.

What to look out for

Head banging, hand biting, hair pulling, face or head slapping, skin picking or forceful head shaking.

NT What to Do

You need to be an emotional detective and find out what the cause of the distress is. Once you have eliminated the distress the self-harming will be alleviated for the short term.

S

1. Acknowledge that you realise they are self-harming but don't make a big thing about it unless they need to be hospitalised. If they are harming to that degree, then mental health services need to be involved.

2. Try and reduce general anxiety.

3. Put into place strategies for the future such as avoidance or using ear plugs if you can't get away from a certain noise.

4. Consider other ways to reduce stress in your life.

What about the other half of the relationship though? What about the mental health of the partners and wives? Have they been driven to self-harm?

In the NT Partner

I have some inkling into this. There was one point, where David was having such a major meltdown and was putting all of the blame on me, that I genuinely did not know what to do. We were not at home and I was trying to stay outwardly calm for our safety and for the children's sake. I didn't want them to realise how serious the situation was. I was genuinely concerned for David's mental health. He was so controlling in that environment that, though I was not scared of him, I was scared for him. I had no option but to wait out the meltdown but, because of the circumstances, I knew it would be a long time coming. Without consciously being aware of what I was doing, I started to scratch my arm with my finger nails. I raked my nails up and down the inside of my arm causing the skin to lift and red welts to appear. I did this for quite some time and now I realise that, subconsciously, it was a form of self-control. What I really wanted to do was run away or scream at him to stop, but I was not in the position to do either. Yes it hurt, though I didn't do any permanent damage, but it was a form of relief as well.

AS What to Do

If your wife is showing obvious signs of this much stress you need to stop what you are doing and calm down. If you find it hard, I would suggest walking away until you do. This is a sign that your wife is completely overwhelmed by the situation and does not know what else to do. It is a way of relieving the emotional pain she is suffering and a visible 'cry for help'.

The Husband Says:

Whilst there might be a low incidence of self-harm amongst male Aspies, I suppose it depends on your definition. To me there is the "high profile" self-harm of cutting and stabbing, but there is a lower form that might easily be mistaken for stimming. When does the repeated action of thumping your head off a wall stop being stimming and start being deliberate self-harm? Younger Aspies, me included (at school - was this attention seeking?), might do this.

Self-Medication

After a long and stressful day, sometimes a glass of wine seems like a great idea. It is a good way to relax but it is often hard to find the balance between relaxing with a couple of glasses of wine and moving on to another bottle. Too much alcohol can lead to depression and therefore you end up in a Catch 22 situation, where you become reliant on it.

There are other forms of self-medication available from health food stores such as St John's Wort or Evening Primrose or Valerian which are said to help with depression and anxiety.

The Husband Says:

There's a fine line between self-medication and an addiction. Stay on the right side of that line, and perhaps, the Aspie can self-medicate with other stress relievers like your special interest? I have found TV box sets to be especially mind-numbing...

The Husband Says:

Quite a lot of Aspies, me included, like some overlap between the senses, perhaps so that we feel that the sensory messages are confirmed and accurate. Some of these overlaps are natural - flavour of food is a combination of both the sense of taste and the sense of smell - try eating a cheese and plain crisp whilst smelling a salt and vinegar one - you will swear you are eating a salt and vinegar crisp. The whole discussion on stimming comes about from these crossovers in senses; I think that touch, balance and kinaesthetic senses all need to work together as somehow "weaker" to be meaningful to us Aspies - perhaps that explains the common dyspraxia comorbidity if that reinforcement doesn't happen?

Sensory Issues

As a child I was fully aware of my father's sensitivities. They always increased when he was stressed or cross with us. He was a very strict and scary man at meal times. I lived in fear of making an accidental slurping noise or worse still, accidentally screeching my knife across the plate whilst trying to cut through some tough meat my mother had cooked. The look my father would give me would freeze me in my tracks and I would apologise. He didn't have to say anything. I realise now that the noises we children made weren't just irritating but actually painful for him, especially the screeching cutlery.

This also reminds me of the fact that my mother complained bitterly that, every time she called us all to the table, my father would suddenly go to the toilet so that he would always appear last in the room. It has only recently dawned on me that this was a sensory thing.

S

I've known for some time about little boys (mostly) who are very poor at getting to the toilet on time. Before my son's diagnosis I put it down to his obsession with video games from an early age, and not wanting to disrupt a game by going to the toilet. 'We now know that many AS people lack the trigger/chemical that tells them in advance that they need to go to the toilet. They cannot assess the situation. I have noticed some (mostly women) deal with this lack of knowledge by going to the toilet at every given opportunity.

The senses are not just the obvious five:

Touch

At first glance you would think that your Aspie does not like being touched. This is true to a point but they are quite happy to be touched and held by family members. My children still enjoy a cuddle or a tickle from me but they do not like people they do not know very well or like touching them at all. I think there might be trust issues involved here.

Taste

Very picky or the opposite. Hyper or hypo. Either hates hot things or can't get enough of them. The first chilli David ever made me was incredibly hot and basically inedible. He added everything from chilli puree to Tabasco sauce without any moderation or tasting it in the process. No subtlety.

Sound

It isn't that they don't like loud noises it's that like don't like unexpected loud noises. Getting in the car after David has been in there on his own and the sound system is always on max volume.

Smell

Smelly people put him off in restaurants or in the queue at supermarkets.

Other Senses

Balance, equilibrioception, or vestibular

- Kinaesthetic, proprioception (the sense of position of the parts of the body relative to each other); often affected Hyper or Hypo possibly leading to symptoms of dyspraxia or making the person prone to travel sickness.

- Temperature

- Pain

Controversially:

- Time - since we haven't found the body's dedicated sensor that can measure this

The Husband Says:

My sensory processing issues are summarised by the whole hypo-normal-hyper thing. NTs have "normal" senses, whereas a morbidity or defining characteristic of Aspergers is to have several out of the ordinary responses to the senses - either seeking much, much more sensory stimulation or much, much less.

Sight

I have excellent vision compared with most of the population, with only a bit of age related long-sightedness kicking in - so slight that I have the lowest possible amount of correction in reading glasses. But I crave the stimulation of changing patterns, but only when they are in focus - my glasses have to be scrupulously clean so I can see exactly what is going on and dust on my computer screen is incredibly distracting.

Hearing

I like it loud to blot out other things. I've probably damaged my hearing in earlier life, but as a youngster I could hear much higher frequencies than my peer group. Now I have slight ringing in my ears at those high frequencies - to slight to be troublesome but present nonetheless.

I have terrible problems picking out one voice in a crowd. I think this is a common Aspie problem. This is probably a processing problem rather than an ear-hearing-mechanics problem. This can be quite disabling when added to my social awkwardness. At a party I feel I can't easily join in the conversation because I'm missing much of it.

Taste

I think I'm hyper sensitive to most tastes and always want to have more. If only taste wasn't attached to calories!

Is hyper sensitivity to things like food-taste and alcohol underpinning of an addictive personality that might be common in Aspies? Perhaps some research is needed here?

Smell

Taste and smell are so connected that it is unlikely that you would be hyper in one and hypo in the other. You can get too much of a good thing though, especially when certain women wear perfume in quantities expected of deodorant and leave a vapour trail wherever they go.

I'm particularly sensitive to the more acrid, sulphurous and vinegary notes of smell. I'll be the first to smell a gas leak with the added mercaptans.

S

Touch

An enigma with me. I either don't respond much to touch (at the pain end of touch), or I'm very ticklish - to the point of not enjoying it after a while.

Balance

I'm very sensitive to balance. I get fearfully seasick when my balance system and eyes disagree about which way is up.

Kinaesthetic

I am that bull in the china shop semi-dyspraxic. I easily lose track of where my body is in space and don't really care until something comes crashing to the ground.

Temperature

I like it cool-cold; not ordinary 20 degrees Celsius office, but on the legal office minimum of 16, if I can wrest control of the thermostat from the NTs around me.

Pain

Another oddity - I register pain rather too strongly (hyper-sensitive) and I'm often considered "soft" or "a wuss" as a result. But sometimes I have no perception of pain until I see my own blood and then it starts to throb and hurt.

Sensory Processing Disorder (SPD)

This is a co-morbid condition where the brain has difficulty sensing and responding to information coming from the senses.

This means that they can be under sensitive or over sensitive to situations in their environment from touch (including pain), taste, light, sound and visual stimulation. For someone with SPD or an AS condition (or both) their environment can be overwhelming or, if they are at the opposite end of the sensory spectrum, go unnoticed. e.g. Loud music or scratchy woollens may be unbearable to some, but make no difference to others; having a heavy coat on can be annoying to one person but have a great calming effect on another; tight bear hugs work for some but, on the opposite end of the scale, others cannot stand to be touched at all.

In extreme cases, some people are even unaware of their limbs.

The Husband Says:

See my comments under Sensory Issues, Stimming, Dyspraxia, Hyper and Hypo. All these things link together.

Serotonin

Serotonin is considered to be what the body produces to provide feelings of well-being and happiness.

Recent research into serotonin and autism has found that those with autism are less likely to produce as much of this which unsurprisingly leads to them naturally having lower, less stable moods.

Interestingly it is a monoamine neurotransmitter which is found in the gut and central nervous system. This could explain why low levels of Vitamin D3 (which helps strengthen the gut lining) can affect mood too.

David has been using this in tablet form but we have recently started using skin patches in lower doses for our teenager.

Sex

As in any normal marriage this is a sensitive issue and, like any normal marriage, there are problems in this area for some. A lot of AS men have an issue with intimacy and in being touched. This is a sensory issue that needs to be dealt with sensitivity and with understanding.

Many AS/NT couples have no problems in this area, certainly in the early years of marriage. As with many marriages, the arrival of children can certainly put a dampener on one's sex life.

Loss of libido by either partner can upset the equilibrium in a marriage. Stress is a major player in libido loss and your AS husband lives on the edge of his stress pretty much all the time. Reducing his anxiety in many ways perhaps with massage or a glass of red wine can certainly help.

Vitamin D deficiency can also cause loss of libido and many people, including NTs but especially those with AS, are deficient in this essential hormone. When you are deficient in Vitamin D one of the symptoms is reduced testosterone. Getting more sunshine to the skin or taking Vitamin D supplements will take the edge of his anxiety and make him feel better in multiple ways as well as reducing his oestrogen and upping his testosterone. You may find yourself with a different man or at least one more like the person you originally married.

The wife too can lose her libido; it may be because you are upset with his every day behaviour that you do not want to have sex with him. He will not be able to connect your reasoning and will take your rejection as a total rejection of himself.

S

Sexual Inhibitors

Some partners literally see sex as a tool for precreation and that is all. After all, that is what they were told at school. They know the mechanics and how to make a baby. Once they have produced children they have very little interest in continuing this just for pleasure alone. Indeed, for some it is a chore that they would rather avoid completely.

Touch

Again, this is a sensory issue and while some partners can be addicted to being touched by their partner, others cannot bear it and even find it painful. For those that cannot bear light, feathery touches, it is best to direct your partner .to use firmer, more massage like touches in certain areas. The Aspie partner should be specific about what areas like touched and what areas they cannot bear to have touched. It may take some of the spontaneity our of the bedroom but still always for loving contact.

Spontaneity

If you have had regular sexual partners in the past you will likely have had those lustful, spontaneous moments of mad passionate sex, especially in your first few weeks and months. This may never have happened with your ASD partner. With David, I thought he was just being a gentleman and not taking advantage of me as I was still very much on the rebound. It turns out the best way to get around the lack of spontaneity is to reduce anxiety by giving fair warning that something may well happen and then if possible, introduce a glass of wine to relax them. Reducing their inhibitions makes for a lot more fun!

Difference in Emotions

We NT women are considered quite emotional by our AS partners and at times they see this as been needy. David has never managed to fathom that if he has upset me that I might not be ready to even be in the same room as him, let alone share his bed soon after. He is able to compartmentalise parts of his life very differently from me. When he has had a major meltdown it also affects me as I am the one that is there as the emotional sponge. I am therefore not ready to switch my emotions to another setting so soon in the way he does. I need time for the adrenaline coursing through my body to go before I can then think of being passionate in another way. I give him time to calm down so he needs to be aware that I do too.

S

Sharing

As any mother with autistic children, or even just strong willed children, will know sharing can be a big issue. An AS person cannot see the viewpoint of anyone else who is competition for an object of their desire: no awareness of the other 'competitors' wants or needs. They see the object and therefore they want it. If a parent does not deal with this issue early on in their child's life, it can make for a very unattractive quality in an adult.

I think David's mother must have dealt with this issue rather well. It may be because she came from a large family (she has 7 siblings), and they just had to share. There wasn't enough money for everyone to have everything.

David is one of the most generous people I have ever met.

The Husband Says:

Sharing is one of the easiest things for an Aspie to put on an act and look neurotypical. Sharing is founded in logic and maths. But watch out for the Aspie trying to share out something intangible - either complex "rules" will be formed and rigidly followed or for some things, sharing might break down altogether - like affection being shared appropriately between wife and children.

Sharing of Household Chores

When we were first married we both worked and didn't have children. Our weekends were our own. We didn't make much mess between us. Most Saturday mornings we would carry out the essential and obvious household chores. It would take about an hour and the house was straight. It was easy and satisfying. Yet when I gave up work to have our first child this all changed. I was tired, worn out and we had so much more stuff! With a child, there seemed to be less routine not more. There wasn't really time set aside for tidying anymore and, somehow, all the responsibility became mine. I didn't want it and didn't enjoy it. I just felt put upon but also felt that, because I wasn't the one bringing in the money any more, I could hardly complain. I find household chores tedious and soul-destroying. The moment you take your eye off the ball, the mess just comes back.

We made the mistake of not discussing our expectations of each other. Perhaps if I had asked him to still help out on a Saturday, he would have continued. But it was the last thing on our minds as our baby was very difficult, I had little sleep and then, due to finances, I had to return to work anyway.

NT
I suggest a chart of chores drawn up by both. Make it colourful and placed somewhere obvious. Also make use of technology and put reminders on both your

phones. Then there is no excuse. If you set a good example by doing all your chores, he may mirror your actions and do his share as he doesn't want to look bad, at least for a week or two anyway.

The Husband Says:

And here we are too alike and, perhaps, less readily compatible for each other. We both hate household chores and will go out of our way to avoid them. Aspies can be quite creative at avoidance. Karen and I form complex contracts where if I end the game of Diesel Jenga by filling up the car with Diesel, she might clean the toilets.

I think that NTs avoid household chores, but not to the extent that I do.

Shooting the Messenger

David is my technical support. I'm happy to hold up my hands and say I don't know how to solve certain problems on my phone or PC. I also think, what is the point of struggling on with something I don't understand when he can quickly solve or fix the problem for me? He is generally happy to do so, it makes him feel useful and he likes to feel useful.

However, sometimes he can't fix things. This will generally not be his fault, but either mine or the fault of someone else. As an emotional neurotypical I cannot but help voice my annoyance at not being able to do or fix something. When I am frustrated I need to vocalise it and, though my words are not directed at David, all he hears is my annoyed tone. He gets upset because he thinks I am disappointed and cross with him for his failure. This is not so at all, but his low self-esteem and negative frame of mind immediately assume that I am having a go at him and he becomes disgruntled, defensive and often asks me to 'Not shoot the messenger'.

I always try and explain to him that I am frustrated with the situation, either with myself for causing the problem in the first place, or for the problem being caused by other people. Yet I can tell he never believes that I am not disappointed in him. This means I try not to ask him for IT help unless absolutely necessary, but this often back-fires: if I asked him in the first place I probably wouldn't get myself into such a mess.

It is a wonder to me that he still thinks I am perfect for him. He obviously sees me in a completely different light than the one I try and portray. I try to show him that I am laidback, patient, kind and forgiving, but the way he reacts to me makes me come across as abusive. He genuinely thinks that I am cross with him all the time for his believed failures. Regardless of the reality, I am amazed he is still here.

I feel sorry for him that he feels this way as surely he can't really be happy, but I am frustrated at the same time that I can't get through to him that he is not a constant disappointment to me. At the same time, it is hard for me to know that I cannot voice my own natural feelings without there being a backlash, regardless of whether my feelings are aimed at him or not. I have to stamp down on them to keep the harmony, and that is not very healthy for either of us.

The Husband Says:

I'm my own worst enemy on this topic. I like stuff to be tidy and finished and to stay that way. But gadgets and technology are forever changing and "improving". I just don't get that most normal people accept that with basic functionality comes a whole pile of technology bugs. The completer-finisher in me wants all of our technology to work properly and, when it doesn't, I get frustrated with the technology - which then overflows into frustration with the users of the technology. I think that Karen should get annoyed with the purveyors of tech that their tech doesn't work properly. Instead, I take on the "annoyed" position, and further, I go out of my way to learn the inner workings of the gadget in the hope of fixing it. These are efforts I could better deploy on other things, like my own special interest. So I start to feel resentful.

Recently Karen has started to find ways of avoiding this stressor. The most successful to date is to spend more money on technology that is closer to being finished before being released on the market!

Shopping

I remember from my days when the kids were tiny, reading up on toddlers and tantrums. The book recommended by my friends was called "Toddling Taming". Grocery shopping, or indeed any kind of shopping, with a toddler or two is a nightmare. I eagerly looked up the author's indexed advice, hoping for some miraculous words of wisdom on this shopping issue. There was only sentence:

"Don't, or do it online!"

With an Aspie man there are two types of shopping. The shopping he wants to do and the shopping he doesn't want to do. The shopping he wants to do is few and far between but can be quite expensive.

The Challenges

Parking

Perhaps I'm a lazy parker, but I always like to park in a quiet spot and walk. I like to park near a trolley bay so I don't have far to walk once I've packed the shopping in the car. When I shop with David, he likes to drive and be in control. He spends ages trying to find a parking space near the shop, especially if its raining. He will squeeze into tiny spaces rather than walk a few extra yards. I feel it's almost like a competition with the other shoppers. It takes way longer to do this than to park somewhere convenient and walk. These days I grit my teeth and let him get on with it. He knows my views. When he is driving, I have decided to rarely question his actions as he is in charge of the car. I don't like it when he queries my driving, so it is only fair. Besides, it's best not to start off the shopping trip at each other's throats. Life is too short.

Sensory Issues when Shopping

If you look online for advice on going shopping with someone who is autistic, they always assume that it is with a child. It is never assumed that the person suffering is an adult. If supermarkets realised that they are preventing a large part of the population from visiting (or at least having a comfortable time in) their store they would, possibly, do something about it. After all, the large stores want you to spend as much time as possible in their aisles falling for their marketing ploys, but most autistic adults just want to buy their essential items and get out of the sensory hell.

The constant barrage of the overly bright lights, Tannoys making announcements, signs everywhere vying for your attention and the constant bleeping from the till area is hard for our overstimulated Aspies to cope with.

Additionally, there are people and lots of them. These require avoidance techniques and having to talk to them if you fail in that area.

As a NT, you will not be aware that you naturally 'tune out' these noises but that your partner is aware of every individual one.

People with Trolleys

David genuinely believes that people are aiming their trolleys at him in the aisles. He must have been clipped on the ankle by a careless shopper once and never forgotten it. He also likes to be in charge of the trolley. If I grab a trolley first I always pass it to him. I think it makes him feel more grounded and, is a barrier between him and other people, and also he has a purpose.

Buying Large Household Items

I dread when a large appliance goes wrong in the house as it inevitably means the initial 'trying to fix it' (and get mad with it) phase, and then the "It's going to cost me" phase. The next phase is a little more pleasant because he suddenly realises that he can go gadget shopping. This is the kind of shopping he likes.

However, woe betide if you try to rush his research. This is a serious subject and all avenues need to be discovered and analysed in depth before any decision can be made. If at all possible, certainly with white goods, I like to use Appliances Online as they give good little video demonstrations of what the fridge etc. can or cannot do. It saves me reading through a whole load of tedious facts and figures. It's even better if they are at a good price and can be delivered the next day. Even if a little more expensive than a local store, David will sometimes go for that option.

If, however, we have to traipse down the road to the retail park to stand in a large store full of people on commission, the atmosphere is very different.

At the Till

Queuing

Each queue has to be assessed for length and quantity of goods. I let him decide most of the time. However, if he gets it wrong he gets quite annoyed with himself.

Izzarding

David and I are both fans of comedian Eddie izzard and this is our favourite sketch. We have given the act of switching between queues at the checkout as 'Izzarding'. We will often look at the queues and each other and say "Shall we Izzard?"

Packing

He never used to help at the till at all though he would always pay. It felt really embarrassing like he was taking the little woman to do her weekly shopping. I complained about it and he did start to help for a bit. If he doesn't know I just ask him if he's going to help or not and then he does. There have been times when the checkout person has been chucking stuff at me way faster than I can pack it and he has just stood there.

He much prefers to put things on the conveyor belt. I think he'd rather I didn't help do this as I probably mess up his order. As far as I'm concerned as long as it fits and nothing spills any order is fine but he like to align boxes to make it look tidy.

Likewise, at the other end, when he does help me pack he only ever grabs things that he has put in the trolley like he has left his aura on it so it is his responsibility alone. I just push things towards him, implying that he should pack them.

Paying

Everyone has their own system. We have a joint account and I also have my own separate account that David pays the household monthly amount into. I use this for most of my grocery shopping and have to eke it out until the end of the month. If he comes with me however, he still likes to pay out of the joint account. Well, I'm not going to complain about that. He likes to appear generous.

Computers in shops still get glitches all the time and I always have my fingers crossed that the card is accepted first time as otherwise he hates people thinking he doesn't have enough money to pay for his shopping. It always has a knock-on effect to the day.

S

Tips for Harmonious Shopping

Advice for both of you:

- Decide what you are going for and try and write a list.

- Let him be in charge of the list and the trolley. He will like being in charge and it will give your freedom to move around.

- Pick a time of day that is fairly quiet. Try to avoid the mad rush on a Saturday. If you have to drive further to get to a more friendly supermarket it is worth it.

- If the kids are likely to play up and get on his nerves try and leave them with a friend of family member.

- Always check you have enough money in your account before you leave the house.

- Don't spend hours chatting to friends you have bumped into.

Stick to the list. Get in, get out as quickly as possible and never take him window shopping.

The Husband Says:

Shopping. It's almost primeval; hunting and gathering to provide for the family. Gladiatorial with chariots replaced by wonky trollies. Little wonder it stresses out the Aspie and that the coping strategies look barely like coping at all in this competitive arena. Shopping brings out the worst in Aspies.

Ordinary grocery shopping is hell. There are so many "opportunities" for social interaction; people don't want to interact, they just want to get on and get the chore of shopping done. Most of all the Aspies. There are unwritten social rules of shopping designed simply to annoy:

- *NTs want to hand over their trolley outside the shop - they chose it so it must be a good one. Now we have the fumble for the pound coin that you "owe" the person who is offering the trolley instead of the token you intended to use*

- *Competition for scarce resources - like bargains - never enough to go around for first come, first served*

- *Trolley pilots who don't understand the highway code!*

- *Having items with no price label when you arrive at the checkout and a store assistant that must go and get a similar item from the far side of the store rather than leave the item behind or look it up on the computer, or make a discount offer.*

S

- People in front of you at the checkout without the means to pay for all their items

- People in a queue with personal hygiene problems

Now high value item shopping is even worse. An Aspie will have already conducted in depth research in the item to be bought and selected the precise make and model with the best mix of features and price. I don't want to be sold a "better" one - the one I chose was perfect. High value items are usually sold on commission so pressure to change to a different item can be high. Don't tell me that if you have one on display that this is a "display model" and cannot be bought and that you have no stock; if you have no stock then take the thing you won't sell off display - you are telling lies by suggesting that I could buy one! And I know the script says that you should try to sell me an expensive HDMI cable, but don't try that with an electrical engineer who has plenty of spares at home and knows that there is no difference between a £1 cable and a £100 cable (other than £99), because the HDMI digital signal is strong enough to be transmitted by wet string. And you don't need my name and address to allow you to send me advertising guff; the law says you only need this if I'm buying a television receiver and that, my friend, is a washing machine.

Rant over. I feel better.

Shouting

This is a major issue for most Asperger Marriages. We all do it from time to time.

Your Asperger husband will take you raising of your voice to him as a verbal attack. He will take it very personally. He may shout back or he may withdraw. What he definitely won't do is forget. I suspect if I asked David to recount every time I have shouted at him; he would be able to do so. Can you remember all the occasions?

Indirect Attack

What is more, in a busy household with children and animals, there can be an awful lot of shouting. On the whole our Aspie household is fairly quiet, but David gets very on edge when the children have friends round and they are caught up with excitement on a Wii game. I can tell the shrieking goes right through him.

He cannot detach himself from the noise and even when common sense tells him it is not directed at him, his body cannot help but react. I liken it to the time when our daughter was a year old and we had a night away for the first time. We had left the children with David's mother and gone into town for a meal and a trip to the cinema. We stayed the night in a hotel and were planning on having a much longed for lie in, then picking the kids up at lunch time. Only I was awoken in the early hours of Sunday morning by a baby crying next door. I was still breastfeeding at the time, and my body just reacted to it even though I knew there was no baby to feed, and until I heard that cry I had been quite relaxed.

I have some sympathy there.

The one person I do shout at is my dog. We have a very close relationship and she dotes on me completely. She also likes to get my attention and sometimes she is quite naughty. I don't believe in hitting children or animals so sometimes the only way to let the dog know she has done wrong (or succeeded in getting my attention) is to shout at her. David never picks up on the warning signs and, therefore, will leap out of his seat as he thinks some disaster has befallen me or that he is in serious trouble.

It is almost comical to me, but not to him. He gets quite upset and can be totally put off his train of thought - which he hates.

On a Serious Note:

Shouting is one of the main things you need to be able to control. You need to try and not voice your anger or surprise quite so loudly. I know this is difficult as it is a natural response to many a situation. However, your husband can get deeply upset and, as I said above can, take it very personally regardless of whether it is aimed at him or not.

These actions have been known to build up to breaking point and the husband has walked out of a marriage never to return. I'm not saying this will happen in your marriage but it is worth noting. Shouting is an action that they cannot understand and cannot find a means to cope with. Sometimes for them, the only course of action is to leave.

The Husband Says:

When I'm shouting at you in an argument, it's not because I'm feeling violent. I'm confused and running out of ways to communicate - I thought my side of the discussion was clear, but you are not getting it; I can't think of any other words to use, so I'll try the same ones but a bit louder.

Put like that in the cold light of day, outside of the heated discussion, I understand that shouting doesn't do any good. But in the heat of the argument with the fight or flight adrenaline flowing, all I can do (because I don't have another viewpoint) is to shout about what I can see. Sorry.

Showing your Love

Words don't mean so much to your Aspie husband. To him, deeds are much more important. He shows you he loves you by the way he does things for you. Apparently, doing things for you that they don't want to do, means that they love you!

S

NT Remember to look out for these unpleasant tasks that they carry out for you, and be sure to reward them sufficiently. Try and look upon it as being as romantic as a passionate kiss or a declaration of love.

Likewise, perhaps you should remind him that all the little things you do for him every day is because you love him too.

Showing your Weaknesses

Is it a bad thing to show the person you love your weaknesses? It will make him feel like he knows you better and feel protective towards you. Letting the person you love, get to know the real you is essential. He needs to know if you are scared of spiders. He will understand and not look down at you, because he might be too.

This is especially needed in an Asperger relationship because he can't always figure out all those little hints by himself. Your refusal to go in the garage to get something might just appear as stubbornness until you explain it to him.

Be careful though. Some weaknesses are good. Some are not. Some weaknesses will throw him into a spin.

How will this make him feel? E.g. he relies on your for social strength to shield him from the confusion and translate a situation to him. How does he feel in a situation where both of you are clueless?

Well, it can go either of two ways and by now you will probably know which one your partner is more likely to do. He will either ignore it and hope it goes away or he will do his research and step up to the mark.

My observations from a couple where both are on the spectrum and therefore both have very similar weaknesses and fears, are that together, somehow, they are stronger. Because they don't have great expectations of each other in this area they are patient and figure it out together. This way lies a more equal partnership in which I have been quite envious as this rarely happens in my own marriage.

Showing your weaknesses can actually lead to a better and stronger marriage in the long run.

Shutdowns

Similar to a Meltdown, a Shutdown is an extreme reaction to the over stimulus of 'Normal' life. They tend to come about gradually responding to long term unresolved problems. However, they present very differently.

S

Meltdowns can often be a violent, angry response to a situation, whereas a Shutdown is more of a withdrawal from a situation that can't be coped with face on.

Shutdowns are linked more to low self-esteem and low confidence.

Your Aspie will withdraw completely from your company, often retreating to bed with the covers over their head to physically block out the world they don't understand.

They may temporarily lose the power of speech and seem almost catatonic and vacant. As a partner or parent it is a scary situation to witness.

However, it is not all bad. This is their way of protecting themselves. Being cocooned from the pressures of the world and taking time out to not think for a while. It is exhausting having to constantly be perplexed.

Eventually, once they have rested, cogitated and evaluated, they will come to and decide to face the world again.

Our son tends to have more Shutdowns than Meltdowns. He is not an angry person but gentle and thoughtful. At times I have carefully cajoled him into facing the world again by applying humour to a situation to make it less scary. Also allowing him to surround himself with the things he loves so that they can distract his negative thoughts. For example, bringing the dog into the room. The dog is always loving and comical and therefore non-threatening, non-judgmental and can often provide him with a lot of comfort.

NT Hints and Tips

- Never get angry

- Never shout

- Don't push him to tell you what is wrong. He may not know himself and he needs time to switch off and later process his thoughts. If left to his own devices he may come to his solution.

- Let him know you are there for him.

- Let him know you love him whatever.

- Be patient

Sighing

He only sighs in utter frustration.

See Intonation for a lot about this one. This is one of my personal bugbears. I am not allowed to sigh. I sigh just at the thought of it.

Apparently if I sigh there is something wrong!

No, sometimes I am just thinking about stuff and sometimes I am just breathing. Sometimes I am groaning at something someone has said or reacting to something on the TV. Sometimes I don't' know why I sigh.

Generally, it's not a sign that you have done something wrong! I just need to breathe! Physically and metaphorically.

The Husband Says:

Perhaps your natural sighs sound like my dad's sighs of "resigned to irritable annoyance". It was a short step from irritated to significantly annoyed, so I always wanted to avoid my dad when he sighed; this could spiral into something more nasty.

Simon Baron-Cohen

Simon Baron-Cohen is Professor of Developmental Psychopathology at Cambridge University and Director of the Autism Research Centre. His work includes the hypothesis that autism includes Mind blindness and delays in the development in the theory of mind.

And yes he is the cousin of Sasha Baron-Cohen aka, Ali G and Borat!

Single Parent

If I could relive the first few years of our children's lives, I would do things very differently. If I had known in 1999 that David had Asperger's Syndrome, and what it entailed, I would have been forewarned and forearmed. We could have come up with strategies in our daily life and especially for parenting our children together.

Though on the outside we may have looked like a normal happy family (and often we were), there was very much a divide where the parenting was concerned.

Before our son was born we never discussed what our roles would be, other than I decided early on in my pregnancy that I did not want to return to work. I wanted to give this motherhood 'thing' my full undivided attention. I didn't know how long for and we didn't discuss that either.

Of course when our son was born, the majority of the role automatically fell to me but, as Morgan grew, so did my expectations of his father. I did make suggestions to David, such as him coming home in time to give Morgan a bath. I believe he did turn up fairly early one evening with the baby-bathing idea in mind, but he didn't really know what to do with his child. I remember feeling disappointed and worried about their bonding. I knew David loved Morgan but it was worrying that he didn't know how to show it.

As I was the 'stay at home mum' I didn't feel like I could ask him to do too much with the baby on top of all the overtime he was working. Yet, when I did eventually go back to work when Morgan was just six months old, David didn't shoulder any extra responsibility for the baby. I still had to get up several times a night and then somehow manage to get Morgan to the child minder, be smartly dressed and on time every morning. It never occurred to David to step up to the plate a bit more, or simply that I would have appreciated the help.

It's no wonder I ended up in hospital (when Morgan was just one) having a major panic attack.

The Husband Says:

I think if we had our time again I would have asked you to be much more direct about what you expected me to do with regard to parenting of our children when they were younger. There may have been the danger, though, that this pressure might have split up the family. Who can tell? There is no reset button.

Situation Avoidance

How can these situations be avoided in an Asperger household? The main answer is to avoid stressful situations as much as possible. However, life is unpredictable and, despite best efforts, often beyond complete control. Not every situation can be pre-empted. The irony is that our house move was motivated by the need to reduce stress. Together we have visualised a larger more private residence, with off-road parking and space for guests, instead of them occupying the coveted study when they stay.

Wendy Lawson believes that the different perspectives of the person with autism and the NT 'explain the challenging behaviours seen in the population'.

With children, it is much easier to control their surroundings. They have less responsibility and there are lower expectations on them. Within an Asperger household, if the parents have worked hard on providing their children with a calm, controlled environment, then autistic behaviour is less likely to occur.

Not so for the adult with AS, especially those who (on the outside) look like they have a normal life. They can be married with a successful career and children. Before getting married and adding to their responsibilities, they may not have displayed autistic behaviour. The autistic behaviour quite often starts as their responsibilities, and therefore anxieties, grow.

S

The Husband Says:

The theory is working. We might not own this house, but the greater space and lower stress is allowing us to put other coping strategies into place. We have managed to de-stress to the point where we can embark on writing this book/app/thing. We have a different type of relationship to that of a few years ago; by avoiding certain situations our relationship is deeper and more fulfilling in the territories we wish to explore.

Situational Non-Transference

This is a theory of mind problem. Some people believe that people on the spectrum do not learn from consequences. This is not true (unless they have additional learning difficulties). They learn that something went badly wrong in a certain situation and will avoid getting into that situation again. However, their brain does not connect in the way our NT brain does and is not able to apply it to a slightly different social situation. One of the current brain function theories is that autistic people are slow to synchronise social cues with social rules.

For example, I regularly find out that David has changed something vital within the home and not told me. I will find this out usually when he is at work and I don't know how to use it. When he gets home I will point out to him that this was a 'Need to Know' situation. He agrees that it was a vital bit of information that he forgot to tell me. I remind him that whenever he changes something vital he needs to tell me about it. He agrees.

The problem is even though he knows that in future he needs to inform me about a change in the situation we just discussed, he does not realise he needs to notify me when he changes something else which in his mind will be completely different.

I need to be psychic to tell him what he needs to tell me.

The Husband Says:

Again this looks about right. I don't want to burden you with things that are largely irrelevant - the minutiae of my day; but what makes a fact or a report of action relevant so that I should tell you? My thresholds are pretty consistently "off" for this - I fear you are glazing over with boredom on something you might later find important.

Sleep

Many men with AS suffer from insomnia. This is often related to stress and they cannot switch their minds off from the happenings of the day. They also manage to worry about the uncertainty of what is going to happen on the following day. They ruminate and obsess over the tiniest details.

S

Anxiety and worry is common to all and, at times, most people find their quality of sleep interrupted by worries. It is how you deal with these worries that makes the difference.

NT
Facing the upcoming difficulties is the best solution. Most problems and difficult situations usually never turn out to be as bad as your imagination makes them. It is finding the courage to face those worries which will help to make them go away.

The Husband Says:

Perhaps I'm lucky, but once I am sufficiently tired or stress has gone away that I can sleep, through a small war, if one is going on. Stress of the unknown can keep me awake for hours though until I come to terms with the likely consequences and form a plan to deal with them.

Social Cues

These are many and various. We NTs don't make it easy for those not in the know.

One of the things that we NTs do to confuse Aspies is to voice instructions as a question. Giving the impression that they have a choice, when they don't. This often leads to the Aspie literally interpreting what the person in authority has said and making their choice, usually the wrong choice. The Aspie comes across as being rude.

For example, my daughter had violin lessons for a long time and I would sit in on most of them. Her lovely teacher would often say to her, "Would you like to play that piece again?" I would watch as my daughter gave this questions great consideration and then made her decision. Sometimes, she would say "Yes." and replay the piece. Most often, she would say "No." Every time I would step in and tell her that her teacher was just being polite and actually wanted her to try again and improve on her last playing. She has never taken these instructions on anything more than face value.

If we NTs said what we actually meant, it would be great help to the AS community.

The Husband Says:

It's here in this self help guide that I'd love to see the complete list of all social cues and how to respond to them properly. But that would take all the "fun" out of NT life where you normal people want a bit of variability and social surprises.

I'd take the catalogue any day and make "fun" elsewhere.

S

Social Norms

Well this could be a very long article indeed. David was the one who came up with the idea for this article and indeed created the page but left it blank for me to fill in.

That in itself describes our whole relationship.

Wikipedia has a page that describes the mechanics of social norms, but not what they might be currently. There seem to be three norms that are obeyed almost universally:

- The Norm of Reciprocity for Concessions: Treating others as they treat you

- The Norm of Commitment: Keeping your promises

- The Norm of Obedience: Submitting to authority

YouTube is useful for looking up the most common unspoken social norms or rules, but be aware these vary from country to country. For example, I was surprised to find out, as a Brit, that winking is considered to be extremely rude in the USA. In the UK it is considered a bit fun or cheeky depending on the context, though it would be frowned upon if you winked at the Queen.

AS

Here are some social norms which are not in any way hierarchical:

- Queuing - in the UK you are expected to queue and wait your turn. Exceptions are letting elderly or pregnant people through.

- Toilet Etiquette - always close the door; most people do not want to see or hear you. Exceptions are drunk girls on a night out sharing a cubicle.

- Personal Space - it is okay to accidentally touch someone you know and love. If you accidentally brush or knock past an acquaintance or stranger, you must always apologise.

- If someone insists on you guessing their age, always guess under by at least three years. It is also considered rude to ask anyone but a child how old they are unless for official reasons.

- It is okay to hold your partners hand in public but anything more than a peck on the cheek is considered vomit-worthy by observers, especially if you are over forty.

- Always look pleased when you receive a gift, even if you hate it. Be careful not to re-gift back to the original sender.

S

- When you see someone in the street you know, however vaguely, you must at least acknowledge their presence with a nod or a smile. If they insist on talking, be polite but tell them you are running late. This a good get out clause and most people will not query it.

- Be aware that most sales people are just doing their jobs and often have to follow a script. It is not polite to point this out to them. You can also politely decline any extras they are offering you without relaying the whole Trade Descriptions Act to them.

- Just because you have something in common with someone, does not automatically make them your friend.

- Never burp at the dinner table but if you do, cover your mouth and apologise.

- Never talk to your in-laws about sex.

- Do not make jokes about sex with your partner in front of people. It might get you a laugh but your partner will be mortified and angry with you. As an adult, it is assumed you are sexually experienced and it is considered uncouth to talk about it once you are out of your boastful teens.

- Always remember your wife's birthday. No exceptions - and it is always useful to make note of the date you met, the day you married and your children's birthdays. It is considered uncaring not to know these dates.

- A conversation is a two-way thing. You are expected to feign interest in someone's health and, in the UK, mention the weather. Always act surprised that it is sunny. Talking at someone about your special interest, without asking them questions or allowing them to speak, is not a conversation but a monologue.

- Being humorous about yourself and your situation must always be self-deprecating.

The Husband Says:

I know I set a task as large as the fifth labour of Heracles - cleaning the Augean stables. But it is the 64-million-dollar question for an Aspie. So, Karen, can you divert a few rivers and give us a complete list? I appreciate that the items listed above are probably just the ones I have broken within the last week!

On a more serious note, social scientists have noted that social norms are not only enforced with explicit verbal sanctions, but violation of the norms are often signalled with body language, facial expression and other non-verbal communication. Perhaps the Aspie problems with recognising facial expression might be why we frequently break these unwritten rules.

About as close as I have seen to a handbook (and this only scratches the surface) is "Watching the English: The International Bestseller Revised and Updated". In this book, an eminent anthropologist sets out to break "the rules" in order to find their true extent.

And before I leave the subject: pro-tip - set a password you use every day to be your wife's birthday; that way you are sure to remember it.

Social Stories™

Dr Carol Gray came up with this simple concept to help children learn social rules and skills. However, these can be applied to adults on the autistic spectrum if done in the right way. Dr. Gray has a website devoted to how best to produce these aids.

Social Stories™ are Carol Gray's Trademark; please acknowledge her hard work if you use the term.

The cartoon strips are a simple visual device to help understand every day activities. If your husband does not react to a list, it may actually be a fun activity if you could draw a stick man storyboard to illustrate your needs.

It's The Little Things That Count

No. 1 How to Make Your Wife Smile:

1. Go to the Kitchen

2. Fill the kettle with water and turn on to boil.

3. Get two mugs out of the cupboard to use

4. Make two cups of coffee; one for yourself

5. Give to your wife and wait for her smile.

S

NT

I admit it is additional work in the short term, but once he understands you are struggling and is fully aware of what you need, he should make more of an effort for you. My warning is this will only be successful if you don't overwhelm him with too much. Take it slowly. Start with topics that will make a real difference like Putting out the Bin.

The Husband Says:

Karen asked me if I felt offended by the child-like simplicity of stick-man social stories. As a visual thinker, I said no. I did suggest though that they would be most successful with adult Aspies if there was an element of humour; even irony in the story.

I got told off for criticising that 'stick-man' was not anatomically correct.

Spatial Awareness

He is often quite clumsy. Yet bizarrely at times he can be quite dexterous. He has these little irritating habits where he over exaggerates his movements when I am around. It is generally to get out of my way. I don't know if this is an inferiority thing, but I have noticed it getting worse over the years and it annoys me because he is my husband and we should be allowed to brush against each other without over-reacting and without having to apologise. I love him and want to be in close proximity to him. For example, when he is driving and I reach into the middle console to find my sunglasses or a mint, he moves his arm out of the way. "What is wrong with that?" I hear you ask.

This sounds terribly petty, but it is the kind of thing you only notice when in close proximity to a person you know well: he moves out of my way, stiffly and too much. In an "I'm obviously offending you by having my arm in this position while you are trying to find your sunglasses and it is making you cross so I will get completely out of your way as much as I can whilst at the same time still managing to stay in control of the car", kind of way. It offends my wifely sensibilities that I cannot wordlessly or accidentally brush his arm while finding something next to him. I don't consider him in my way. He is in exactly the right place for driving the car and it is me that should be careful not to knock him or interfere with his concentration. If I need him to move so I can lift up the lid of the arm rest to rummage around in the box between us, I will ask him. He just doesn't get these subtleties.

I think he finds it hard to tell the difference between a deliberate or an accidental touch. He doesn't realise that, these subtle bumpings and touches that happen in everyday life between those who live and love together, are part of the intimacy of the relationship. It isn't something you realise you had until it is gone. A neurotypical in a 'normal' relationship may not understand this at all until it has happened to them.

S

What to do about it? Perhaps write a book and get your husband to read it?

The Husband Says:

Once again I think your analysis is spot on. I'm not at all sure what the social convention is for a loving social contact outside of the bedroom, so it's something I'm going to need to learn. In fact, I'm going to have to un-learn my usual response of getting out of the way which is the correct response to having your social space invaded by a stranger or a work colleague, and what I have learned as a coping strategy.

Special Interest

Some AS men have managed to hide their obsessions or special interests because they are so common they are not thought of as unusual. If you are a football fan, no one calls you weird. If you collect empty beer cans and arrange them chronologically and have to move house to accommodate them, then people start to notice and talk about you as eccentric or obsessive.

Most people have a special interest. Some have that interest for life and others will discard and pick up new ones as they go along.

Should a special interest be considered a problem? It can make a partner more interesting, especially if you share the interest. It is quite possible you met because of your special interest.

A special interest becomes a problem when it turns into an obsession that takes over not just the obsessive's life, but affects the whole family as well.

Work as a Special Interest

David is the Asperger type that does not have an obvious interest. It was however, the first thing I noticed about him. His life is his work and his work is his life. He has a job that generally he loves and keeps him interested. There are many positive aspects of this type of interest. Because of his good eye for detail and his natural talent and interest in all things engineering and anything related to his current engineering project, he has always been in work and very much in demand, and is well respected in his field. Having a good job and a good job title helps with self-esteem and knowing who you are.

His job also, of course, helped us meet. I was very much taken with the fact that he was the complete opposite of my last boyfriend. He had a good job, house and car and was able to impress me with his knowledge of the world courtesy of his travels with work.

I wasn't consciously looking for a man with a stable job and good future prospects, but it was certainly part of the attraction I felt for him. I was at an age where, unwittingly, I was ready to think about settling down. The money, support and reliability of such a man does not at first ring alarm bells. You only see that he is a hard worker. I didn't seek to change that. I knew instinctively that it was part of him.

To this day he does not really have any other special interests. He seeks relaxation by watching TV and having an ever ready glass of wine by his side. He, in fact, recently asked me what his hobby should be. I could not answer that for him. It has to be something that piques his interest. I have tried to get him into a more healthy life style. We have spent a considerable amount of money on bikes for the whole family, bike carrying apparatus and tow bars and we have only used them a handful of times because work is always a priority. He cannot relax until he knows all problems are solved. It is a persistent problem.

I can only wish David had a special interest outside of work.

Speech

AS is a Social Communication Disorder. Aspie's don't understand the message behind the intonation in your voice. They take words literally. They don't understand that NT's have an unspoken language e.g. Use of approximate time - "ish". Not an exact time.

They are rule followers but they don't expect that rules can changed or be bent.

Social and emotional development as a child can be anywhere between a third and two thirds delayed e.g. a 12-year-old AS boy may have the emotional capacity of an 8-year-old boy. They have not managed to steady their emotions from being either too high or too low, they have not yet found a happy medium. I would say that actually this reaction is never really learned or developed. David is very much an 'everything is wonderful' or 'everything is terrible' person. He used to drag me along on this emotional roller-coaster ride before I realised it wasn't real, so now I have learned to step back from it.

For example, he worries constantly about finances, usually whether we have enough. When he gets paid he can be extremely generous and will suggest I can have anything I want. He will suggest that we can buy the biggest house that I want. Towards the end of the month he is terrified of spending any money at all as it starts to run out and, if the subject of moving house comes up, he usually doesn't want to discuss it but, if he does, he will only discuss it in a negative way. That we shouldn't move, that we can't afford the size of house that we want, that there is nothing wrong with the house we are currently in.

Spontaneity

Lack of spontaneity in a marriage can lead to a dull and predictable existence. For the AS man this is safe. He likes his routines and feels the need to know what is happening next. To the NT wife, though she can probably admit that some routine and predictability is a good thing, she will soon crave spontaneity in their life.

Spontaneity happens when you just go with the flow. Let your emotions out and act on them. This means that when you feel love for your partner you act on it. Those little gestures, the sudden hugs and kisses. It is rare for the AS man to do any of these. He may well like it when his wife and children show their appreciation of him but, for some, even this small amount of touching is too much of a sensory overload and unpredictable. It is awful to feel rejected in this way, knowing he doesn't want you to touch him.

The Husband Says:

...and from this problem comes the compromise solution planned spontaneity.

Stages of Grief

When our son was first diagnosed, I was told that I would go through stages of grief for the child I thought I would have. The same can be said for the marriage I thought I would have and, though I have never asked him, perhaps David's own expectations of our marriage have not been met. Perhaps he has also had to grieve for the marriage he thought he was getting on 18 October 1997.

There are a few popular versions of the stages of grief model but the one I most related to was:

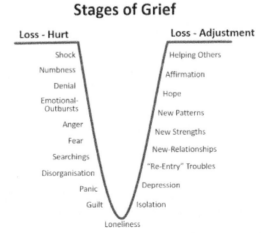

Stages of Grief

Loss - Hurt	Loss - Adjustment
Shock	Helping Others
Numbness	Affirmation
Denial	Hope
Emotional-Outbursts	New Patterns
Anger	New Strengths
Fear	New-Relationships
Searchings	"Re-Entry" Troubles
Disorganisation	Depression
Panic	Isolation
Guilt	
Loneliness	

S

Kubler Ross Model

Elisabeth Kubler-Ross hypothesised five stages of grieving:

- Denial
- Anger
- Bargaining
- Depression
- Acceptance

Note that Kubler-Ross did not mandate that the stages would always occur in this order or that the stages might not over-lap - these are common misconceptions; although the order presented is a "natural" one.

It took me a while to even realise that I was grieving for my marriage. This was long before I knew David had Asperger's. I certainly went through the shock and denial process and the loneliness part lasted for a long time. Every now and then it still hits me but when it does I reach out to others that understand.

I'm not sure whether I ever really entered depression or not. I certainly had some very low moments but luckily I am one for getting myself out of situations. I try not to carry my woes around with me too much and I can park them to one side when I leave the house.

I'm surprised to not see Acceptance on here. Maybe I should write a chart specifically for Asperger wives including acceptance. I feel without acceptance it is hard to move on.

Both David and I are now at the stage of helping others. It makes everything that we have been through more worthwhile.

The Husband Says:

I hope that the fifth stage of acceptance can be subdivided into two alternate paths of "growing" and "moving on"; Karen and I are now growing and improving a Version 2.0 of our relationship; some couples may choose to separate and move on following separate paths.

Staring

David rarely switches off from work. I often find him staring into space or at me and I ask him if he is okay. He just tells me he is thinking about work and trying to find a solution to a problem. He often says he should charge them thinking time. I believe his thinking is most effective as he always does come up with a solution in the end. He does however, have no idea he is staring blankly at me. It is a little unnerving.

The Husband Says:

And if you think staring blankly into space gets me into trouble at home, its ten times worse at a workplace. What's going on is that I'm trying to access a visual memory or a "mental blackboard" on which to work on a problem, so I've chosen to look in the direction of something that isn't changing so as to reduce the physical stimulus but without appearing to be asleep. You just stepped into my eye-line. I'm as startled that something changed as you are concerned that I'm now staring blankly at you.

There's another danger to gaze being misinterpreted by NTs and Aspies. When does an innocent glance turn into a flirty exchange of eye contact and then an unwanted stare from an Aspie in a stable marriage in an already uncomfortable social situation?

Staycation

It is okay to stay at home during the holidays.

There is tremendous social pressure to conform to the social norm of going away.

What if going on holiday is just too stressful or too expensive?

This year, before we even moved house we decided we were not going to have an expensive foreign holiday. We had so much going on with the stress of the move and exams and work and all the expenses involved we couldn't even consider adding to it with the stress of dragging everyone on holiday. It was a relief to say "No. We are staying at home to relax."

Who cares what everyone else thinks? If your kids just want to stay at home and chill out and see their friends occasionally and your husband come back to a house he is familiar with every night, then why stress? Put the money you would have spent on an expensive holiday in the bank and save it for when you are more relaxed and ready to do so. Ignore the queries from your friends. There is even a term for staying at home now.

Stigma

I cannot deny there is a stigma around autism and Asperger's Syndrome.

Many people wrongly consider this a mental illness. This is not so. Autism and Asperger's is often comorbid with depression or bi-polar but it is not a mental illness. It is a different way of thinking; the way the brain is wired. They are not broken.

Unfortunately, many professionals especially GP's do not understand autism or AS at all. They have had little or no training. I was told by my family doctor when I asked for a referral for our daughter that there was a stigma about autism and surely I didn't want my daughter to have a label.

I told him that I would prefer her to have a label if it meant she would get the help and understanding that she needed and didn't end up with meatal health conditions when she was older. I had recently attended a conference on women and girls on the spectrum and the statistics regarding additional mental health problems were astonishing and scary and I didn't want that for my daughter. She needed a diagnosis.

What is the Answer?

The answer is to be brave and be proud. Public opinion is slowly changing to understand more about autism and AS but there is a long way to go.

Stimming

The Husband Says:

I think that Aspies grow out of, or are talked out of childhood flapping and stimming activities. But there are still some adult stimming behaviours that go on.

I feel like I work better in my home office with a bit of noise going on. It doesn't matter what it is - I'm not actively listening to it, but the burble of conversation from the BBC News channel or a musical rhythmical beat seems to be the sort of positive stimulus I need to help to maintain a train of thought.

Some Aspies find the label in clothing irritating and have to cut them out. I find them comforting; like a stress relief ball. I don't think NT people notice much but I will lift up the left side of a pullover and rub a shiny fabric label back and forth over itself, just for the feel of it. From an expert: Marks and Spencer have the best labels.

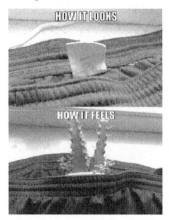

S

Strategies

I cannot tell you precisely what strategies will work for your Aspie. I know what does and does not work with mine, and these experiences I have shared with you. As the saying goes once you have met one Aspie you have met one Aspie. They are all different, yet they do have character traits in common and those I can make suggestions for and have written articles about.

NT I have mentioned previously that you have to be an emotional detective. It may help to keep a diary or, if you can, make a mental note of when he has had a meltdown and what was the run up it. The difficulty is that there are different types of meltdowns triggered by various events. There can be long or short term causes and it may be hard to distinguish whether the attack was triggered by a long run up of stress, or whether some unexpected news has set off a panic reaction (or quite often, a combination of the two).

The Husband Says:

AS *In writing these articles, I've "confessed" a few of the strategies I use to cope and hoped to remain hidden from the NTs. I hope you might find them useful in your relationships. Or if not, at least help you to see the range of strategies that us Aspies play out to "appear normal".*

Stress

Anxiety and its Effect on Social Behaviour

People with AS are aware of their social inability and tend to act out a role in public in order to appear 'normal'. This self-awareness is a double edged sword. In the first place, it can help them to act normally and be initially accepted into society but also, due to the extreme pressure they put on themselves to perform and get it right, it is both exhausting and stressful for them. The level of anxiety created by the AS individual is extremely high compared to the NT and especially compared to a classically autistic person with severe language and communication disabilities.

Impairment of Judgement Under Stress

When stressed, the body goes into a Fight or Flight reaction. This releases adrenaline, making the heart work faster, but also reduces the intelligence of the person temporarily. This will make them less reasonable whilst they have an increased heart rate.

S

Bauman and Kemper, suggest that 'high functioning autistic individuals may have more pronounced abnormalities in the amygdala (a part of the brain responsible for processing emotions and behaviour).' (Bogdashina, 2006)

Baron-Cohen (2008) reports that the 'regions of the brain that are bigger in males than females, and in autism are even bigger than in typical males, are the amygdala, overall brain size and head circumference. Not only is the social brain affected by the size of the amygdala, but research has also discovered that hormones have a part to play. Oxytocin levels have been found to be lower in autistic individuals.'

'There are large numbers of oxytocin receptors in regions of the brain such as the amygdala ventromedial prefrontal cortex, both regions that are underactive in autism, during certain kinds of social stimulation.' (Leslie & Martin, 2007).

These behaviours can display in many ways including irritability, anger, aggression, withdrawal and depression.

Every AS individual has their own calming strategy. This is their special interest or obsession. The process of intense concentration and study on their special interest calms them and blocks the stresses of the day. The NT wife needs to appreciate that her husband needs his own space and time to calm down. This goes against the grain for any NT (who is generally pleased to see her husband return) who would expect some demonstration of affection or acknowledgement upon their entering the home. I have learned over time to stand back when David returns from work, or even to let him find me in his own time. I witness the dog gleefully welcome David home every day and see it as a metaphor of my own feelings as, every time, he ignores her advances.

Style

Relates to Awareness.

When I first met David it was at work, so the fact he always wore a white shirt and black trousers was not noticeable. He did wear a black pullover as well though - which made him look like a Sixth Former from my old school - but I dismissed this matter as unimportant.

It wasn't until we arranged a first date that I noticed he wore exactly the same clothes and his trousers were way too short for him! When I managed to get a sneaky peak into his wardrobe it reminded me of the 1980's film "The Fly", where Jeff Goldblum's scientist character (that poor man's rather typecast isn't he?) had the same identical outfits hanging in his wardrobe as "it saved time".

To cap it all, when his mother came to visit she brought him some new shoes. He stuck one foot in without tying the laces and told her they were fine. He had one pair of black shoes that he wore for everything. He had no imagination, no interest in clothes at all and just played safe with the basics.

Well I changed all that. I dragged him into town and forced him into a pair of jeans and bought him some colourful shirts. Bless him, he desperately wanted to please me and didn't complain. He is actually better with clothes these days and has decided he actually likes colour, but he still manages to make fashion faux pas on a regular basis.

The Husband Says:

Fashion and style are complex subjects for the Aspie. Let's just get one thing straight though, which will help. Style never goes out of fashion. Karen, as an NT, has a gift for selecting clothes for me (and wallpaper for the house) that is smart and timeless and will never go out of fashion.

Us Aspies can go horribly wrong if we put on an act and try to be fashionable. We are followers not trend setters and, by the time we have followed the fashion of the time, it is no longer fashionable. Also, we try to get "value for money" out of our clothes so our clothes have to hang around for a good few years, not just the one event of wearing for the paparazzi.

But don't bully us into wearing uncomfortable clothes. I want jeans with zips that get to my waist and don't hang precariously off my buttocks. And uncomfortable means not only the sense of touch when wearing the clothes, but the emotions they summon up. I am not a walking advertising hoarding, so I don't want my clothing plastered with logos. Timeless and elegant does mean just a little bit anonymous.

Sunlight

We have been told for the last few decades that sunlight is our enemy. Yes, we know that certain skin cancers are caused by over-exposure to sunlight but, actually, these cases are pretty rare. The benefits of sunlight outweighs the benefits of avoiding it.

We all need vitamin D to function and, though we can take supplements of this vital hormone, simply getting 10 to 20 minutes of sunshine every day is beneficial for many reasons.

Recent research also states that: though supplementing with Vitamin D is good for us, we cannot get all the nutrients we need just from the supplement. Scientists recently published a paper saying that our body produces Nitric Oxide when exposed to the sun - this research is in its infancy, but it seems that this can only be activated by introducing our bodies to the sun (not vitamin supplements) and that it is vital to our existence.

S

Support

An Asperger Marriage needs more than the traditional kind of support. If your Aspie partner cannot reciprocate with the emotional support that you crave, then you may have to turn elsewhere for this.

I know of women who have turned to other men for the type of love and acknowledgement that is missing in their marriage. This may work for them, but I am not advocating it. I can't see how infidelity is constructive to a good marriage. I think it would be preferable to end the marriage and then seek that type of love and support elsewhere.

NT Try to confide in a good friend or a close family member (careful not to open a BIG 'Can of Worms' if you are confiding in someone from his side of the family - don't forget the genetic links with Autism disorders). However, you may be better talking to someone with a greater understanding of the subject matter.

Try to find out if there are local support groups in your area. The National Autistic Society has local groups advertised on their website.

Try approaching your GP and ask for counselling. It is good to be able to talk confidentially to someone who will not judge you.

The Husband Says:

I don't see a whole lot of external support for Aspie males in a relationship. It's not the sort of thing you might talk with work colleagues about. It's not a "blokey" thing to talk about either. And talking with any (probably rare) female friends would be so close to infidelity that it would be impossible.

So yes, us Aspies in relationships do acknowledge that we might also need professional counselling and therapy help but this is simply unavailable at the moment. I hope that changes soon, led by people like Karen.

But very much, I hope you can find help from within your relationship if your NT partner is strong.

Surprise!

On the whole, we NT's love a surprise, a good one at least: flowers for no reason; a loved one turning up unexpectedly. The most romantic thing David ever did for me was to trade in his business class ticket to Canada and buy two economy tickets so I could fly with him. I only had twenty-four hours' notice and I had never flown so far. Even though it was a work trip for him, we still had an amazing time. British Columbia is beautiful and we have always meant to go back and 'do it' properly.

S

For your Aspie though, generally, surprises are not good. They are not planned. They don't know what reaction to give. They haven't had time to think it through!

Even having a loved one turn up on their doorstep can be taken badly. Family members will have learned over the years not to do this.

The Husband Says:

Ah, the sound of a surprise being sprung; and the image of carefully laid Aspie plans being ripped to shreds.

Us Aspies "do" surprises very badly; often with bad grace. The one proven strategy to overcome this is planned spontaneity.

Switching Tasks

This is one of the questions my sons' consultant asked for the ADOS diagnostic questionnaire. "What is he like switching from one task to another?".

I believe "Terrible!" was my answer.

It does not come naturally to your Aspie at all. Often they are deeply involved in their current task. They are single minded and like to carry out one task well and to the end. My son's form teacher once asked me why Morgan would not put his book down immediately, when she asked him to. I asked her what was wrong with asking him to get to the end of the paragraph and giving him advance notice that she wanted him to listen. She had no patience for this at all.

As a NT, we are easily interrupted and distracted, but we also have the ability to pick up where we left off quite naturally. We leave a mental marker to come back to. Not so for your Aspie. They have to mentally wrench themselves away from their task and recalibrate their thinking every time. No wonder they get cross when interrupted. It is no good saying, "Well, he just needs to learn to do it." They cannot learn to do what comes naturally to us. They can fake it in part, but that is different and also mentally exhausting meaning there will be a backlash later on.

NT Strategy for Switching Tasks

- If at all possible, plan and communicate when it will be time to switch tasks.

- Try not to demand they switch tasks unnecessarily.

- Wait for a natural break in their work.

Always be patient and don't over react if they seem grumpy when you interrupt them.

The Husband Says:

THIS! ALL OF IT! Take Note!

If you take away one piece of advice from this book, take this one.

Sympathy

It can be hard at times to be sympathetic to your husband. He is very good at making the most of an illness and often appears to have 'man flu'. If anyone around him is ill, he will assume that he too will get the same. He will immediately take steps to avoid it whilst letting you know, by coughing, that he is probably coming down with an even more deadly version of the illness.

This really does not help if you are the one with the illness and you are genuinely much more poorly than he is. All activity on his part is most likely to have stopped. While you know that though you don't feel up to everyday tasks, life goes on.

It is very frustrating when you do not get the sympathy you need (and deserve) and he inevitably turns your illness into a competition.

NT The best thing you can do is offer him plenty of sympathy and remedies and hope he gets better soon while trying not to lose your temper with him. It seems like he is committing a very selfish act but he cannot help it. It is the way his psyche works.

The Husband Says:

I don't like feeling unwell. It's really hard to keep up an act with even a relatively minor cold or flu. I suppose when I'm stomping around with a sniffle, I'm trying to warn you that, if I don't throw off this bug before it becomes a full blown illness, I'm going to become quite unbearable.

You have gradually educated me, though, that by a joint reduction in the stress of our lifestyle, that the incidence of illness in the family has greatly decreased. A genuine win-win.

Synaesthesia

I discovered I have Synaesthesia whilst watching a documentary about it. The person whom the programme was about was able to 'taste' words. It basically means that your senses get their wires crossed. Synaesthesia is quite often a comorbid condition with ASD, but bizarrely it frequently goes unrecognised by the person with it. As in my own case, people can live with it all of their life and never realising that virtually no-one else has these feelings.

So what is my super power? Well it is pretty useless really. I relate particular colours to certain moods and when I think about people I know, their name appears in my mind in bubble writing and always in a colour personal to them. I do not consciously choose this colour. I have tried to work out why certain people like my best friend Charlotte is always in brown with a blue background. I don't even like brown as a colour, though I do like blue. It may pertain to people's characters or how much I love them.

- David is always RED.

- Morgan is always BLUE

- Sioned is always YELLOW

If I don't know the person their name appears in basic Arial black font. No distinguishing features.

I have realised that if I am introduced to someone new and told their name, unless I visualise their name, I forget it almost instantly and then I have to confess (or spend the rest of my life pretending I know what their name is). I suspect my Synaesthesia is an Aide Memoire but whether it is meant to be I have no idea.

Tactfulness

This is a skill we all have to learn but it comes easier to the Neurotypical than to those on the autistic spectrum. If as a child, you do not realise you have upset someone with your thoughtless words because you do not recognise their facial expressions then you will not be able to adjust your own behaviour to circumstances.

it is quite common for people on the spectrum to be told that they are rude or tactless but it is less common for people to explain to them why this is so and how to change it. The offended person or observer may just assume that the person knew they were being rude. It is likely the ASD person who has been berated for their behaviour will just be downhearted and confused rather than enlightened.

How to be Tactful

`AS` I have never asked David 'does my bum look big in this' though he lives in fear of the day as he believes it is a trick question that he will come out of badly.

If my bum does indeed look big in the new outfit I am asking him to judge, how indeed should the poor man answer?

This is where he falls down in his social skills. Most NT men would skilfully avoid the trap and would either have their fall-back statement of "Of course not, you look beautiful," or the cleverer ones may have prepared a stock answer for such an occasion such as "I like that dress, but I love the black one you wore last time."

How not to Offend

Look for the middle ground where everyone will come out happy. This is hard for Aspie's who are not skilled in moderation, but it can be learned.

Major No-Nos

If Someone is Overweight:

`AS` Never refer to someone as fat, especially to their face. It is better to use a more factual but less insulting term such as 'a larger lady' or even though it is downplaying it and possibly not even true 'a bit chubby'. Always understate not the other way around.

Annoyingly, the same rule does not necessarily apply when in a group of lads or men. It is practically considered rude not to mention that your best friend is a 'Porker'. This is called male camaraderie.

T

Asking Someone (not in the First Flush of Youth) Their age:

AS It is okay to ask children their age. Unless you are a professional and it is relevant to your job, it is not acceptable to ask someone outright what their age is. It is acceptable to imply that someone is older and within a certain age category such as middle-aged. Beware you will seriously offend anyone under 40 by referring to them as so.

Do not say Unkind Things About Someone Just Because you Think it is Funny:

AS Not everyone shares your sense of humour. People are generally sensitive about their appearance, jobs, finances etc. and even if they do laugh off your joke, they are likely to dwell upon it and be upset. They may avoid you socially after that.

The Husband Says:

There are certain challenges to tactfulness. The rules are different between business and social life and beware the difference. In business, "telling it like it is" can be considered an asset. In your social life this is seldom (if ever) the case.

There are so many traps for the unwary in social circumstances that it can seem difficult to have any sort of conversation at all whilst being tactful. Neurotypicals are so very sensitive about so many subjects that there is little to talk about once politics, religion, people's appearance, ethnicity and sexual orientation are taken away even if blindingly obvious because you have to be tactful and not run the risk of offence. Aspies are some of the first to complain about political correctness going over the top.

This constant battle with yourself to be tactful in the face of fuzzy rules can lead to a desire to avoid social situations like parties altogether. I dread having to come up with small talk that avoids the 'elephants in the room' of the obvious but tactless conversations about people at the event and its setting. Aspies often invent a whole new persona for parties that is "safe". I heard a story about a wedding guest who declared himself to be a Chocolate Biscuit Designer - he claimed his best work was the Jaffa Cake; his fake persona was interesting (to say the least) and I can't think of a way that a biscuit could be considered offensive or their discussion tactless.

Taking Things Literally

A common scenario - almost an urban myth, is when the teacher is lecturing the AS child for not doing well in class: "You are going to have to pull your socks up,

Sam." Sam looks down and, even though his socks are fine, he reaches down to adjust his socks to please his teacher. His teacher, believing Sam is being insolent, then punishes the child with a detention. Poor Sam is totally confused and distraught as, no matter what he does, he cannot do anything right. Sam is a literal thinker.

We NT's lay verbal traps wherever we go in our language and communication. We pepper our conversations and writing with metaphors and idioms and slang. We rarely ever explain what these things mean, we just assume that everyone else knows what we are talking about. Sometimes we NT's know instinctively what these phrases are roughly about, but often, if a child asks us to explain what we mean, we ourselves don't know the real origin of it. Commonly, it is something we were brought up saying because our parents did.

Most adults with AS will have traversed this linguistic minefield for quite some time before you have met them, and they are pretty good at recognising and remembering the actual meaning. Some go to the extreme, probably to fit in, and use them almost indiscriminately themselves.

For example, I noticed my husband uses phrases like 'Give the cat another goldfish' quite regularly. I never knew whether phrases like that were a Northern thing or not, but I certainly hadn't heard it and I didn't understand it at first.

I have since found it written as: "Blow the expense, Give the Cat Another Goldfish!"

The Husband Says:

Interesting. "Give the cat another goldfish" has a soothing prosody and rhythm (intonation) to it. Perhaps that's why I like to use it in conversation.

Business, especially that in the public sector, seems to be littered with management-speak. Why use three words when ten is more and obviously better. As an Aspie, looking to fit in, rather unconsciously I adopt these little NT-in-business sound-bites and incorporate them into my communication. Not knowing all of the time where these things come from (their etymology), I can make occasional hilarious mistakes - especially mixed-up-metaphors.

Highlights from this week's buzzword-bingo: "We must adopt a common direction of travel."

Now does taking thing literally explain my rather coarse sense of taste in the arts? The simplest explanations are the best aren't they, so no reason to view literature, music or a painting as having some sort of deep inner meaning? I have to consciously invent some 'feelings' towards the arts in order to fit in and be middle class. That might be a very nice pile of bricks, but it's still a pile of bricks. I'm much more likely to respect the skills of the craftsman who made the bricks than their arrangement as a sculpture.

T

Talking through a Suspected Diagnosis

NT You have to give this much consideration before you approach the subject with your partner. It may be he already has suspicions himself or he may be completely unaware of his differences or at least that they add up to a condition or even a disability.

The worst thing you can do is blurt out in anger, in the middle of the supermarket, that you think he is autistic.

Preparation Do's

- Choose a mutually convenient time.

- Find a quiet place you will not be interrupted by phones or children.

- Do your homework. There are recommended resources throughout this book. Look on the NAS website for helpful information and to find your local branch and support group.

- Make a list of reasons why you think he might be on the spectrum.

- Start by telling him that he is a wonderful person.

- Say how worried you are about him and about your relationship.

- Say you have done some research and you think he may have a social and communication disorder.

- Give him a chance to ask questions.

- If he doesn't want to talk about it do not push him. Left alone he will think over what you have said and probably do his own research.

- Be prepared for anger and denial.

- This will be very difficult for him to discuss and he will feel you are criticising him so keep your language as positive as possible.

- Offer him help and emotional support.

Preparation Don'ts

- Do not use negative language.

- Do not immediately tell him you think he is autistic. David visibly flinched when this term was used. He is much more comfortable with the term Asperger's Syndrome. AS has more positive connotations than autism. There is still much stigma around autism, the implication being that they are lesser people. We know this not to be true and that autism is a difference in the wiring of the brain but, unfortunately, many people (including some professionals) still need to be positively educated.

- Do not be impatient or cross if he denies it.

- Do not get angry or rise to any of his negative comments. He will only take the negativity away from this conversation otherwise.

- Do not push him for an answer one way or another.

Good Luck

The Husband Says:

Once you realise that Asperger's is a state of being - a collection of character traits - rather than a disability, then there are no real down-sides to accepting a formal diagnosis. There can be significant up-sides; what was considered eccentricity or quirky behaviour can now be associated with different (not lesser!) brain "wiring".

In particular - and a key reason for seeking a diagnostic "label" - it can be tremendously beneficial to be able to explain some non-NT behaviours to your partner by explaining that you have Asperger's or autism and that the behaviours stem from the condition, or are the side effects of putting in place 'coping strategies' to help you get through each day. What is, to the Aspie, perfectly logical and optimum behaviour, often comes across as unexpected or eccentric to the NT. Your Label will give your NT partner an understanding and a new viewpoint. Part of making Aspie coping strategies work, is to share the burden out. By letting partners and close friends into the reasons why you 'put on an act', and showing them the difficulties you experience living in a 'social world' that seems to be actively trying to trip you up at all times, you can start to feel a release of pressure.

"Coming out" as an Aspie can be beneficially cathartic.

Taxi Driver

I have a wonderful group of friends that I like to socialise with. David is always supportive and never resents me going out with my friends. He doesn't particularly enjoy sitting in a drunken group of people and talking about nothing (see Chit Chat), but he does like to get involved in his own way.

He is very happy to make sure I get home safely by offering to pick me and my friends up from pubs and events. It gives him a role that he is happy to play, and it means he is appreciated by all. He quite enjoys seeing and hearing the results at the end of an evening.

This way he fills his 'social cup' but doesn't let it overflow.

The Husband Says:

Like a real taxi driver, being the sober driver allows you to hover on the edge of someone else's social group. It's the perfect "cover story" to infiltrate a tight knit social group of NTs - you get to listen to the gossip, can throw an opinion in with impunity, but if the social going gets tough you can shut up and drive and blame the traffic for why you have had to leave the conversation.

Team Work

Contrary to popular belief your Aspie can be good at, and indulge in, team work. Before marriage I felt that David and I worked very well as a team as we never fell out and we listened to and respected each other.

The problem with team work is when he is not empathising with his team (or wife) at all. He cannot see their point of view and, basically, believes that they are wrong. However, when you and your Aspie are on the same wavelength, having the same goals and ideas as you, they can be a fantastic support.

I have noted from our AS daughter's school report that she has difficulty with team work. The problem with school is that often you are not allowed to choose who your team members are. If she was able to choose her elite team with like-minded people she would be formidable. As it is, when she does not agree with her classmates, she loses interest or gets angry with them for not being able to see what, to her, is obviously the best way.

As a family we recently had a day out that I knew would appeal to their logical minds. We went to try the Escape rooms where you get locked in for an hour and have to work out all the clues to find the key hidden in the room in order to escape.

I thoroughly enjoyed this experience but on a completely different level to my little family. Though I did make suggestions and help look for clues, mentally I was standing back and watching how they all interacted together. Even though we were under time pressure with the clock counting down on the screen, no-one got stressed and no-one fell out. They knew what the end goal was and nobody was at an advantage over any other. Their logical minds clicked and ticked and calculated and mused and we escaped with 18 minutes to spare. I was so proud of them.

(T)

The Husband Says:

Us Aspies can do team work. But for it to be successful we have to set boundaries:

We struggle to communicate in the initial design process of a team task. Our social conversation timing can be affected by our condition which means that we can struggle to find a gap in the conversation to make our point known. This makes it look like we are talking over, or down to, other valid opinions which makes us look domineering.

We are very logical - this can oppose some "off the wall" creative processes; our creations tend to be linear, logical and bounded; we recycle what we have seen and heard before and worked on another occasion.

We work best on a sub part of the project that can be well defined with neat and tidy interfaces.

Woe betide anyone that changes the fundamental premise of the team effort without communicating the change with extraordinary clarity and gets full buy-in from everyone that the objectives have changed.

Can the NTs in the team, PLEASE define what success, completion, closure or "finished" looks like? Otherwise you NTs will abandon the project when you consider it "done" and us Aspies will continue to slave away until it is perfect, often needlessly so, becoming increasingly upset that we seem to be the only one left working on the task.

Technical Support

This is not true of every Aspie but with their logical thinking they often have an innate ability to engineer, solve problems and provide good technical support for computers and gadgets at home and in the work place. Their advice can be invaluable though it is often taken for granted.

The Husband Says:

We like logical puzzles. Technical support is logical, puzzling to NTs and something we excel at. There is always a reason for a technical failure. We might not be able to fix it - it might be out of our control, but we are also really good at figuring out work-arounds. But also watch out that once the "proper" solution becomes possible and known, we will remove the work-around and substitute the "proper" solution. Perhaps unexpectedly!

Teeth Cleaning

Up to a quarter of the population do not clean their teeth twice a day. Though there are no statistics to say whether these people are on the autistic spectrum or not I suspect that many of them are.

T

This is a sensory processing disorder. David knows all the reasons why he must clean his teeth but he very much dislikes doing so. I often have to remind him. This does not sit well with me as it makes me feel like I am his mother, and that is not conducive for a good marriage. On the other hand, neither is bad breath.

The Husband Says:

 Dentistry has a number of challenges for me, all sensory issues or matters of habit:

When I was younger, state school dentists didn't feel it necessary to explain to their clients what was going on. When I was young I had eight teeth removed all in one go with no warning this was going to happen. Little wonder that I went out of my way to avoid dentists

There are lots of sensory issues; I don't like things in my mouth that I didn't put there. Especially the current need to be rubber gloved as a dentist to prevent spread of infection.

The feel of stiff bristles on gums is unpleasant. I now know that I should be brushing my gums as much as my teeth.

Toothpaste in general tastes awful; mouthwash even more so. Some medicated toothpastes make me gag and retch.

Tooth-brushing's a thing that is best if it is a habit. None of the above encourage the habit.

Some tips for other Aspies - but you will have to experiment...

Corsodyl® toothpaste comes highly recommended for those with gum disease, but it makes me retch. Curasept® is an alternative and tastes of aniseed and is available from Dentists and the Internet.

Sensodyne® toothpaste is good for sensitive teeth and perhaps the market leader, but the Oral B™ toothpaste does the same job and doesn't taste quite so bad (for me at least). Double up the sensitive toothpaste with the gum disease toothpaste for best effect

I can't get away with the little between teeth brushes, so I make do with a decent electric brush.

Explain that you are an Aspie with sensory issues to your dentist. Sack your dentist if they don't understand and accommodate.

Try to persuade your NT partner not to "tidy up" your toothbrush and toothpaste - the key is to have it there silently nagging you into making dental hygiene a habit every time you are in the bathroom.

Temple Grandin

Temple Grandin had developmental delays when she was a child and did not speak until she was four. However, she had great support from her parents and teachers.

Temple does not have Asperger's but autism but she is a great example to all on the autism spectrum. She has an amazing eye for detail and has written books, gives talks on autism and has even had a film made about her.

Thank You

It is such a small thing to say. Thank you for making my breakfast every morning. Thank you for working all day and walking the dog and making tea and dealing with the kids' school and doing the dishwasher and pouring me a glass of wine while I sit on the sofa.

Just a little smile to let me know I exist would be nice.

 The easiest and nicest form of reciprocation. Saying "Thank You" to your partner doesn't take much but it shows that you really appreciate the little things they do for you. It is debilitating to be taken for granted on either side of the marriage.

AS Say "Thank You".

The Husband Says:

Whoops! The above should not be taken lightly. I've been slipping and forgetting to do those things recently.

Here's an important way in which our Aspie social communications blindness is a disability. NTs use these little pleases and thank-yous as conversation filler and a way of maintaining social rank and order. An interaction where something thoughtful is done and a thank-you and a smile is missing in return opposes the expectation of NTs that even small gestures are thanked. It might be logical that something needs to be done by Aspies like you and me, so it just should be done, but NTs expect a thank you in acknowledgement that even duties have been done.

AS *Say "Thank You" and mean it; even for the little day to day stuff and stuff you assume should be done because you think it is a duty. Make it sincere. Don't devalue the 'Thank You'.*

T

The Big Bang Theory

The Husband Says:

First of all, is "The Big Bang Theory", a TV show that centres on a group of friends where one or more are clearly Aspies: offensive, affectionate, parody or nature study?

I love the programme. I'm an Aspie and I think the subject is handled with such sensitivity in good humour that it could be considered a documentary. Jim Parsons playing Dr. Sheldon Cooper is a delight.

Favourite Episodes

Season 2

Episode 11: "The Bath Item Gift Hypothesis"

Sheldon worries about the approaching Christmas holidays and his indecision about what gift to get Penny. After deciding on a basket of bath items, he discovers a wide selection available; unsure about what Penny is going to get him and what he should get her in return, he buys an entire array to cover all contingencies. Penny's gift to Sheldon is a napkin both autographed and used by Leonard Nimoy. Sheldon is overwhelmed; he responds by giving Penny all the gift baskets and then a rare "Sheldon" hug.

Season 6

Episode 21: "The Closure Alternative"

Amy decides to teach Sheldon to overcome his closure obsession. She leads him through a series of activities, forcefully stopping him from completing the activity just before he is about to finish it. These events make Sheldon furious at Amy, but he hides his true feelings from her and lies to her that he has been cured of his closure obsession.

Season 7

Episode 19: "The Indecision Amalgamation"

On the subject of decision making, Sheldon is torn between different games consoles. Sheldon's decision ramblings really annoy Amy both during their dinner date, where she fakes exaggerated interest, and spending hours at the shop contemplating his choices. Sheldon has a Bonio moment.

T

The Elephant in the Room

David and I have been married since 1997. Although in some ways we have a very strong and certainly a very faithful marriage, in other respects, there have been many communication difficulties and misunderstandings. Realising that my husband is on the autistic spectrum has saved our marriage by allowing us to establish ways to avoid certain triggers that lead to meltdowns. I have also been able to develop strategies for both my family and myself to cope with difficult situations. I would like to prove, using this app to share my experiences and research, that divorce is not always the answer.

There is a significant diagnostic gap for adults who are probably on the autistic spectrum but have never been referred to clinicians to be assessed. Asperger Syndrome was recognised as a condition only as recently as 1981, in the seminal work by Dr Lorna Wing, Clinical Psychologist and founder of the NAS.

Thirty years ago, AS was considered very rare and, therefore, many of today's adults who were young children at the time of this revelation have fallen into this diagnostic gap.

Having spent several years attending support groups and meeting other parents with children on the spectrum, I gradually become aware that I am not the only parent who has difficulty understanding AS children's behaviour but also with communicating with their husband.

As a committee member of the local NAS branch, I set up a support group for partners of people on the autistic spectrum. Using the NAS mailing list, I had a good response from people who were interested, proving that I was not alone. Unfortunately, the group was not successful as we live in a rural area and due to the nature of the condition, these (mostly) women found it difficult to attend. I started searching online and found many forums, particularly on Facebook, which had been set up for women to support each other through the travails of life married to a man on the autistic spectrum.

This proved to me that my situation was not unique, but also that the need was there for research to be conducted and disseminated using my insight and position to ameliorate, support and justify the experiences of numerous, anonymous and despairing women. My intention is to let them know that they are not alone and that they are believed.

Theory of Mind

Theory of Mind occurs naturally in Neurotypicals which means they can empathise with people or 'put themselves in their shoes' to understand a little about their lives.

T

They can consider what it would be like to be them. Our husbands have great difficulty doing this.

In a 2001 research paper, Simon Baron-Cohen describes Theory of Mind as "...being able to infer the full range of mental states (beliefs, desires, intentions, imagination, emotions, etc.) that cause action. In brief, having a theory of mind is to be able to reflect on the contents of one's own and other's minds."

A deficiency in Theory of Mind is called mind blindness.

Theory of Mind Test (The Sally/Anne Test)

I tried this on my children when they were young. It worked on my daughter who was eight but not on my son who was eleven. He was able to logically work out what would happen whereas my AS daughter leapt to what she thought was the right conclusion.

The Husband Says:

The whole Baron-Cohen Theory of Mind stuff has elements in it that I believe and some weaknesses in his theories. The theories are generalisations and have to be quite simple and adults can mask the symptoms by preparing the 'Aspie-act'.

Where Baron-Cohen suggests an absence of applying an emotional state to a person, thus the person is little more than another object, I think that us Aspies can be just slow to tease apart the signs that point to an emotional state, primarily because emotional state is transmitted first by facial expression to which we are not particularly sensitive.

Thinking about Your Own Language

NT

What you say, and how you say it, will make a big difference to the way he feels about himself, and also the way he thinks you feel about him. If you are positive about him, you will raise his self-esteem. With low self-esteem he will get increasingly defensive and will stop listening to you altogether.

Consider how to approach a subject. It doesn't have to be an important subject, it may just be a small task you would like him to help with.

Instead of nagging him to do something, explain how it is important to you that this task is done and that it is something that you cannot do by yourself. He will immediately feel more important and useful, because he can show his love for you by doing something for you.

Once he has carried out the task, make sure you take note that he has done this. Praise him for doing a good job and thank him. He will be much more willing to carry out the task for you next time.

The Husband Says:

Karen hints at this, but I'll be more explicit. It is not the content of the message that might be difficult or might offend, it is all about the delivery. A careful choosing of the location where the message is delivered, and the state of mind of the Aspie recipient, is important. Choosing a gap or pause in what your Aspie is doing (or not doing by procrastinating) or choosing some time where the message will be relevant, is key to how the message will be received.

Difficult messages are those about familial stressors like employment, money, moving house, how the kids are doing at school. Really difficult messages are about relationships, friendships and partnerships; particularly if relating to change that is required to improve any of those.

It sometimes works to 'make an appointment', but set this some hours (to days) into the future so that your Aspie can choose to do some fight or flight response. Rehearse some of the discussion, choose which parts will be constructive, and dispose of those parts that might be accidentally destructive - because they are blurted out without warning or being properly thought through.

Please don't start a difficult discussion or debate when I'm devoting a lot of brain power and emotional intelligence to driving the car. That's not fair.

Expect debate and logic even though you will be talking about something emotional. Be prepared to leave the topic and come back to it. But be careful not to do so, because if the debate is becoming argument that you think you are "losing" you may need to re-run the whole thing again to try to turn a loss into a win. Logic, even twisted Aspie-trying-to-be-emotional logic, doesn't work like that - you put the same data in, you get the same result out.

Thinking He Told You

This is a very common problem in AS/NT relationships. There are two reasons for this and one of them is Theory of Mind. He knows what is going on, therefore you should too. His brain doesn't always make the leap and connect its thought processes in a way you would expect and he just assumes in his own Aspie way, that you know what is in his mind.

Some autistic children are very confused by this and accuse friends and family of lying when they say they do not know something. The child is convinced they DO know what has happened and actually believes their parent or friend to be lying. This is not because the child thought she had told them about what happened, it is because they assume that they know, because she knows.

The other reason is easier to understand where your Aspie has thought about something so much he has actually forgotten that he hasn't told you about it.

T

Strategy

NT   Well other than having a rewire, it is quite difficult to get them to think differently. There are steps that we can take to help remind them that we cannot see into their brain:

First of all, in a calm moment, and not in the heat of just finding out something vital, you need to sit down and point out some differences between you two. It helps greatly if he has a diagnosis or is accepting that he has Asperger's, but it may be possible for you to carefully word that you think differently and require certain information from him without using the term autism or Asperger's Syndrome.

It may help you to write out what you want from him and how you are going to approach him.

Explain carefully how you do not know what he is thinking unless he tells you. Likewise he does not know what you are thinking unless you tell him.

Additionally, you are completely unaware of his actions outside of his house, at the supermarket, or at work, because you were not there. If he wants you to know he had a bad day because a client was late or somebody shouted at him, then he needs to tell you.

He may not want to tell you what has happened to him during the day the moment he comes through the door - as he will most likely feel the need to decompress. Once he has decompressed he might be distracted by the gadgets in the house and then forget to tell you important information.

You need to agree when and where you can discuss his day, and anything of note, that happened. Be respectful of his need for space and try not to be too impatient to hear news. Usually, if the news is truly momentous (good or bad), he may feel the need to tell you the moment he steps through the door. It tends to be the smaller inconsequential news (to him) that he forgets to pass on.

A list of news that is important to you, even if not to him, would be useful. He will probably like something to refer to, to check whether it is worth his time telling you what he sees as boring social information.

For example;

- Whether someone in the family has died

- If someone at work has been sacked

- If a friend or relative has got engaged or is expecting a baby

- Whether the baby has been born and what sex it is (don't push for too much information)

- Whether someone in the family is ill

T

- Whether a friend or family member is getting divorced or separated

- Money troubles

- His own health worries

Impress on him how important this information is to NT's and, especially, women. It is useful to know this in order not to make social gaffes and to know how to react when meeting people. There are certain expected conventions, such as birthday cards and gifts for new born babies, which, if they are missed (due to lack of awareness), it can be embarrassing to find out about after the event.

The Husband Says:

Part of the problem and confusion does come about from Theory of Mind - Mind Blindness issues. I spend significant 'processing time' trying to understand people's behaviour and particularly the group behaviour of the people I work with and meet - how their interactions work (or don't). I build up a mental model of how this system of relationships behaves and what I think the group might do in response to some new stimulus. It's cold and calculated and frequently wrong. Now because of my mind blindness, I think that you neurotypicals do the same thing, just that you are faster and better at it than I am. Us Aspies can't believe that you NTs are just "wired up" to be able to make sense of these relationships without having to do the same amount of analysis that I have to do. My Aspie logic says that if you are doing the analysis the same way that I'm doing the analysis, that's logic and we will both come to the same answer. So perhaps I don't have to tell you about my perceptions of a group social state, because you are an NT and you have figured it out already.

Except you haven't... and you need me to communicate my perception of the situation but, for the logic above, I think I already have because such communication will be a waste of time - because you have already come to the same social conclusions as me, yes?

And then it all goes horribly wrong...

Oh yes, one more thing: I have a great memory, and sometimes (only sometimes) you just completely forget to tell me something that I would have thought was important, and you assume that I already know. And then THAT goes horribly wrong...

Thinking Time

Your average Aspies like to think carefully before they speak, especially when it is very important to them. This can be a little unnerving to the NT who likes to have an answer to a question within a short, unspecified amount of time. In a job interview it can be considered quite odd not to answer straight away but, I know generally, the interviewer is always impressed with the 'correct' answer when it comes.

T

In some ways it can be good to be a little different, to take time over our thoughts and to get them right. Indeed, I have learned to be a bit more circumspect with my thoughts over the years and not just blurt out the first thing that comes to mind. David doesn't always understand what I mean, so I have to ensure that I phrase it in a specific, unambiguous way.

Waiting too Long

A few years ago I went with David to see the GP and it was suggested that he should return to have some tests. He was to arrange this with the receptionist. He spoke to the receptionist and she offered him some dates. He took out his phone (with his work diary on) and spent some time staring at his phone. The receptionist felt that, because he had gone past that unspecified amount of time when he should have answered, he was having difficulty fitting that date into his calendar. She helpfully offered him another date. He practically bit her head off and I was thoroughly embarrassed. Worse, he told her "not to bother" and promptly walked out of the surgery leaving us both standing there with our mouths open.

I made some excuse to the receptionist and quickly made an appointment that I hoped would be okay. I made my way to the car park hoping that the car was still there and that he hadn't driven off. He was waiting quietly in the car and, when I told him I had made the appointment for him, he said that it was fine.

The Husband Says:

Karen is correct that, as an Aspie, I can require significant processing time to come up with an optimal solution. Don't get me wrong, my 'knee-jerk' instant reaction to situations can be quite good - almost as good as that neurotypical sixth sense of what is right in any given situation; I probably out-perform you NTs on science, technology and matters of fact. Empathetic decisions? - you beat me hands down on social and emotional decision making.

I spend significant periods of time "checking my own work"; mulling over these knee jerk reactions to see if they can be improved by applying logic. Now emotional issues don't yield very well to applying logic hence processing times can be somewhat extended. Taking Karen's appointment example, not only was I trying to make a gap in my work diary, I was also trying to fit in the emotional needs of others, like if Karen would want to accompany me, whether I would like Karen to accompany me, if Karen was picking our daughter up from school for a singing lesson (not in my diary, but held in my memory), and so on...

It is interesting that I think my business clients respect and value me spending overt thinking time. I am often asked what is so interesting outside the window where I am staring, but it is the blank stare of rumination on a complex problem. My Aspie model of team dynamic and relationships is valued by clients because I do apply it analytically, and if necessary, I can provide a documentary commentary on the decision making process. Further I can tackle the business "paralysis of fear" - I am willing to make a time sensitive knee-jerk decision on a complex technical matter and then refine that decision through logic and debate when my peers are paralysed by the fear of the magnitude of the decision. Bizarrely, that makes me a great manager in a crisis.

This thought and decision process on all matters is also why these "write down the first thing you think of" psychometric tests just don't work properly on Aspies - if they work properly on anyone at all. Do you want my socially inept first answer or do you want the answer that fits in with the social model of the role I am projecting towards and putting on the act for? Is your test so sophisticated that it can "see through the mask"?

Tics

What are Tics?

This is a comorbid disorder with an ASD. Tics are rapid and sudden movements of muscles in your body and also vocal tics such as involuntary noises. Tics are more noticeable in childhood but adults with ASD can still be affected. Many have learned how to cope with and reduce their effect over time, at least in public.

Some adult's tics are so subtle they go unnoticed or people believe that the noises are voluntary expressions of opinion. This can give the impression that the person is being rude or disrespectful and can be embarrassing for those who can't control their tics. The embarrassment and stress can compound the situation making it a whole lot worse.

Difference between Tics and Stimming

A tic is like an internal pressure that builds up and has to be released at some point, like Tourette's Syndrome. When you have been stressed you have probably experienced a facial tic that you could not help.

Stimming is different and though they are not always aware they are doing it they can be stopped by giving them a stress toy to play with. However, it is a sensation that they enjoy and it is a way of coping with excitement. My son no longer flaps his hands but he spins on his computer chair constantly and he used to flick his earlobe. I had to point out to him the ear flicking made him look odd and he shouldn't do it at school. On the other hand who can resist spinning on their chair?

Transient Tics

These are tics that appear for a short amount of time but disappear as suddenly as they started. This most often happens in childhood.

The Husband Says:

Some tics might be a sign of a neurological condition. Go and get checked out by your doctor to eliminate this and feel relieved! Otherwise don't stress about these repeated behaviours -

T

they are probably responses to stress so if you try to deliberately suppress them you will probably become more stressed in the effort - a vicious circle.

Time Keeping

As the Aspie wife, I am in charge of organising and planning in the household. I am good at prioritising and getting myself and the children to their destinations on time.

I feel uncomfortable if I am running late for appointments and therefore I get quite tense and anxious when other people make me run late. I feel it is a sign of disrespect for the person waiting for me and a sign that I myself cannot manage.

You can put your Aspie into one of two time keeping categories. Those who are consistently early or on time and those who are not. There is a sub-category here. Your Aspie will always be on time If the destination is important enough to them. They will keep an eye on the clock and plan down to the minute when they will organise themselves and when they will leave to get there on time. If however, it is not a situation of enough import to them e.g. it is not about them; they will not prioritise it in their minds and will delegate responsibility to you or worse ignore what is happening.

To be fair, David on the whole is the former type of Aspie and does not like being late but he also fits neatly into the "It's not about me," subcategory and there have been times when his priorities have superseded our family obligation; to the point where I have left him dealing with a work call and gone without him. The first time I did this, I was utterly furious with him and his incapacity to understand my concerns about how my lateness would look to the school. These days, I prepare myself mentally for such disappointments. It is doubly annoying when you know that they married us for our superior executive skills, yet they will only take on board our advice when they feel like it.

Habitual Lateness

It is their lack of social function that makes them very late at times but there are also many men on the spectrum who have the double whammy of an ADHD comorbidity. They have little sense of time keeping and often don't realise they are late until it is too late. They always believe they have plenty of time. Their internal clock is slightly out of sync.

The Husband Says:

There's (at least) three factors at work here:

Perception of Time

I have quite poor perception of time. I become task absorbed and forget what time it is, and I'm poor at predicting what time it might be. A big clue is that clock watching staff start shuffling off from their desks, but that may mean I've already missed an appointment.

The 'cure' is a comprehensive diary on my phone with timely alarms. Beware, however, having put your phone on silent in a meeting (rather than vibrate) and forgetting to turn the reminders on afterwards. Beware also fellow Aspies hosting meetings that over-run for no good reason and no one feeling able to explain the social convention that I'm now late for another, more important, meeting.

Aspie Desire to Follow Social Convention

The social convention is to be punctual, so Aspies will, whenever they can, be punctual; but...

Communicating Priority

When two events are close to each other and seem to have equal priority, which one should the Aspie choose? Or will he be like Buridan's Ass, equidistant between hay and water, unable to choose and so dies of starvation?

This paradox is solved by clear communication. "My work client who has phoned me is very, very important so, even if the phone conference over-runs, I will stay at work to entertain him; can the school meeting be postponed or can you cope with it without my direct support of being there?"

Tiredness

When our son was tiny he was a terrible sleeper. He didn't sleep through the night until he was eight months old and that was a one off. I have never been the type of person to party all night. I like to be in bed long before midnight and get up early instead. I am often described as a lark.

I found it very hard to cope with the loss of sleep that a new baby created. However, due to Morgan having undiagnosed Asperger's, he was a very clingy baby and never wanted me out of his sight. It was hard to have a shower unless I sat him in his seat in the bathroom.

David never once volunteered to help me with Morgan's crying at night. Though I can't remember what conversations we had about it 16 years ago, my lasting impression was that David had to work and I didn't, therefore I was the one who always had to deal with him. When Morgan was six months old, I was forced to go back to full time work and this 'single parenting' situation still continued. I would pick Morgan up from the child minders and it would just be me and Morgan alone in the house for several hours until David got back from work.

T

This situation became untenable as, when on holiday, I ended up having a major panic attack and had to be taken to A & E. They couldn't find anything wrong with me other than low potassium. I had heard of panic attacks but had no idea how severe they could be. I literally thought I was going to die. It took me quite some time to get over it as, ironically, I would panic that I would have another panic attack. I worked for another month and then handed in my notice as I was getting very ill.

Being an Aspie wife means you carry on beyond exhaustion and your husband doesn't even notice.

The Husband Says:

How can I defend the indefensible? Well things did change - they had to. The strict division of duties worked but made us both quite lonely; Karen at home raising the children and me out at work, bringing in the cash and avoiding coming home because I was performing my special interest as what I was being paid for. All changed for the better when I moved into self-employment (with Karen's blessing and encouragement) because, as a team, we were better able to control when I would be at home and some of the money compulsion went away - now that I'm self-employed, if I want more money I can work a bit harder.

The subject of tiredness has another facet. Us Aspies get very tired not only trying to have a "normal" life (whatever that is) but putting on this act of normality. Perhaps I don't spend as much time as I should be enjoying home life because I'm spending time recovering from the tiredness of work-life?

Tolerance

NT
To survive an Asperger Marriage, as the wife, you must have tolerance. It is not an option. It may not be there at the start but it is something that you can build upon if you really want your marriage to work.

Ingredients to make Tolerance

- Understanding
- Patience
- Strength
- Support
- Compromise

T

The Husband Says:

Sadly, us Aspies are not very strong on support and compromise. You also have to work hard to make us understand an issue so very complex, but we do eventually. You might not think so, but we can be patient and strong. It's the whole package on the right proportions we have difficulty with.

Tony Attwood

I have had the pleasure of attending a few conferences where Tony has been either the main or sole speaker. Even though I have read his books I still learn something new every time I attend. For me he is the 'go to' guy for Asperger Syndrome and the person who cast light into my world when I read his book "The Complete Guide to Asperger's Syndrome". It was the first book I read after I was told of the educational psychologist's suspicions about our son, and I still refer to it. It is a well-thumbed copy and I even have it on my Kindle™ so it is easy to travel with and search through.

At a small conference in Birmingham in 2014 I was lucky enough to have a few minutes' chat with Tony and to thank him for his innovative work in this area.

Professor Attwood has specialised in autism spectrum disorders since qualifying as a clinical psychologist from London University and gaining his doctorate under supervision from Professor Uta Frith. Tony now lives and practices in Queensland, Australia.

The Husband Says:

In conferences, Tony has the ability to talk about common sense explanations and solutions to problems. His books are more practical and accessible than others in the field. In Australia, where Tony practises, there is a much more enlightened approach to adult Autism and Asperger's, I suspect largely through Tony Atwood's leadership in the field. All his works come highly recommended by me.

Top Down Modulation

This is the ability to filter our thoughts for the right occasion. Many people on the spectrum are actually handicapped by having a phenomenal memory but they become overwhelmed by the amount of data they hold within their brains and are unable to make the right choice. We NTs have an innate ability to quickly sort through our mental storage facility to find the right answer - if we have to. Our Aspie partners have the information, but are less likely to successfully access it immediately, especially in stressful situations.

T

This is a major problem for our son who we know has an incredible mathematical ability but, despite this, was held back in a lower maths stream at school because he could not get his thoughts down on paper. However, if you talk to him in a calm environment he can show you exactly how much he knows.

Our cognitive processing has two main schemes:

Sensory input from our surroundings demands our attention based on stimulus characteristics - such as novelty or salience (bottom-up processing), e.g. being unexpectedly prodded: this demands immediate attention.

We are also capable of directing attention toward or away from encountered stimuli based on our goals (top-down modulation). So we can set ourselves goals and work towards them, ignoring the "noise" of unwanted stimuli.

Aspies often have poor skills of top down modulation - an inability to work towards goals when information to reach the goal is "noisy"; perhaps there is no immediate clear answer and a debate on which is the strongest argument is called for.

The Husband Says:

When Karen first told me about theories regarding top down modulation, certain Aspie behaviour traits became obvious. On the immediate conscious cognitive processing front, I could understand how, with reduced or inhibited top down modulation, I could be swamped with noisy information and not be able to see the wood for the trees. Very careful overt and conscious planning and prioritisation can make up for a failure of the unconscious and automatic modulation that I am missing.

But there is another subtle mechanism at play here. A neurotypical (with fully functioning top down modulation) "primes" their cognitive processing with regard to emotion and social expectation. For example, a neurotypical expects sadness and unhappiness at a funeral and is even more sensitive than usual to those emotions at such gatherings. This is considered to be a desirable social norm. Without top down modulation, Aspies have their usual poor levels of emotional surveillance and measurement, and appear cold and disconnected at a time of NT high emotion. Worse still, this top down modulation driven sensitivity in NTs makes the stimulus of happiness, enjoyment and frivolity appear as a massive bottom-up stimulation for the NT, meaning that deviation from the social norm at a funeral is genuinely shocking in its unexpectedness. Thus the "wrongly" behaving Aspie is caught in a trap both ways - not emotional enough and emotional for all the wrong reasons according to the NTs.

Tourette's Syndrome

This is quite a rare and misunderstood condition where people suffer from uncontrollable physical and verbal tics.

T

It can be a comorbidity of Asperger's Syndrome. People with Tourette's have great difficulty fitting into society as they are often considered by the public to be rude, threatening and violent.

Traditional Marriage

I always thought I was a modern girl, not bowing to the traditions of life. I was a little rebellious in my youth: I was a Goth and my parents let my boyfriend live with us. Never did I think I would end up in a traditional marriage, where the man goes out to work and I would stay home with the children.

When David and I first met, I was single and career oriented. I knew what I wanted to do and I was not going to let our fledgling relationship get in the way. Even though I moved in with him for a while, I didn't hesitate to move away when I was offered my dream job in London. I was selfish enough to not worry about how this would affect David because, although I was happy to stay in the relationship, my career came first.

As it was, the dream job didn't turn out quite as I hoped and I missed David dreadfully. We made the decision, after a year, to get married and that I would return to the North East. I quickly found temporary (but unsatisfying) work to help pay the bills and, nine months later, we were married. We had no intention of having children at this time, and I was still intent on finding the right job for me.

I fell into a good job as Child Protection Registrar for the area but shortly after I became pregnant with Morgan. I did consider going back to work after having Morgan but by then my attitude to having kids had completely changed and I wanted to be the best mum there was to him and he really needed me to be around. So before I knew it we were a traditional, nuclear family with the dad going out to work and the wife staying at home looking after the children. There were good points and bad points to this. I adored being a mum despite its difficulties and Morgan was the most gorgeous blonde haired, blued eyed baby but at times it was quite boring too. When he was eighteen months old we moved from the city to the rural village we live in now and our daughter was born. I didn't have time to go back to work and I also became very ill with severe migraines and headaches, lethargy. I didn't have the time and wasn't well enough to even consider getting a job.

In hindsight I can see where things were going wrong. David was the sole breadwinner and he had an ill wife and two lovely children to support. He had a stressful job with a lot of responsibility and all this on top of his Asperger's that we didn't know about. Yet, bizarrely in some ways this is what he wanted. He needed me to be at home to look after the house and the children so it left him to concentrate on being provider. Modern life is a paradox because we want everything but we can't really have it. I wanted to stay at home with the kids but I also wanted a fulfilling career. I was both happy and dissatisfied with my role as traditional wife and mother.

The Husband Says:

I'll wager that most Asperger Marriages are 'conventional'. Why? Well the Aspie side of the relationship is trying to figure out the set of social norms for marriage so, by definition, the result will be very conventional.

I suspect that there may be higher than average failure of Asperger Marriages when the Aspie partner realises that, like in other areas of life, the conventions of marriage from the rule book are not the end of the story. There are many, many, unwritten rules.

It is easy to dwell on what might have been rather than making the most of what you have got.

Transactional Analysis

The Husband Says:

I went on a training course with one of my clients about how to be a tutor and presenter of technical material. There was a lot of good advice on "crowd control" and how to manage myself and my tutor group if conflict started to occur. The advice was based on Eric Berne's Transactional Analysis theories with a bit of game theory thrown in to establish an optimal strategy.

The theories seemed to play out very well in class-room role-play, so I have extended the ideas to account for how I think my Aspie brain works, applied the game theory again, and found some strategies and explanations of my behaviour that seem to ring true and have the potential for improvement in my social communications, bearing in mind that communications is one of the principal keys to relationships.

Eric Berne's Transactional Analysis Theory

This theory seems to be very popular in the practise of modern psychology and is quite accessible to us lay people:

In any conversation or communication, even an argument between people, each "unit" of the conversation is a "transaction". Those transactions might be a sentence, just a few words or a whole paragraph. Each transaction invites another transaction, unless there is nothing left to say and both parties are happy that information and opinion has been communicated and agreement reached.

Further, Berne said we each possess three voices or "egos"; the inner child, the inner parent and the adult.

T

The Parent ego speaks with authority on rules that must not be broken - commandments like "Thou shalt not commit murder". These are social imperatives; if these rules are broken the consequences are inevitably serious.

The Child ego speaks of our emotional state: seeing, hearing, feeling, and how the world makes us feel.

The Adult ego speaks of logic, thoughtfulness and is based on the measurement and perception of the data gathered of the moment around the person.

Berne theorises that the most successful transactions that come to a natural close with satisfaction to both parties are when "adult" speaks to "adult". "Parent" speaking to "Parent" is successful, albeit less of the time, and "child to child" can work out too. Conducting transactions from dissimilar egos tends not to work out so well.

If a crossed transaction occurs, there is an ineffective communication. Worse still either or both parties will be upset.

Berne's Ego State and Brain Development

Could it be that the different ego states of a person develop at different times and are processed in different parts of the brain?

Some of the "Parent" ego is so deeply ingrained that perhaps it is inherited or at least conditioned very early after birth - imperative concepts like an outright "no" to murder or incest. The remainder of the imperatives are so strong they are "wired" into the brain in many parallel paths and reinforced so that they are immutable.

The "Child" ego is a result of early learning and conditioning, again "wired" into the brain in early years, but more loosely and with interpretation of the environment and experiences of those early years.

The "Adult" ego state is not pre-ordained and hard-wired in the brain. It is the product of applying logic to the here and now with significant and time consuming processing required to get a result.

Now if the Baron-Cohen theories of brain development in Aspies are true, then perhaps in us Aspies the "Parent" ego is reasonably well formed and wired up into our chain of response to transaction, and our "Child" ego is poorly formed but still "wired" into the decision making chain, but much slower to respond - on the same timescale as the "Adult" ego, leading to us Aspies having to rely mainly on our calculating "Adult" ego state to make sense of the here and now.

Transaction Processing

Others have theorised that brain processing is organised in a hierarchy depending on how critical it is that a timely response is made to an incoming transaction.

If the brain is organised and prioritised by ego state then the "Parent" ego will finish processing and come to a decision as to how to respond first; this "Parent" response will be either blocking (e.g. don't murder the person sending the transaction) or one of ambivalence, allowing the next layer of processing to yield a more finessed result.

Next to complete (in the neurotypical), with its slightly weaker "wiring" is the "Child" ego state based on experiences of being and feeling, and how things worked out previously. Again the result is either a strong and conditioned response or ambivalence.

It is theorised that in the neurotypical brain the "Adult" ego is the last to complete processing on the incoming transaction and the information to hand. If the Parent and Child ego states have not yielded a high priority response, then the Adult ego is the final decision maker producing (hopefully) a logical response that might be balanced but perceived as "cold"; some call this lacking in emotional intelligence (EQ).

So what if in the Aspie brain the speed and quality of response from the "Child" ego processing is slow and uncertain - not through any lack of opportunity in early years to develop, just that "wiring" of that part of the ego system is a bit shoddy? Moral imperatives will continue to be met (assuming this is hard-wired in multiple redundant pathways in the brain), but the neurotypical instinctive and intuitive emotional responses could be at best delayed and at worst ambivalent to absent leaving only the cold calculating "Adult" part of the decision making chain to make the transactional response.

Putting it all Together as a Strategy

Applying a bit of game theory for optimal outcome to Berne's theories leads to the following strategies:

Where the incoming transaction is from an adult ego state, the Aspie adult ego state will cope perfectly well, like the neurotypical.

Berne's optimal transaction exchange is the best strategy; respond using the Aspie adult ego. This describes business communications - we are all "using our heads" and calculating our positions and following a well-defined set of rules of business ethics, so these transactions usually end up being complete and satisfying.

Where the incoming transaction is from a parent ego state, an order is being given.

An Aspie brain should spot a high level imperative of this sort and respond with the parent ego state of compliance very quickly.

If this doesn't happen, the best strategy is to try to move the transaction chain into the Adult ego state. Only a well thought out and logical argument presented calmly will win the day for the Aspie, and this will depend on the instigator and transmitter of the transaction chain being willing to move to the Adult ego state too.

It might be hard to do, but if the instigator will not move to the Adult ego state, then leave the instigator at "Parent" and also move to the Parent state and agree to follow the imperative, allowing time (and it might be a lot of time) for the instigator to choose to come to the Adult state and perhaps finesse their imperative to something more acceptable to you for a win-win situation.

There is a very high risk strategy sometimes used by neurotypicals when there is conflict between two parent ego states - switch the dialogue into the child ego state. This means throwing a childish tantrum and turning on the tears. This very, very occasionally works for neurotypicals if both parties end up in their child ego, but for Aspies with a poorly performing child ego, this route is fraught with danger and not at all recommended.

The final state of the instigating transaction being from the child ego is the most complex. This is the whole field of discussion and communication on emotion and feeling.

The normal best scenario of answering the child ego from the child ego is quite high risk for neurotypicals - for responses to be acceptable and transaction to continue the child ego conditioning of both participants has to be compatible and equivalent. Sooner or later one of the neurotypicals bends the conversation round, usually to the adult ego state and hopes that his or her partner in the conversation will follow.

The normal best scenario of answering in the child ego is difficult to impossible for an Aspie - essentially there is no "reliable" child ego, so the results can be rather random leading to conflict and breakdown of the communication.

Responding in the parent ego with an imperative is doomed. Don't go there.

So the remaining choice is to respond in the Adult ego, but with a twist. Try to think and calculate what a response from a neurotypical in the child ego might be. Pretend! Neurotypicals would be taking a risk here on an emotional response; try a few rounds of a fake-child-ego response and hope that your partner's child ego becomes confused and less reliable and their adult ego state kicks in to match yours.

So the game theory outcomes show that us Aspies have a clear disadvantage if the communication starts from the child ego. Your best bet is to pretend and "go with it", thinking "What would the neurotypical do?" before responding. But don't take too long to respond or the moment will be lost to your partner's child ego. I'm afraid that you have to gamble. Take heart that the more often you repeat the gamble, the more often that it will give the desired outcome making us look more neurotypical, just a bit "emotionally slow".

Transitions

AS **NT** Transitions are very tricky for your average Aspie. They are leaving the familiar behind and starting with something new and unknown, e.g. changing job, going on holiday, or moving house. The nature of the transition, and even the amount of desire they have for moving on, is almost irrelevant as they still need to deal with the change before all else. The motivator is that the change is, theoretically, for the better (a job with a higher salary or a nicer house with more space), but when they are in transition they do not enjoy the unsettling change one bit.

T

The kind of behaviour you will see during any type of transition, even with a certain amount of preparation, will be catastrophizing, exhaustion and panic.

If at all possible, to avoid the worst of these occurrences, it is worth having a dry run. For the new job, you can go with him and try out the new commute and look into all the pitfalls that may happen and prepare him for them. Going on holiday, you can now use Google Earth and Street View to find out exactly where your hotel is and use the Sat Nav on your phone or in your car to get there.

Moving house is trickier, but allow him to pour over street maps and floor plans to his heart's content. David has been known to get out his engineering drawing package to draw up floor plans and pieces of furniture so he can visualise where to put them. This eases his distress remarkably.

The Husband Says:

All good advice that, when put into practise by Karen, helps me greatly. And a calmer me co-operating with the transition, instead of fighting for the familiar, is a happier Karen.

Triad of Impairment

To currently qualify for an ASD diagnosis the patient is expected to show this. Lorna Wing, the founder of the National Autism Society in the UK, came up with this formula for impairment:

Social and Emotional

Difficulty with:

- Friendships
- Managing unstructured parts of the day
- Working co-operatively

Language and Communication

- Difficulty processing and retaining verbal information
- Difficulty with jokes and sarcasm
- Difficulty with social use of language
- Literal interpretation
- Difficulty with Body Language, Facial Expressions and gesture

Flexibility of Thought (Imagination)

- Difficulty with change

- Difficulty with empathy
- Difficulty with generalisation (abstraction of concept)

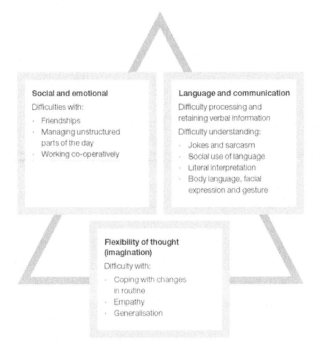

Social and emotional

Difficulties with:
- Friendships
- Managing unstructured parts of the day
- Working co-operatively

Language and communication

Difficulty processing and retaining verbal information

Difficulty understanding:
- Jokes and sarcasm
- Social use of language
- Literal interpretation
- Body language, facial expression and gesture

Flexibility of thought (imagination)

Difficulty with:
- Coping with changes in routine
- Empathy
- Generalisation

Triggers

NT These are the situations which cause enough stress to trigger a meltdown. The strategy to recognise and avoid them is a 'must' for an Asperger Marriage to stand a chance.

NT Make note of them when they happen and then plan around them for the future. Many triggers can be predicted and avoided to help your partner. His calmness and happiness is the key to your happiness.

NB: Not everything can be predicted or expected, no matter how well you plan. Volcanoes explode and people get ill. Sometimes you just have to accept that 'sh*t' happens.

The Husband Says:

There are various topics of discussion or social situations pretty much guaranteed to trigger an unwanted Aspie response from me. But note that every Aspie is different, so my personal list might not chime with someone else's.

- *Talking about money and social ambition*

- *Being invited to a party where I don't know a significant number of the people present and I have no excuse to play host*

- *Having a surprise sprung on me, especially surprise parties*

- *Being required to sing or dance like some sort of performing seal*

- *Having to make a large and significant change to a long standing (and well thought out) plan*

- *Being required to go on holiday somewhere hot with 'nothing to do'*

- *Being forced into a boring and repetitive task that should have been automated or abolished long ago. (e.g. filling in a tax return)*

NT
Karen can be very good at lessening the impact of such things with a combination of careful planning and good humour.

Trust

When women get together to talk about their AS husband's, there can be a lot of negativity flying around. After all, why would they feel the need to get together to celebrate how wonderful their lives are?

Yet, we do also talk about the positive sides. We often ask ourselves why this relationship is worth it. Why are we still there? Those reasons are the ones that made us fall in love in the first place. The man who initially wooed us with his devotion and generosity.

Why did you decide to marry him? If you were like me, it was that he gave you a feeling of security and being wanted and loved unconditionally. I knew I could trust David. He had never let me down. He was supportive and selfless with me. I very quickly realised how loyal he was to me and I grew to trust him very quickly. Despite all our emotional traumas I have never once, not trusted him.

In previous relationships I have not always been able to completely trust that person which was the main reason for those relationships ending. How can you give yourself to someone who you are not entirely sure will always value you and be there for you?

T

Above all else I hold trust, loyalty and fidelity to be the crux of a marriage, whether it be one that was performed in a registry office, a synagogue or a church. It does not matter whether God was present or not, it is the vows that you say and mean to each other that count.

When David is late home I know it is because he has been held up at work or the traffic is bad. I never have any doubts in that respect.

The Husband Says:

As slaves to the social norms, it should come as no surprise that us Aspies can be trusted.

Karen tells me that it's OK to go 'window shopping', but I won't even do that because I don't necessarily trust myself not to break the great trust that Karen has in me. Would I want to take it further? I just don't know, so I just avoid the situations where the risk might be there.

This whole trusted through avoiding temptation can make us Aspies in relationships look very prudish.

T

- ✧   Ulterior Motive
- ✧   Uncertainty
- ✧   Understanding each Other
- ✧   Understanding your Wife
- ✧   Unpredictable Behaviour
- ✧   Unrealistic Expectations
- ✧   Unreasonable Statements
- ✧   Unresolved Situations
- ✧   Unwritten Rules
- ✧   Uta Frith

Ulterior Motive

HE DOESN'T HAVE ONE.

Uncertainty

Not being able to use past experience to predict the future, can be a major issue for someone with ASD. This uncertainty adds to their anxieties, which is why they crave control and routine.

See Intolerance of Uncertainty

Understanding Each Other

 This is vital to salvaging your marriage. Without communication and trying to understand each other's point of view you will have difficulty carrying on long term.

- Learning and knowing each other's strengths and weaknesses.
- Acknowledging and supporting each other.
- We both like to be in control but not always of the same things.
- Sometimes we make a great team.

Leaping to Conclusions

NT We have to remember as NT wives that we do not have the same thought patterns as our husbands. We are very good at seeing things just from our point of view and leaping to conclusions. However, we need to be aware that we have a talent that our husbands do not: that of theory of mind and good empathy. We are able to put ourselves in someone else's shoes and try to work out why they did such a thing from the clues given by their life style, routine and habits.

The Husband Says:

If I have one ambition for my contribution to this guide, it is that it may help each partner to foster a better understanding of the other in an Aspie Marriage. The Aspie team member has difficulty communicating outwards and receiving communication inwards. I hope that, to help communicating outwards, fellow Aspies can borrow my words under "The Husband Says:" items, and just say "this" to their partner. Likewise, I hope that the NTs can communicate better with their aspies by pointing at Karen's words and simply saying "read this".

If we haven't used the right words in this edition of this digital guide to help you understand each other better (either scientifically or empathetically), please give us feedback and we will fix that very quickly and update everyone.

Understanding your Wife

AS   This is a tricky one because, though we may come under the label Neurotypical, we are many and diverse in character.

On the whole your NT wife is likely to be more naturally and outwardly caring and outgoing, but possibly not extrovert. She is likely to be patient and tolerant and sympathetic to the Aspie cause. Or at least she was when you met, I hear you cry!

What happened?...

Well, 'Life' happened. Marriage, children, and the pressure of work can all divert her exclusive and loving attention from you. It doesn't mean she doesn't love you as much as when you got married it just means there is only one of her, but her attention is demanded and divided by other things that are also priorities in your family life.

Points to Consider

- Your wife can multi task. She can listen and cook at the same time.

- Your wife has a big heart. She does not love you less every time you have a child. Her heart just gets bigger.

- Your wife loves her children because they are also part of you.

- Even though you treat your wife in ways that you would like to be treated, what she really needs is for you to treat her how she would like to be treated. She may not want another complicated gadget for her birthday. She may want a bracelet to wear that you have thoughtfully bought for her. That bracelet will remind her how much you love her and she will treasure it.

U

Unpredictable Behaviour

AS We NT's do not help situations with our unpredictable behaviour: our impulsivity; fickle ways; and love of change.

We find routine hum drum, dull and predictable. To us these adjectives have bland, negative connotations.

We must seem like butterflies to our Aspies, brightly coloured and flitting from pretty flower to pretty flower. There must be part of this behaviour that appeals to an Aspie or they would never have been attracted to us in the first place.

But it's like we buy dictionaries from separate planets, where the definitions of the same words are ever so slightly different.

To Aspie's, routine is reassuring, comfortable and safe. They have control.

To be fair, we NTs do like a certain amount of routine and control in our lives, but we have it as a central core that we revolve intricately around, like a Waltzer, flying in and out. Never quite knowing where or when life is going to stop. It's exhilarating.

Unpredictable Behaviour in Asperger's

We NTs don't own all the rights on unpredictable behaviour though. We find it hard to predict Aspie mood swings or understand why they happen. We need to be patient with each other's foibles.

Unrealistic Expectations

NT Having expectations is not a bad thing. Expectations keep me motivated and full of hope. They get you up in the morning. However, having your expectations badly dashed can quickly lead to the opposite, more negative feelings of disappointment, despair and even depression.

You need to consider whether your expectations about your current marriage are realistic or not.

Don't be afraid of lowering your expectations. You will be surprised how this can actually lead to happiness.

U

Unreasonable Statements

This subject was suggested to me by a lady on a Facebook forum. She described how her husband complained to her that someone at work took HIS parking spot - even though they do not have assigned car parking spaces.

This relates to his Theory of Mind and how he expects other people around him to know what is important to him, even though he has never informed them. The ownership of a certain place, just like Sheldon's Spot (his specific seat on the sofa) in The Big Bang Theory, provides them with comfort and routine. When this gets disrupted they take it personally as it genuinely does upset their equilibrium.

Unresolved Situations

As a NT I am annoyingly slap dash in my attitude to life. It drives David mad. It's not that I don't want to finish what I started, it's more like I just haven't got the time or I have been so distracted I have forgotten what I was doing.

We are way past our original deadline for doing this digital version of the guide. I would have launched it ages ago but David has been insistent that we get it right. It has to be perfect. I don't disagree with him really and in fact I admire his determination but at the same time I really don't want to be this stressed.

What it comes down to is that I can cope with imperfection and he can't.

See The Big Bang Theory for an example where lack of closure leads to Sheldon having a meltdown (Season 6, Episode 21).

Unwritten Rules (The Big Secret)

We neurotypicals are a dreadful and uncaring lot. We have these unwritten rules that we just assume everyone knows. We don't tell people about them. We just expect them to know what to do when they get there.

Our natural ability to walk into a room and sense the atmosphere, be it tense, relaxed, welcoming or excited, is something that those on the spectrum just do not get. There are so many different rules, and it would be impossible to list them as we really don't know them consciously ourselves, but I will have a go...

This one is for the men only and one that my tutor Lynne Moxon is very fond of talking about: Where to stand at the urinals. This relates to the 'Unwritten Rule' of Personal space. Nobody tells you that you should stand further away from people you don't know than people you do know.

See David's detailed rules for this below!

Social conventions: For example, unless you are in a mood with your loved one or friend, you should always say goodbye, even if it is just a wave. It is not enough for your NT wife or loved one to just drop you off at the station: they expect a kiss, a verbal acknowledgement of your leaving, and possibly your return time, and at least a wave as you walk away. This makes them feel appreciated and wanted and will keep them going until they next see you. Just knowing that you care for your wife is not enough for your wife - you have to demonstrate it.

The Husband Says:

Some of the unwritten rules may seem complex, but they are, on the whole, very logical - just the outcomes have been pre-computed for you. Take Lynne Moxon's urinal problem. The response stems from two simple rules: "Maximise the space between you and any fellow user" (don't be tempted to peek), and "Maximise the opportunities for further urinal users to benefit from maximum space". In practise it works like this:

- *First in: choose the end furthest from the door, but not so far as it might be a route march (for large facilities)*

- *Second in: As far away from the first user as you can get*

- *Third in: split the difference between the existing users trying to leave an empty stall between you and each other user (splashing issues)*

- *Congested: take any free stall, be quick, don't shake excessively, but move out in a timely fashion. NO PEEKING!*

- *Complicating factors: With luggage, wait for an end urinal.*

Generally, you can formulate social rules and conventions if you think about it long enough and perhaps do a little research. A friendly NT might even give you a clue.

Uta Frith

Professor Uta Frith is a German developmental psychologist at University College, London. She has mentored both Professor Tony Attwood and Simon Baron-Cohen. She has pioneered much of the current research on autism issues and has written many books and papers on the subject.

U

- ✦ Vagus Nerve
- ✦ Validation
- ✦ Velcro Brain
- ✦ Venting
- ✦ Verbal Abuse
- ✦ Vertigo
- ✦ Vestibular
- ✦ Victim
- ✦ Violation
- ✦ Visual Thinker
- ✦ Vitamin D3
- ✦ Voice of Authority
- ✦ Volume Control
- ✦ Vulnerable

Vagus Nerve

The Vagus nerve is the longest of twelve pairs of nerves that originate in the brain, serving as the brains central command in the fight against stress, inflammation and toxicity. The vagus helps regulate our 'fight or flight' response, digestion, detoxification and blood pressure.

Recent research by Dr Steven Porges from the University of Illinois was published in a book and paper showing that the Vagus nerve also regulates our immune system and provides us with a neurological infrastructure that determines many of our emotional responses, enabling us to empathise and communicate with others.

This essential nerve provides up to 90% of the body's sensory neurons which provide information to the central nervous system.

This results in the Vagus nerve being in charge of what we hear, see and oxytocin receptors in the brain which influence how attracted we are to other people and our ability to feel and love.

Validation

For an Asperger/Neurotypical marriage to work it is not always vital for the AS partner to have an official diagnosis but both partners have to acknowledge and agree that it is extremely likely.

Usually it will be the female, neurotypical partner who will push for the AS partner to acknowledge that they think differently to each other. This is a first major step for both. With validation, you can move on and forward together.

Validating Within Counselling

When I counsel wives of Asperger men, I always have a box of handkerchiefs close to hand.

To have someone to confirm to them the misery and tension and loneliness that they have been going through unnoticed and unsupported for years, can be quite overwhelming for them. Tears of relief are inevitable. To know that they were right all along and they are not alone in their thinking is a wondrous thing. Yet, paradoxically, this feeling also brings with it sorrow as you realise that yes, you were right, that your marriage is in great difficulty and your husband is a difficult man.

Just to have someone listen and understand is like having a great weight lifted from you.

The Husband Says:

Whilst Karen suggests it will be the NT partner who might push for a diagnosis (or validation) for the Aspie husband, such a move might be instigated by health professionals investigating the cause of Autism or Asperger's amongst the children in the family. This is no bad thing if the adults in the family unit are coping with the situation and can lead their children by example.

Velcro Brain

I have always felt the dumb one in my family when I was growing up. I had parents, both with multiple degrees, and my brothers, who were good at maths and the sciences. I lost my confidence with maths early on and lived in a world of books and writing. I felt this was easy and enjoyable, but not on a par with the rest of my family. I didn't understand at the time that this was my forte, and that not everyone has such a mathematical /logical brain. In fact, I have a very creative brain.... it just didn't feel appreciated very much by some people at the time.

So again, in my own little family, I am the odd one out: Husband and two children on the spectrum. It was evident from an early age that both the children had phenomenal memories just from their recall of past events, but these days they will quote to me vast swathes of newly learned science, verbatim.

I admire this quality in them very much and am quite envious of what I call their Velcro brains, where facts just seem to stick.

Venting

 For the Wife:

There is so much we have to put up with as Asperger wives and often we cannot share our feelings with our husbands. However, it is unhealthy for us to keep our feelings locked up. When he has done (or not done) something that annoys me, I calculate whether it is worth mentioning it to him. A lot of the time I don't. So many things seem so petty and it is easier just to do it myself (and also do it the way I like it done). Yet, sometimes he will behave in such a ridiculous or despicable way, I am left in disbelief. At times like this I need someone to talk to who understands my situation.

I never publicise anything about our relationship on Facebook as that is not fair. I do however belong to a private group of (mostly) wives where there is always someone there to listen. I know that once I have typed my grievance, or even my funny story, and pressed Post, that I will relax and will be able to get on with my day. David is aware that I do this though I rarely involve him in the posts. Just having someone validating my thoughts and saying, "My husband does that too," is so helpful.

I occasionally will vent in person to friends, but usually only to very close friends, or friends in support groups who are in similar situations. The worst thing that can happen with acquaintances is that they will try and temper your vent by telling you how all men are like that.

As yet, there is no support group locally that is specifically for spouses affected by Asperger's but I know they are being set up, not just around the country but around the world.

To be listened to and to know you are not alone is invaluable.

Verbal Abuse

This is difficult to write as I think it will upset David to read it. I know he does not intend to speak to me the way he does at times, but it is still nasty and it still hurts.

When we were first courting, and over the two years before we got married, David was never rude or disrespectful to me. In fact, he was quite the opposite. He was generous and deferential, and supportive in all ways. I did not go seeking a man who treated me with such respect and, in fact I was very cool with him at first. I was almost uncomfortable with the amount of attention and money he lavished on me.

The day we married, he was trembling so much in the church that I held his hand to calm him down. He was wonderful that day but, almost literally, the next day I started being treated differently and started having regrets.

When I once pointed out that he was in the wrong driving gear, it was humiliating to be told that I could only tell him what to do when I had passed my test. This I remember distinctly as it was a very low blow to me. I had taken my driving test several times and made silly mistakes because I was so nervous. He, himself, had told me I was a good driver and he was always happy for me to drive him around. He knew how desperately I wanted my independence and how it affected my self-esteem. He too knows what it is like to be terribly nervous about something. My helpful remark was thrown back at me and his words cut me like a knife. At least it wasn't said in public.

And what to do in a situation like that? Sit there and allow him to talk to me like that, with no respect at all? It makes me so angry to be treated like a downtrodden woman by the man who professes to love me. I have always known I am worth more than that and, at times, I have only stayed with him because of the children and my ill health. I knew however, it was better to seethe than to escalate an argument - no matter how much it hurt my feelings. I didn't want the children to witness it and I needed the day to go ahead as planned. I knew if I kept quiet that he was likely to calm down and it would be forgotten (by him).

Now, however, we know the reasons why he treats me like he does during moments of stress. Most of the time I am glad that I stayed with David as we have been able to turn our marriage around, and I know there is a future for us even when the kids leave (which I suspect David is very much looking forward to). It is still hard to take, and it is still not worth pointing out his transgressions in the heat of the moment. I can't change that, but these moments are fewer and fewer these days and, mostly, I have back the man I first met twenty years ago.

The Husband Says:

Our 'debates', over what is predominantly my condition and the effect it has on our marriage, can get quite argumentative and heated. I don't intend for these discussions to get so ugly, but tempers flare easily, blame is laid and this pattern of angry response to Karen's imperatives to change, can look to be an abusive side to our relationship - thus the topic of verbal abuse rears its head.

Karen has said before that it is not genuinely abusive unless I am arguing and damaging our relationship with an intent, a pre-planned malice towards her. This is not the case and very far from my mind. My possible verbal abuse of Karen comes from me being affected by the adrenaline of a heated argument - that fight or flight response. I lash out unintentionally with words.

Vertigo

When our son was a toddler, we hired a car to go on holiday. It was the first time we had encountered satellite navigation and we thought it would be fun to use it. Unfortunately, it was set for the 'shortest route', which is fine for city navigation but not in rural Wales. This resulted in us going along a narrow gravel track, up a very steep mountain pass, in order to get to Bala Lake and go on the steam railway. It wasn't too bad going up but, it was on our descent, I discovered for the first time my husband's fear of heights and steep drops.

At first I thought his protestations were just in jest but, when I looked to see how pale he was and that his hands were shaking slightly, I too got a little nervous. Generally, I had trusted his driving up until this point, but seeing his nervousness and how he was convinced we were going to fall to our deaths at any moment was a little unnerving.

It turns out that vertigo is quite common in those with ASD due to dysfunction in the vestibular system. My father also has it, again discovered whilst on holiday in a high unprotected place. Me, I would scamper up anywhere as a child, and my brother Nick and I would always have competitions to see who could climb the tallest tree. Our other brother preferred to stay on the ground.

It turns out that our daughter gets vertigo when disembarking a train. I have learned to be more sympathetic.

The Husband Says:

Yet another unexpected co-morbidity of Aspergers that is explained by hypo or hyper responses to stimuli (sensory disorder), this time the sense of balance.

This doesn't explain, however, why my vertigo can be suppressed if it is me who has built the tall thing or has tied the knots in the rope that I'm using to hang from the high thing. There's clearly more to it than a sense of balance; perhaps I don't have true vertigo and more just a fear of falling.

Vestibular

The vestibular system is responsible for posture, balance and the body's ability to know where it is in regards to its surroundings.

This complicated system is connected to the central nervous system. Leo Kanner, the American autism expert, recognised that autistic children had an abnormal modulation of sensory input. This meant that the their bodies were either over responding to sensory data or under responding to it.

The amount of vestibular input differs depending on the child. It can be noted that while some crave movement, others are motion sensitive.

If you watch an ASD child, you will see that they are self-treating as they love to bounce, swing and twirl around. They do this to feel grounded and know where their extremities are. In fact, our son loves that spinning sensation so much that it resulted in a trip to casualty when he was younger: shortly after getting out of the bath, he was twirling around the room with a towel over his head; unfortunately, I did not discover this until he had crashed into the wall and I heard him screaming because blood was pouring out of his nose; it was so swollen I had to take him to Accident and Emergency where the doctors carefully questioned him as to how he had done it. These days he tends to limit himself to swinging ceaselessly on his desk chair.

This behaviour is less apparent in the adult Aspie, though you can see it in their dislike of climbing ladders (vertigo) and other high places. Another feature of this that David has mentioned is that, when he has been on a long journey, he will say to me he needs to wait until he feels like he has stopped moving. I always assumed this was a figure of speech but now I realise he really does need time for his body's central nervous system to get the memo.

Victim

 Who is the victim in your relationship?

Unless you're in a 'traditional' relationship of abuse, there is generally more than one victim in an Asperger Marriage. Neither partner wants to be the abuser or the victim but both, after some time, start to feel like this.

An Asperger wife is often a very strong woman who would never, at first, consider herself to be a victim in her marriage. She will stand up for her rights and not back down when her husband is dismissive of her concerns. The irony is that her husband will see her dissent and escalating argument, not as defence but as aggression towards him, and he will also feel the victim whilst feeling very isolated.

As time goes by, both will start to feel unhappy, unappreciated and unloved. I have seen so much bitterness coming from the partner who feels like this. It is very sad. They will automatically be defensive before forgiving. They are more likely to blame than to forgive. They will feel resentful and angry towards each other. Yet all this is due to misunderstanding and lack of the right kind of communication.

Most couples in this situation are not aware that their partners are on the autistic spectrum when they meet, and so they have no understanding for their differences. Instead, the differences are seen as arrogance, laziness and disrespect and, when this happens on a daily basis, it feels like you are both falling out of love.

Some couples will have tried to revive their failing marriage by seeing a marriage counsellor, but often this makes a situation worse, especially for the AS partner who comes across as uncaring, or even narcissistic or abusive. An untrained counsellor (despite their professional impartiality) is likely have sympathies that lie with the NT (usually female) partner which can result in validating her own feelings that she is being abused.

It is not surprising, therefore, that the wife feels the victim here and, with validation, will likely look to separate or divorce.

But here, sadly, there are two victims. The poor, confused AS man who is even further misunderstood and now disliked by more than just his wife, or so it seems to him. This is a devastating situation for him to be in. We must not forget how vulnerable our AS partner is. It is easy for an NT woman to vocalise being the victim (and I am not saying that she isn't), but her husband, who she once loved, is left confused and vilified with no support when he needs it most.

Hopefully, with help and growing understanding from this App, or finding the right counsellor, this situation can be averted.

Violation

A violation in a relationship is when your partner has gone a step too far where boundaries are concerned. He needs to know what these unseen boundaries are, but until you tell him he will continue to be oblivious.

We all have Expectation Violations, but we NT's usually shake our surprise off and deal with the change. Not so much our partners, who may take whatever the surprise is as a personal affront.

Visual Thinker

Your husband is most likely a visual thinker which may result in him often misinterpreting your speech or not remembering what you have said. A lot of women in a NT/NT relationship may say scathingly that 'All men are like that', but it is not so.

NT To communicate an idea successfully to him you need to know that he has not only heard you, but actually understands what you have said. There are tools you can use to aid you both in this.

- As a visual thinker he will remember more once he has seen instructions written down.

- Write a list with clear instructions

- Send an email with your thoughts, feelings and, if necessary, instructions

- Show him what you want him to do and how to do it. Make sure he is watching and listening and not thinking about something else. Make him repeat it back to you.

- Draw a diagram. They are good at working things out from diagrams and actually appreciate having something to refer to. Who doesn't love a picture?

The Husband Says:

It's that last one. Curiously for people who struggle with non-verbal communication through facial expression, we can gain so much more from a diagram or a picture than a jumble of words. I have to comprehend and construct a picture from the words - if you draw a picture, you have done that work for me and removed the ambiguities of interpretation.

There are loads of Aspie Engineers. We have formalised this 'drawing pictures as communicating' by making it part of our daily ritual to carry a day-book (a note-pad in which we can write words) - but if you look inside, you generally find many more pictures than words.

Vitamin D3

NB: Please note that I am not advocating this as a cure for autism but as a supplement to overall physical and mental health.

In the last twenty years we have been advised by our governments and health agencies to cover up whenever in the sun with hats, long sleeves and sun cream. This well-meaning advice was to prevent burning and its long term effect of skin cancer or melanoma.

Autism and Vitamin D

There has been significant research regarding the use of Vitamin D and autism. Accidental overdosing of children with Vitamin D3 by parents who were meant to give their children three drops a day but gave their children three pipettes a day saw no harm come to the children. The children who were accidentally overdosed were the ones who showed significant improvement in their overall behaviour and health.

Signs of Vitamin D Deficiency

Muscle and Bone Weakness, feeling Unhappy, Pain Sensitivity, Chronic Gum Disease, Hypertension, Sleepiness, Mood Swings, Decreased Endurance, Head Sweating and Psoriasis.

Sources of Vitamin D

Sunlight, sunbeds (it turns out they aren't that harmful if used correctly), oily fish and vitamin D3 supplementation.

The Vitamin D Council (a lobbying group) also recommends that people that supplement with Vitamin D3 would further enable absorption by adding Magnesium, Boron, Vitamin K2, zinc and Vitamin A.

The Husband Says:

I was sceptical, but as Karen's guinea pig, I'm proof. I was told there were lots of mystery ailments afflicting me during a mid-life health check at the GP. Most things, including a nasty patch of psoriasis seem to have cleared up now that Karen gives me a hefty dose of Vitamin D every morning along with some other vitamins and minerals that help it work. This seems to be the antidote to our sedentary office bound lifestyles.

Read up about it and make your own mind up.

The Wife Replies:

I haven't been able to get him on a sunbed yet. He likes the pale look.

Voice of Authority

We had a bad experience with a volcano in 2010 and were stuck in Florida for an extra two weeks! So when, just before our holiday last year, I heard mention on the news about another volcano erupting, I mentioned it to David. I said "It's probably nothing to worry about but we'd better keep an eye on flight information." He dismissed my fears and it wasn't mentioned again.

The following morning, I was making coffee when he came running into the kitchen saying, "There's a volcano erupting in Iceland again, I'd better check the flight information," and he continued into the study where I could hear him tappity-tapping on the keyboard.

I stood there open mouthed with a cafetiere in my hand, wondering to myself if that had really happened. It was like the conversation we'd had the day before had never existed. He had dismissed my fears as irrelevant until he himself heard the Voice of Authority on the BBC news the following day. In previous years, before diagnosis, I would have been left wondering if I was going insane or whether he had early onset Alzheimer's. Now I realise that it isn't my sanity at stake, it is just the way he receives information and files it in his brain. I am learning not to take it personally.

The Husband Says:

Us Aspies live in a world of noisy data, where scraps of information need to be assembled into a whole to make sense. In particular, social information is especially noisy and often contradictory. What Karen describes as "the voice of authority" is my judgement of how, on a particular subject, a particular source might be more authoritative and might need to be taken more notice of. I believe in the wisdom of crowds - if I hear the same thing from lots of sources then I'm much more inclined to believe it and take more notice.

Volume Control

You may have noticed that your partner shouts when he is on the phone. Mine does. Despite the fact he has an engineering degree, he doesn't seem to have grasped the fact that you don't have to shout down these devices. He is not deaf and, as far as I know, neither are most of the people he works with.

The reason behind this is a little hard to say for sure, but I'm sure at times it is assertiveness and getting his point across to the other person. It is a need to control and take charge of a situation. He has learned that the more noise he makes the more likely he is to be heard.

It could well be more than that though and be related to how Aspie's perceive their surroundings. I know, for example, the children always raise their voices when they use their headphones. I have given up telling them there is no need to shout, that I can hear them. I think they are less able to gauge the subtleties of language, including volume control in this way. When in a state of high excitement or enthusiasm, you may notice your Aspie getting increasingly loud, as if their emotion gets in the way of volume control.

Of course, as in many cases within our ASD group, the opposite is always true and that many will talk far too quietly. See Hyper/Hypo. This is possibly down to lack of confidence or not realising that, just because they can hear themselves, others can't necessarily hear them. With our son I started to wonder whether I was going deaf as I was always having to ask him to repeat himself. He is a little improved these days.

The other more complicated answer is that it is connected to the dysfunction of the vestibular system which controls their internal moderator.

Vulnerable

As a Couple

Being in a partnership should make you stronger together but, when you unknowingly end up in an AS/NT marriage, you both become vulnerable.

As the wife, you have invested everything into your relationship, your physical presence, your spiritual presence, your money and time and, most of all, your heart. You have given it to the man you thought you wanted to spend the rest of your life with. So, when he starts to reject you, it feels as though he is rejecting the very things that make you "You" and the things he had been most attracted to in the first place. It leaves you confused and vulnerable. It can be very lonely.

On the other side of the coin, however, your husband or partner is equally feeling that you are rejecting all the things he holds dear, the things that you had admired about him. Trying to change his habits or telling him what to do means you are rejecting who 'He' is. He too feels vulnerable. It can be very lonely.

Walking on Eggshells

NT One morning you wake up and you realise that you are not the person you used to be. You are more tentative, timid and not as spontaneous and you think about what you say before you open your mouth.

You question whether you are in an abusive relationship. You never expected this to happen to you. You question your own sanity and whether you love your husband anymore. How did this happen?

It was probably gradual, the occasional falling out, maybe not very long after you were married. Before you married, you hardly ever disagreed. Perhaps you can't even remember an occasion when you had an argument. Looking back, is this because things always went your way? Is this why your relationship felt perfect? Everything you suggested he thought was a great idea?

These days however, it feels like any suggestion you make, any sign of spontaneity gets stamped on and shouted down. Every thought you have is made to feel unreasonable and possibly selfish. When things go wrong it turns out it is always your fault, regardless of whether you had anything to do with it or not.

Life becomes so unpredictable, you try and anticipate his moods and his every need. You stop inviting friends around as you never know how he is going to react to their presence. You don't socialise as much and rarely together. You tiptoe around your husband, trying to support him as much as you can with his stressful job and the aftermath of it.

Simple tasks at home go undone because you are too afraid to bring up the fact that the washing machine is making a strange noise or that a tile is loose in the bathroom. You find yourself deliberately not asking him simple questions like, 'Have you seen my keys?' because you know that the next thing will be an explosion of frustration from him and he will ransack the house until they turn up. It is not worth mentioning the little irritations in life because he blows them all out of proportion.

You wonder: how did this happen? Where has the man that you married gone? Is it your fault?

For my dissertation I was asked to write my autobiography about my life with David so far. I recently decided to publish this separately. I have called it Walking on Eggshells.

The Husband Says:

This article from Karen, taken at face value, is quite depressing. It paints a picture of a relationship cul-de-sac from which there is no turn-around or escape.

What Karen is describing is our marriage state a few years ago, before she decided to turn it around, figure out what was broken in our relationship and to coax me into participating in a repair job. We are part way done; the cul-de-sac turned out to be a narrowing of the road but we are past that and beginning to make things as they should be in a healthy relationship. It's a work in progress though, with that progress measured in months and years and small gestures.

The job begins with understanding.

Walking through a Minefield

For the woman, every day is like walking on eggshells but what does it feel like being the AS partner in this marriage?

The Husband Says:

I suppose it's another metaphor for what I'm feeling some days. Not a very accurate metaphor though - it would be improved if there was some way to describe how the mines are moved every few days. Now we are getting mixed up metaphors with moving goalposts - not quite accurate either.

Warning Signs

How to Spot the Warning Signs

Some Aspie children have 'service dogs' who become aware early on that the child is going to have a meltdown and take evasive action. Unless you have a clever dog like that, you will have to sniff out trouble yourself. Your husband is not as aware of his feelings as you are.

I have mentioned before that there is no moderation with your Asperger husband. He doesn't really understand or know how to experience a 'grey area'. You will find he is either completely relaxed or totally stressed. They are not aware of anything in between. You will have to watch out for the warning signs. My Aspie family describe this area of non-feeling as Meh.

David was driving the car the other day when I noticed that he went from relaxed, one hand driving (like a van driver) to being really intense and hunched with both hands on the wheel at 'ten to two' like we are told to do in our driving lessons. Whatever had caused it (probably an impatient driver not keeping a safe distance) was beyond my control, but I had immediately noticed his body language and took pains to be calm and sympathetic.

The Husband Says:

Watch out also for me butting in to your conversation - cutting you short. If that's happening, then it's because I MUST be heard - there's a crisis brewing and I need your help.

We are Liars

AS NT We Neurotypicals lie all the time. Half the time we don't even realise we do it. Our language is sloppy, laid-back and inaccurate. We tell our children to be honest but we lie to them constantly.

We are vague with our language and don't think that our Aspie partners or children take every word we say as truth. When we say to them "I'm just popping into the supermarket for a pint of milk", we know in our heart of hearts that it probably won't be just the milk we are going for. We will suddenly remember there's only one slice of bread left in the breadbin and dash off to the bakery aisle to get some more. To us, this Is natural and necessary, flexible living. To the AS husband or child it is further proof of our tenuous hold on the truth.

It must be so frustrating for them when we plan ahead what we are going to do and then completely change tack without any warning. I have done this to David so many times. I have got frustrated with his meltdowns and his inflexibility and couldn't understand why he couldn't see that a change to the plan was necessary.

Now as I am starting to figure out how his mind works, I try harder not to deviate from the plan. It makes everyone happier in the long run.

See also Expectation Violation and the fictional character Dr. House and his observation that everybody lies.

What am I for?

Or perhaps I should ask 'Why did he marry me?'

Another common misconception is that those on the autistic spectrum do not want, or need, relationships. There are those, such as Temple Grandin, who prefer not to have the complications of relationships in their lives and are fulfilled by their work. I would lean towards these people being more high functioning autists than Asperger's. Those with Asperger's, though they like their space to recharge their batteries, do very much like to socialise, to love and be loved. Both my husband and son are extremely affectionate people.

I haven't asked David at what age he started wanting a relationship with a member of the opposite sex, but I don't remember him mentioning any girls that he liked before going to university. Those with AS tend to mature at a slower pace than their NT counterparts. Often in school, teenage Aspies are confused and confounded by the courtship rituals amongst their peers. They often see school as their time for educating themselves and setting themselves up for life, so they can't understand why other teenagers waste time and energy on excessive emotions. It may be to their advantage, as they don't let the ups and downs of NT courtship distract them from a good education. By the time they are mature enough to cope with a female counterpart, due to their high level of accomplishment in education and career, they have become more attractive to the twenty-something female who is looking to settle down in life.

So, what am I for?

Firstly, I believe for companionship. At aged 26, I think David was not entirely fulfilled by only having work in his life when we first met. He saw in me someone who had a good sense of humour and, presumably, he was physically attracted to me. I believe those were the main items on his conscious level of agenda. What about subconsciously? Had he pinpointed my natural social skills and wanted a piece of it? Did he realise I would be able to smooth his way in life with my high emotional intelligence? Quite possibly yes. This has certainly become one of my main roles.

Lastly, and I think he has admitted this one to me: my purpose is to make him look 'normal'. He can go to work and talk about 'the wife and kids'. It is a sad truth that NT people generally 'feel sorry for', or even look down upon, someone who cannot hold down a long term relationship, and David did not want anyone's pity. He just wanted to be normal. My presence makes him look normal. He often talks about me to people, and it is his way of wearing an invisible badge that says, 'Normal'.

Perhaps I should bat this one straight on to David.

The Husband Says:

I don't disagree with any of your detective work. Principally you make me and us (as a family) look pretty normal. That's part of the reason why, at work, you are usually referred to as "Mrs. Slee"; normal but formidable - the power behind the throne.

What is 'Normal'?

I grew up in a loving household. We lived in a middle class area of Cardiff and sang in the church choir. I had two older brothers, a father who worked at the university as a lecturer in statistics, and a mother who mostly stayed at home to look after us.

On the surface, a fairly conventional childhood. In fact, when we moved to the North East of England, my naive eyes were opened very wide indeed. I realised I'd had a good, stable upbringing and, though we didn't have much money we never really went without. No divorce, no social workers.

Yet, once it eventually dawned on me that I was brought up in an Aspie household, I started to analyse my childhood a little more.

Looking back, I could see that my father had his obsessions: work; rugby; and his pipe. When I was seven he received his Ph.D. in statistics. I was very proud of him (though I had no clue what it meant) but I liked his mortar board and robe and I used to look at them with great pride as they hung in the wardrobe next to his every day clothes.

As a Welshman, it would be wrong if you were not obsessed with rugby. Surely?

His pipe? Well it was an annoyance, but then smoking was rife and at least it wasn't the acrid smell of cigarettes. I still occasionally get dragged back to my childhood by the lingering smell of my dad's preferred tobacco in the street, though it happens less and less these days.

I considered all my father's behaviour perfectly normal. It was all I knew and no one ever questioned it, at least not in my hearing. That is, except for him wearing his coat in the house, regardless of temperature or time of year.

So if I was brought up in a household where quirky behaviour was the norm, them it was no wonder I was accepting of David's behaviour when we first met.

The Husband Says:

Sadly, there is no book of social norms - the answer to the question "What is normal?".

In any case, since 'normal' changes as fast as the seasons and women's fashion, the book would always be being reprinted and would always be wrong.

This app does document a few social norms that are less likely to change and might represent the largest faux-pas if ignored.

Update:

I have discovered that Normal is a town in Illinois, USA.

What is the Autistic Spectrum?

The above term is bandied around a lot but do you actually know what it is?

See Autistic Spectrum for a modern interpretation of the term.

When Aspies Marry Aspies

This is very common but you don't hear about it so much as these are generally harmonious marriages. These couples think the same way and are therefore not offended by each other's direct speech. Indeed, they find it refreshing. After a day at work where they are trying hard to fit in it must be a relief to get home to your partner who won't ask you about your day or play mind games with you.

Of course, this is an over simplification of the situation as there are varying types of Asperger Marriages where perhaps one is 'more' autistic than the other and possibly prone to more anxiety than the other. They will of course have their own difficulties but I don't believe that they will have such miscommunications as in an AS/NT marriage.

Further work needs to be done on this. Watch this space.

When Things are Going well

Don't be afraid to mark the good moments.

NT Tell him you are happy and that he has made you happy. Don't however, refer back to less happy moments or he will start to think negative thoughts. Try very much to stay in the moment.

NT Later, after the event, don't be afraid to ask or say why it went well. Take note of the circumstances such as good planning and add it to your toolbox. When questioning your partner about his good mood or actions, keep the tone light and don't refer back to any negative situations. Instead of feeling praise he will feel criticism and fixate on that.

The Husband Says:

And feel free to feed-back to us what went well for you. If it's not too personal, we will share in the next edition of the book and App. We are all learning and improving.

White Lies

We NT's are very good at this and we use these lies in order to get out of an awkward situation.

- Santa Claus
- The Tooth Fairy
- "I had a migraine"
- "I've got a headache"
- "What, this old thing?"

The Husband Says:

Everybody lies; NTs and Aspies alike. It turns out to be an essential social lubricant - to gloss over some of the ugly truths so that people can just get along by ignoring what we all hope to be petty irrelevances.

It's just a shame for us Aspies that a key tool of the NT, the little white lie, is difficult for us to pull off. Probably because we over-think it, and also because we are poor at interpreting other people's facial expressions, we fail to control our own whilst 'in the act'.

Why did he get Married?

I know very little about my grandmother's life before I was born. According to my father she got married relatively late in life. My grandfather (whom I never met) was persistent and kept asking her to marry him. She gave in eventually, more or less to shut him up. Not very romantic. I think she probably would have been very happy as a spinster and being able to live her life as she wished, working, using her intellect and not raising a family. She was not afraid to be different, or indeed to offend anyone in her path.

Why does a man with Asperger's get married?

He knows he is different and wants to appear like everyone else. Everyone else gets married. It is the norm and expected.

Does he Really Want a Relationship?

Does he regret getting involved with a woman who is disorganised, organic, spends his money and wants noisy expensive children that she has to devote all her time to instead of him?

The Husband Says:

So many questions grouped under "W". The root cause and answer to most of them lies in what is considered the social norm; the expectation of NTs as to what normal should be and the Aspie struggle to appear "normal". It is expected of you to marry, settle down and have kids. It even says so in the standard marriage vows.

Why does he Never Say Sorry?

Does he realise he has done something wrong?

If he is unaware of his mistake he will not say sorry. If you have pointed out this mistake or criticised him he will not say sorry. This is because you are pointing out his failures. This is the worst thing you can do to someone with AS. Their whole self-esteem is based around their achievements, no matter how big or small. They know they are inept at social situations but they do not want them pointed out.

It is excruciatingly embarrassing and painful for them to make a mistake. They will become paranoid and believe that, not just you, but everyone else is aware of their mistake. Yes, to us it seems like they blow things entirely out of proportion, but to them it is perfectly reasonable and logical to behave like this.

Be careful of criticism. Do you really need to? Can you reformat your language in a more positive way?

Saying Sorry too much or inappropriately

This is a sign of insecurity and lack of confidence or not wanting to offend but being unsure whether they have or not.

It is a very British thing to bump into someone and apologise, whether it was your fault or not. Do we all have a problem with Spatial Awareness?

The Husband Says:

I can't get the balance right. I want to apologise for my most significant shortcomings, but I struggle to sound sincere (to my own ears). I over compensate and apologise for everything, and I know that annoys you.

Perhaps the answer is to encourage behaviours that mean I don't have to spend much (if any) time apologising? This would be the best of all worlds.

Why does He Reject Me?

Why does he cut off his nose to spite his face?

Why when I am kind, does he reject my actions?

I've often suggested that I do him a packed lunch for work like I do for the kids school lunches but he always rejects the idea. The only time he has taken food in to work was when he was on a diet and he would take fruit in to sit on his desk. He says he ate it.

He is so disorganised and never eats properly as he prioritises work over everything else. Why is he always surprised when I do something nice for him?

He always looks surprised when I bring him a cup of coffee. Does he assume he isn't worthy of such thought? Or is it because he almost never brings me one? Let's not go there right now!

Yet sometimes he doesn't even look at me when I hand him something, he is so engrossed. I have learned (mostly) not to take it personally.

The Husband Says:

It's a fine balancing act and I'm not very good at it. It's also not personal. It's a response to a perception of an office social norm and a coping strategy that defuses that particular problem.

One of the advantages of working from home is that I'm generally less tired because I don't have to put on the "work" act so much. I'm preoccupied by work because I'm working, so that means I'm not putting on the "family" persona.

On the question of the surprise of a cup of coffee - at work there are elaborate rituals designed to make the workload of refreshment "fair". These rituals are so complex that I seek to avoid them - I'll buy in a soft drink that is clearly uniquely mine and I'll make a point of serving myself or I'll drink decaf cafetiere coffee from a pot made for one to show that I don't want to participate in these group rituals. So at home I don't expect coffee to be made for me - I'm not expecting it so I'm genuinely surprised.

Perhaps we need a strict curfew between home-work time and home-time. I don't think that will fully work either. This working from home lark is still a work in progress.

On the taking food to work situation - again there are office rules and rituals to be aware of. Some people are criticised behind their backs for bringing leftovers or pungent food and re-heating in the microwave; I don't want that to be me. Further my main client has its roots in the civil service with a thriving quality, health and safety "police" in the office - about the most dangerous thing in office life is the extremely remote possibility of food poisoning through poor food preparation and storage; there is an under-current of office muttering that somehow packed lunches are dangerous! Again, I just avoid the situation altogether - lunch comes from a reputable outside source and waste is disposed of within the lunch hour or lunch is not consumed at all.

You know the reason why I "cut of my nose to spite my face"; Aspies hate being wrong so will carry out an illogical course of action if it is what they said they would do at the beginning. We back down with very poor grace.

Why has He stayed with Me?

Well this is one question that I can't really answer but I can tell you why I am asking the question.

His perspective is so very different from mine. He can never relax and he thinks he is 'in trouble' constantly.

He misunderstands my body language, facial expressions and the intonation in my voice. He always assumes that I am feeling negative towards him.

When I am angry about a situation outside of the house and I raise my voice a little to show my frustration, he still assumes I am attacking or accusing him in some way. So far I have tackled this from my point of view but, if we look at it from his point of view, I must come across as an irritable, heartless, moody and an aggressive person.

So why does he stay?

Apart from the fact that this makes me sad, that he doesn't really know the real me, I worry that his perspective will take him to Breaking Point one day.

The Husband Says:

I can't really answer the question. A few times (a little while ago) we had some spectacular arguments, and you quite clearly left, but after a few hours you came back again. Likewise, I've been tempted to leave, but never summoned up the courage to demonstrate my failure in this relationship by leaving for any recognisable length of time.

It's an Aspie trait not to give up on something until it is finished properly. Leaving a relationship part way through is not "finishing it off properly".

Why have I Stayed?

I had to give a presentation to my fellow students about my work in autism. Everyone else on the course was doing this to enhance their careers and getting their fees partly funded to do so. I was there because I wanted to learn as much as I could to help my family. So while everyone else presented about their places of work: hospitals, mainstream schools or special needs colleges; I was the only one to stand up and introduce them to my family.

Why did we get Married?

The reason I stay is because, in many ways, he is still the man I married. Admittedly he disappeared for a while, but he is beginning to emerge a little more now. I married a man who was immediately smitten with me, who was hard working and generous. He was loving and reliable and wanted to do anything he could to make me happy. We shared a love of films, music and comedy and he was open to me showing him things he had not tried before. I was attracted to his confidence, intelligence, his humour and I liked the way he worshipped the ground I walked on. What woman wouldn't? I knew he would always be there for me and I could trust him with anything. Okay, he had his quirks, but who doesn't?

We were married two and a half years after meeting.

Why would I Consider Leaving?

The first two years of marriage were pretty great. Yes, I did have a few doubts on the honeymoon itself. In hindsight, the lack of structure and too much down time was very hard for David and, as we were living out of hotel rooms, he didn't have any time to himself. He obviously couldn't voice to me that he needed his own space. What bride wants to be told that on her honeymoon? Once we got home, life got back to normal and so did David.

There are too many things to go into, but life became very difficult and very lonely after I gave up work and the children were born. Of course I was a full time mum and loved it, but I hadn't expected it literally to be 100% full on without a break - ever. He never got up to help feed the baby, even when I stopped breastfeeding. It wasn't worth faking sleep (he was much better that it than I was), and my hormones would not let me lie there whilst my child cried. Even when I went back to work he didn't help out any more. I ended up having a full blown panic attack whilst on holiday, which I think was brought on by sheer exhaustion. The more I needed him, the less I saw of him.

But that didn't make me want to leave him. It was the sudden unpredictability of his behaviour, the verbal outbursts, the uncaring and tactless words. The accusations. The worst times were when he behaved like that in front of other people. I was mortified, but I never wanted to cause a scene so I would just play it down or walk off. I don't think he ever knew how much he hurt and humiliated me.

It came to a head one day when he accused me, without any reason or warning, of doing something quite despicable. For once I lost my temper ... I mean I really lost it! I screamed and I shouted and I kicked things, and he stood there in astonishment wondering where MY behaviour had come from. I told him that was it and I packed the kids into the car. They had obviously heard it all and Morgan turned to me and asked if "I was leaving dad"? That brought it home to me and stopped me in my tracks. I went back into the house and found David sitting on the stairs looking absolutely dejected; despairing and confused. We still didn't know he had Asperger's but I knew something wasn't right. In a way, I knew it wasn't him. My heart softened a little and, after we dropped the kids off at their grandmas, we had a very long discussion. I was adamant that I was still leaving, and I told him so. He didn't beg me to stay. He didn't try and persuade me at all. I think he felt I was right and he didn't deserve me. It was heart-wrenching. Instead he got all practical and started talking about how he would still support us financially. I think it was easier for him to think about that than what was actually happening.

I felt so sorry for him and it also started to dawn on me how much he did love me and the kids, even though he still hadn't said it. He still wanted to look after us and felt we were his responsibility, even if I was leaving him. This was the kind hearted, generous man I had married.

Eventually, after lots of tears from both sides, I suggested we give it another go.

So, when one of my fellow students asked me why I stayed, this is what I told her.

Besides I couldn't bring myself to 'break' another human being.

Window Shopping

We neurotypical women have a tendency to shop. This is a necessity for life. Some enjoy it and others don't. David understands that we do have to shop (occasionally) and he is okay with that. There is a point to it.

What he cannot comprehend is the hobby of window shopping that many women (or men) have. I thought at first it was because he couldn't see the point in it. As in, what is the point of looking at something you can't have? There is logic in that.

However, I noticed he actually got quite agitated whenever he found me window shopping. This doesn't have to be the traditional, nose up against the pane of glass shopping, however. These days, of course, it is virtual. It is actually quite hard to avoid virtual window shopping, as we are bombarded with it daily on our TV's, computer screens and phones. Some I solicit and some I don't.

What makes him agitated is he believes that: whenever I look at something, I must want it. You can't just admire something from afar or check it out to see whether it might be suitable. He gets anxious that I might want something and either will spend our money on it, or he feels we can't afford it, or he feels guilty for not being able to provide me with something I would love but cannot have.

What he doesn't understand is that it is simple 'escapism' that I derive pleasure from, for example, I like looking at other people's mansions on line. I love nothing better than to drool over other people's houses and wishing we could afford to own such a place. What he does, by his anxious attitude and accusations, is not allowing me to dream.

The Husband Says:

I've said elsewhere that I think us Aspies have old fashioned values. We believe ourselves to be the male hunter-gatherer-provider. Seeking something like a big house that is financially out of reach for us is fine, but you have to preface it that you are just window 'gazing' and

not window shopping. If you are shopping, then I can't provide - you are setting me up to fail. That's where the tension and conflict comes from.

We really need those little flags with "JOKE" and "WINDOW GAZING" written on them so we can fly them next to our computers when we are not really serious.

Us Aspies are really bad at telling a subtle hint from a red herring.

Withdrawal

I've had a number of clients who have come to me and asked for help with this. A meltdown they can weather through, but complete physical and mental withdrawal is hard for any spouse to take.

This behaviour seems like a complete rejection from the AS partner as they can't, or won't, turn to their life partner for love and support.

What causes Withdrawal?

Most likely, your partner is overwhelmed with anxiety caused by an external influence beyond their control. Often it is pressure of work or a family situation they can't control. Sometimes they are putting so much effort into getting their work life right they have no time or energy left for you. They come home only to rest and refuel.

It may even be a health problem that they are concerned about, preventing them from getting on with their life because they can't face up to it.

For example, our son was very withdrawn and would not settle down to any revision for his exams. He eventually confessed to me he thought he had cancer. This is because at school they had been given a talk about teenage cancer. Most kids will listen and then dismiss most of the information they have been given, but our son took it very much to heart. He found a lump between his nose and his eyeball and decided it was cancerous. He worried about it for weeks before telling me. I checked it out and told him I was pretty sure it was just a hard spot but I could see he wasn't reassured. I made an emergency appointment with the GP and explained the situation. He checked him over thoroughly and assured him he was fine. He was able to get on with his life without the overriding fear of illness. To us it may seem trivial but to him it was an enormous obstacle he just didn't know how to deal with.

NT Unfortunately at times like this, if you can't get them to communicate at all, it is often a matter of a waiting game. Make them aware that you are there for them when they are ready to talk. You may want to preface it with a warning that you won't wait for ever.

AS I have come across couples where the AS partner has withdrawn from their partner as they feel that they are not understood. When the suspected AS partner has looked into the symptoms of Asperger Syndrome and recognised it in himself, after some thinking time he has felt a profound sense of relief that there is a cause for his problems. On further educating of himself and his wife they have been able to communicate effectively again as there is no longer any blame.

Women and Girls on the Spectrum

Until recently it was assumed by professionals that the vast majority of people with autism were men, at a ratio of 4:1.

Now, with better understanding and diagnosis, people have started to question this figure. In a recent conference I attended Tony Attwood suggested the ratio could actually be 2:1 if not 1:1.

One of the reasons why this has escaped psychologists attention for so long, is that women tend to be better at hiding their feelings, have more supportive networks and are great mimics. They learn what is acceptable behaviour is and then try to replicate it. Underneath the calm exterior however, the anxiety remains.

Asperger Wives

NT These Asperger girls turn into attractive, intelligent and loving women. They often come across as naive and sweet and princess like. Non-threatening and they look up to the men in their life, perhaps even looking for that reassuring father figure they had at home.

Other Asperger women are very different to their 'girly' counterparts and think more like the men, but they too are attractive to NT or AS men in a 'hard to reach', challenging way.

The men who fall for them are similar to the women who fall for the male Aspie. They tend to be outgoing, caring and full of ideas. The women are attracted to this personality which fits neatly into their jigsaw of strengths and weaknesses. Like their male counterparts, the Aspie wife relies on her husband to define who she is.

The Husband Says:

There's a few more chapters needed in this guide to tackle the issues of an Aspie-Aspie marriage. If a few years ago the conventional wisdom was that Aspie men don't marry, and this is now clearly wrong, then in a few months and years we need to acknowledge that there are Aspie-Aspie marriages out there. Goodness knows how that might work out (or not?)

Wooing

The Oxford Dictionary definition of Wooing is "Try to gain the love of (a woman), especially with a view to marriage."

I think our Aspies may take this dictionary definition rather literally, not surprisingly given their Theory of Mind. However, we need to let them know that the Wooing should not stop just because he has succeeded in his mission.

David told me once that, before we met, he had been teased at work about how unfit he was. One of the Directors would go jogging at lunch time and invited David to join him. David decided he would to prove that he could do it. He doggedly ran through the countryside chasing after his Director for a few weeks until he got fitter. One day he overtook his Director and got back to work before him. He had succeeded in proving he could run, and was better than his work 'superior'. From that day on, he did not go jogging again. I think he is treating his marriage in the same way. He can't see that the whole point of marriage is to enjoy the benefits of it the whole time. To keep his wife and children happy by treating them well (and I don't mean financially), he can't see that this would benefit him too. He put all that effort in to succeed, but did not sustain it and, therefore, lost the benefit of it.

The Husband Says:

I'm taking this bit to heart and waiting for the day, when the kids are self-sufficient enough, that I can do again with you the sorts of things we did before we were married. It's going to take a little while longer than perhaps we thought because our kids are Aspies too - they will take longer to be able to make their own way than perhaps NT adolescents would.

This is another time of transition.

Work Place Etiquette

This subject may not seem entirely relevant to your relationship at first glance, but often your partner is the main bread winner it is vital he does well in his job.

This is for a number of reasons, such as self-esteem but if you are at home with young children, or are working part time, his income is vital and I have come across many occurrences where the man gets into trouble at work due to misunderstandings.

There are two ways of approaching this:

1. Keeping the diagnosis/suspected diagnosis secret but learning and implementing the correct work etiquette.

2. Talking to Human Resources or your boss about your diagnosis/suspicions of diagnosis. Often Occupational Health can help you get a diagnosis.

In the first case it can be understandable at times why you would not want employers to know you have a condition or are disabled by that condition. It is true there is still a stigma and ignorance around autism and Asperger's Syndrome but employers are becoming much more enlightened now. You cannot be sacked for having a disabling condition but human nature can at times be mean if they understand a situation.

On the other hand, anecdotal evidence from men with Asperger's Syndrome who have been open and honest with their workplace and colleagues have always given positive results. The colleagues are much more understanding. Where once they just thought someone was rude or at best shy, they now know that sometimes that person is just unaware of how they come across. Many colleagues actually learn to appreciate a no nonsense approach to work.

In certain cases, where colleagues have been aware that a member of their team has a hygiene problem, they have only ever muttered about it to each other. If they start to understand that this might be a sensory issue for their colleague, they may be more understanding. They may also gently take them to one side and point out that it is an unspoken rule in the workplace that people maintain a general level of hygiene and appearance. Many people on the spectrum would actually appreciate being told this by a colleague, especially one that they look up to.

General Standards Expected in the Workplace

- Hygiene. You should shower or bathe before you go to work.

- Clean shirts should be worn every day. Trousers can be worn for longer as can jackets.

- Appearance depends on the type of job that you are in but for an office job smart trousers, formal shirt and tie are often expected. Take your cue from others. It is better to overdress than underdress. you can always take your tie off.

- You can never offer to make tea or coffee for your colleagues too often. Unless you are their superior then doing it occasionally for them is considered a nice treat. If you do it too often you will be considered a walk over.

- Always be polite. Smile at people's jokes even if you don't get them or you don't think they are funny.

- When thinking, if you need to stare into space try and stare at an inanimate object or out of the window rather than at a colleague. They will find if very uncomfortable. If you get caught staring, apologise and say, "Sorry, I was miles away." Telling the truth, even if a little embarrassing will make people think more highly of you than if you tell an awkward lie.

- Try and take your lunch rather than working through. Your colleagues will expect you to do this. Your body will need a break and will need to refuel throughout the day. Be kind to your body.

- Show polite interest in your colleagues lives outside of the office. Safe topics are what you did at the weekend and how well your children are doing. Never talk about sex or make dirty jokes (unless you work on a building site where it is considered essential).

- In most places of work, it is okay to take the occasional personal call from family as long as it is not a long chat. This is not a sackable offence unless specifically mentioned by your bosses.

- Always try and be on time and give reasons if you are not. However, do not berate people for being late unless it is your place to do so and they are making a habit of it.

- If you are a manager do not be scared to delegate. That is what your staff are for.

- Always praise your staff for doing well.

The Husband Says:

I agree with Karen on all of the above, and have direct experience of all of them.

In my first few jobs, I was either in the Civil Service or working for very small family firms. In both cases I was uncomfortable and knew I was different but I didn't know what it was. It felt like I would be admitting to a weakness that would make me less valuable as an employee. Once I became my own boss, I found it much easier to be able to tell selected clients and explain how I use my personality traits from Asperger's as an advantage in business. I don't put this on my CV or in marketing brochures - there is still a significant stigma.

Adding to Karen's points:

- *In an office environment you can send subtle non-verbal clues to colleagues. Choose a shirt with a pocket and fill it with pens and pencils to look like an Engineer or Scientist. Choose a shirt without a pocket to look like a "money man" - it's a form of power dressing.*

- *Again in the office - choose a less formal jacket and leave it on a peg or the back of your chair with a tie that matches your shirt in a pocket. That way you look (and feel) more relaxed. This is the way that the high flyers from the Mediterranean countries dress. But for the first meeting with a client use the tie and jacket until at least the opening hand-shakes are done with.*

- There might be some sexual and otherwise offensive jokes flying about. Play it safe and go a bit quiet if others choose to be less discreet.

- In public service there is still a silly level of political correctness. It's coffee with milk (not white coffee), making a note on a chalk-board (not black-board), and thinking outside of the box (not brainstorming).

- Whilst the office hours for professional grades might be 9 to 5, expect the working day to over-flow.

- Share any gifts given by suppliers with the whole team. Public servants have to declare significant gifts anyway.

- If you work on the shop-floor, get decent and comfortable Personal Protective Equipment, Human Resources can help with this. If you are, like me, on the larger side of normal, get extra sets of coveralls, boiler suits etcetera and put them in the laundry more often to help with hygiene issues.

- Befriend (subtly) the ICT and administrative staff. They often have to set and police what you might call the "petty" rules that make the office operate smoothly, and being on their right side can smooth away any minor transgressions. Don't forget it is the administrative staff in the finance department that make sure you get paid on time!

- Put your mobile phone - even your work-issued 'phone - on vibrate during office hours. And carry your mobile phone with you - it's called 'mobile' for a reason. If you leave it behind on your desk, even when getting the teas in, how will someone else answer your locked 'phone (it is locked, yes!) and stop that annoying ring-tone or vibration? I have seen (once) someone return to their mobile phone submerged in their cup of tea. Otherwise expect to play "hunt the mobile that has had its battery taken out"

- In general, no one is **that** important; that includes you.

- There is usually a staff hand-book that the Neurotypicals didn't bother to read. Read it, understand it, check any questions you might have with Human Resources, act by it, **but don't quote it to colleagues**. Silently knowing you are right is enough.

- Staff appraisals are hell for everyone. Unless your boss (who will usually be doing the appraisal) has specialist human resource training, he or she will be dreading the appraisals as much as you are. Appraisals are genuinely meant to be helpful. Nearly all bosses are not at all vindictive and will not stand in the way of your career progression and pay rises, and will often act as mentors and confidantes. If you don't think their criticism is constructive, politely say so.

- *Workplaces will insist in organising "social" events, often without your partner (and safety net). Since you have already spent much of your day working with these people and exhausted all avenues of chit-chat, then you might find yourself very uncomfortable extending the working day for further socialisation. I have found that the best way of dealing with this is to pay the contribution, but then find some important business engagement or family reason why attendance at the social event is not possible.*

- *In a professional office, flexible working time is the norm. If anxiety is getting too much, go for a walk, either on the premises, disguised as business or a "comfort break", or out of the office, bringing back some biscuits or something else that your colleagues (who covered for you) can share. Better to reduce anxiety than to blow-up or meltdown.*

There's scope for a whole new book just on this subject.

Worry

This will form a large part of your husband's day. It will keep him awake at night and employ him while he is driving to and from work. The only time he is not worried and working out how to fix something is when he is concentrating on something he enjoys, usually his obsession.

Strategy

NT A good way to reduce his worrying time is to occupy his mind. You are unlikely to be able to stop him from planning and worrying about his day before he gets to work and in fact he probably needs that time to psyche himself up and get into work mode and be mentally prepared. However, if you and the family are going for a day out in the car, a good way of keeping him calm is to occupy his mind with something interesting or amusing. David often downloads podcasts from the BBC of the highlights of his favourite radio programmes, usually comedy. We have often bonded over comedy so it makes for a happy occasion in the car. Another suggestion would be listening to audio books on a subject that you both like. The radio can be okay if it is talk radio, but it might have a subject that could get him worked up, and music only radio gives him a good chance to worry about potential problems ahead.

Work

Since I met David at work, I have always known how talented and hardworking he is. I never felt it was my place to change him and ask him to do less than he wanted. I know how important it is to him. Yet there comes a time when, occasionally, you have to impress on him how important family life is too and that occasionally it would be nice for him to come home from work at a reasonable hour to spend some quality time with me and the children. This has to be finely balanced because, if he doesn't want to be there, if his mind is on some vital piece of work that he feels he is missing out on doing, it is not worth putting up with his company. He cannot switch off until he is satisfied that the essential work is done.

Self-esteem related

Planning a holiday and getting away from the desk at work and at home, is often the only way they can really relax. These days of course with mobile phones, laptops and the increasing availability of Wi-Fi it is harder to do, but it is possibly a blessing in disguise. David knows that in an emergency he can be contacted by work but he is not in the office or at his home desk to be contacted. Most colleagues will read his diary entry and see that he is on holiday. He can relax safe in the knowledge that he is officially 'off work' but that he can also deal with any emerging difficulties that can't be dealt with without his input.

The Husband Says:

All good advice. The challenge is in finding ways to implement all this good advice. Aspies fear change so it will be for the NT in the relationship to lead the way.

Writing

As Therapy

When I had my first supervision meeting for my dissertation and I told my supervisor my idea, she told me I had to write everything down. I had from time to time kept a diary but this one was to be retrospective. It was hard work, and at times emotional, but very cathartic.

It wasn't the story of my life, but it was the story of my relationship with David. I have stopped writing it now, but I do have a considerable autobiography which shows how pervasive his behaviour has been in my life and its effects, good and bad, upon it.

The Husband Says:

Writing something down makes it documentary, makes it real, turns it into data that must be acted on. It is solely because you started to document our dysfunctional relationship of the time and showed me the evidence, that we have started to change my expectation and behaviour for the better.

Written Communication

NT
You may have noticed with your partner (and indeed David has readily admitted) that he doesn't listen.

When important issues need to be discussed, then your best chance of getting his full attention is by writing to them. This is a useful tool as they can get to it in their own time without pressure or interruptions.

Putting information in black and white, simple font, gets the information across clearly and without any unnecessary emotion getting in the way. As visual thinkers they are more likely to remember what you write so be careful to make it positive.

- Xanthan gum
- Xanthippe
- X Factor
- X Rated

X Factor

The wife of an Asperger's man will have been auditioned as harshly and strictly as a contestant on the X Factor. All her pros and cons would have been weighed and considered and found acceptable or even perfect. She has the X Factor for him.

For an amusing fictional account of this audition I recommend you read 'The Rosie Project' by Graeme Simsion.

X Rated

Your Aspie is generally completely obsessed by taboo subjects or just won't go anywhere near them. They may even be very embarrassed by the very mention of sex. On the other hand, they may view it as just another bodily function and nothing to be embarrassed about at all.

For example, when our Aspie son was eight he came home from school having learned some inappropriate and factually incorrect information about where babies come from. I bought him an age appropriate book and gave it to him which he read from cover to cover.

A few days later I had friends round for coffee and we were discussing in a light hearted way why we didn't want more children. Morgan overheard us and came into the room to announce that, "I had better be careful that daddy didn't put his penis in my vagina then". He walked out of the room to a stunned silence.

So sex is often at the extremes of a couple's boundaries and experience. In this day of easy access to pornography, it is not uncommon for a wife to feel rejected while her husband obsesses over unrealistic women and situations. The wife finds it hard to compete with fake women who never answer back. I am aware of a number of marriages that have broken down due to this obsession.

The Husband Says:

This can cut both ways as Karen has suggested. Our Aspie son might have been able to use all the right language at age 8, but at age 16 we were watching "True Lies" (one of mine and Karen's favourite films) and he could do nothing but cringe at the humorous scene where Jamie Lee Curtis does a striptease for her husband. I was cringing for him at the same time. He had no language to describe what he was seeing, thinking and feeling and I had no language that would be helpful.

Xanthan Gum

For those on a gluten free diet this can be useful in baking as it helps with the structure of the food once risen which is normally the role of gluten, which makes wheat products light and fluffy.

Xanthippe

NT   Xanthippe was the young wife of Socrates who was supposed to be shrewish, scolding and argumentative. Socrates describes his own wife Xanthippe as "the hardest to get along with of all the women there are." Yet, familiarly, he admits that he actually chose her for these very character traits he now dislikes. He portrays his wife as difficult and argumentative, yet she is described by Plato as nothing more than "a devoted wife and mother".

I have sympathy with Xanthippe, perhaps Socrates was on the Spectrum?

X

✧   You

✧   You are not Alone

✧   Youth

✧   Youthful Appearance

You

NT You are very important. You are crucial to this marriage. Without you there would be no marriage.

NT Take time to think about yourself. To reinvigorate your self-belief and refresh who you are. You will always be different from the younger version of you who so naively and sweetly fell in love, but that girl is not necessarily gone forever. You just have to find her.

NT Take care of yourself. Find the time just for you. It may be that you have found yourself spending time alone and lonely, but when you plan good quality "alone time", it is different. You can indulge yourself in your own pleasures. It could be to book yourself a facial or it could be to read a book you just haven't made time for. It is important to consider yourself. It is not selfish to put yourself first sometimes.

Indeed, anecdotal evidence suggests that if you spend less time doting on your husband and pandering to his every whim, that eventually he notices and starts wondering why. It may be worth a try to enjoy a little 'You' time.

You are not Alone

NT You and I are here because we have married, or have long term partners, who have a diagnosis (or you suspect he is on the autistic spectrum). It is likely that you met and made a commitment without knowing this. The fact that you did not recognise your partner is autistic means that he is most likely to have Asperger's Syndrome.

The reason that you may have thought he was an interesting, quirky and attentive guy, is that from the moment he met you, he knew he wanted you and worked hard against all his instincts to get you.

You were most likely flattered by the attention, and felt you were well matched. Fast forward a few years and you are married, possibly with kids and things are very different. He has shown his true colours. Every day there are misunderstandings and irritations. At first you may have thought every marriage was like this, but eventually you will have realised that you don't understand him at all and he certainly doesn't understand you. Believe me, not every marriage is like this.

Y

However, most marriages where one partner is on the autistic spectrum tend to follow this formula.

The NT woman feels very let down, used and unloved. There is no emotional reciprocation and no support from the partner. In some cases, there isn't even any financial support and the woman is also the main breadwinner. There are no statistics for Asperger Marriages or Asperger Divorce, but if you look at the statistics for marriages of parents with autistic children that end in divorce - they are much higher than average.

I want you to know that YOU ARE NOT GOING MAD. That the strange and unexplained events happening within your marriage are explainable. Remember, THIS IS NOT YOUR FAULT. You are married to someone who, at best is living with a major difference in the way that he thinks, and at worst has a disability. You both need help.

I am here to share my experiences of my tumultuous marriage to David over the last 20 years and how we have so far survived. I have a Masters in Autism and wrote my dissertation on my marriage. I interviewed many women who I first came to know as parents of children with autism. As we got to know each other better, they confessed to me how difficult their marriage was and how they suspected their husbands were also autistic. Most of these men have still not been diagnosed. However, with the wives accepting that their husband is different, it has helped them to treat them differently and more tolerantly. For the husbands who have either agreed they are on the spectrum or received a diagnosis from a professional, it has made a huge difference to their marriage. They can be more open and honest about their feelings and feel safe in the knowledge that the person they love is trying their best to understand and support them.

Youth

It is often said that those on the spectrum are emotionally more immature compared to their peers. Physically they develop at the same rate but they are soon left behind socially.

They appear innocent and naive compared to others even into adulthood. They are often not ready for a relationship until they are in their twenties rather than their teens. This means that their first girlfriend may have to relive teenage dating scenarios rather than those she has experienced in the more mature relationships she has been used to.

However, this naivety can be endearing and it is no bad thing to have a willing partner who is keen to learn and hasn't picked up any bad habits or emotional baggage along the way.

Youthful Appearance

Tony Attwood mentioned in his book "The Complete Guide to Asperger's Syndrome" that children on the spectrum are often described as having the faces of angels and they often look younger than their years.

Y

- ✧   Zeal
- ✧   Zenith
- ✧   Zoning Out

Zeal

This is one of your Aspie's best qualities. Their zeal and enthusiasm for certain areas of interest. When they are interested in a topic, especially a new interesting one, they are like a dog with a bone and will not let it go until they have discovered practically everything there is to know on the subject.

This can be very endearing and also very useful. Indeed, before we started writing this App, David knew nothing about the programming and application of it all. He has plenty of experience in programming but not in this area and indeed all his programming is self-taught. When I first suggested writing a book about this subject he was mildly interested but he never really had any zeal for it.

When I discovered that no one had ever attempted to do a digital, interactive version of an Asperger Marriage help guide, he was suddenly filled with zeal and found out all he needed to know about the subject. There are definite advantages to his enthusiasm, logical mind and eye for detail.

Unfortunately, like a dog with a bone he can suddenly become very aggressive if interrupted and not willing to let the subject go! It can become annoying for everyone else after a while, but at least he is happy and interested.

Zenith

Many an Aspie spends their lives trying to reach the Zenith. The Zenith is considered the highest point above an imaginary celestial sphere and so really it is pretty impossible to reach.

Some Aspies spend their lives trying to reach the Zenith (of their education, careers, sport etc.) and, when they just don't quite make it, are disappointed in themselves and the world around them. They may blame others for their failure or, most likely, blame themselves. To them 'good enough' is just not good enough. These are often candidates for depression who cannot accept that they are, in theory, not infallible human beings.

Other Aspies, with perhaps lower esteem, would like to reach the Zenith but don't believe it is possible and never even try. These Aspies can be particularly negative in their thoughts and are also candidates for depression. Some come to the odd (but for them the rather satisfying) conclusion that, if they cannot reach the Zenith and be better than all the rest, they will do the extreme and reach the more easily achievable Nadir.

Z

Zoning Out

Depending on the Aspie and their perception of this, if you ask them about zoning out, you will get a myriad of answers.

For some it is taking time out to calm their overstimulated brain, where they glaze over and are less aware of their surroundings and what is going on in them.

Our sixteen-year-old Aspie confesses that he has missed large parts of his lessons because he was, in his words, "Daydreaming" about some vital part of a game he is currently obsessed with playing. He is so deep in thought that he is unaware that the teacher has come in and started the lesson. He may give the impression of listening when he is not.

David likes to give the impression he is always on duty even when it looks like he has switched off. He will stare into space while trying to decipher a problem at work and not notice he is staring directly at someone. It can be a little unnerving. He believes that this is quality thinking time and it is very effective. I have seen the results and can confirm this to be true.

Other times, I just catch him snoozing on the sofa whilst he is pretending to watch the TV or read a book.

Zoning out is different to Shutdowns.

Z

ENDNOTES

Picture Credits

Images have been specially commissioned for the App and this book, licensed from image-banks, found copyright free in the public domain or free of charge licensed through Creative Commons.

Creative Commons Images are licensed CC-BY-SA:

In the order of appearance in the book:

- Signing the Register: Original work by unknown member of the Rowlands family, used with the permission of Jim Rowlands

- Plate Spinning: By Henrikbothe (Own work), via Wikimedia Commons: Creative Commons CC-BY-SA

- Dog with Mountain of Biscuits: Image: dreamstime.com/Gvictoria/RF-LL

- Grass Cutting Pie Chart: Original work by David Slee January 2016

- RACI Chart: Unknown, via Wikimedia Commons: Creative Commons CC-BY-SA

- Facial Expression Examples: Visual Cognition (1997) Vol. 4 Iss. 3, p311 to 331: "Is There a Language of the Eyes?": Baron-Cohen / Wheelwright / Jolliffe.

- Toasting the Bride photo: Karen Slee original work Jan 2016 – photo of a cut out from a magazine.

- Personal Space Diagram: Re-drawn by David Slee Jan 2016 from Edward T Hall's research.

- Putting out the Bins Social Story: David Slee original work Jan 2016 using royalty free clip-art.

- Romantic Poster: Unknown – found on internet as royalty free clip-art

- Aspie Romantic Poster: David Slee own work Jan 2016, from royalty free clip-art

- Making a cup of coffee Social Story™: Karen Slee own work Jan 2016.

- Cactus Label: Unknown – posted on Facebook
- Stages of Grief diagram: David Slee own work Jan 2016 from Karen Slee sketch
- Triad of Impairment: National Autistic Society

Printed in Great Britain
by Amazon

48739526R00271